Partial denture
construction

Second edition

Partial denture construction

Principles and techniques

WILLIAM L. McCRACKEN, D.D.S., M.S., F.A.C.D., F.I.C.D.
Professor of Dentistry, Department of Prosthetic Dentistry,
University of Alabama School of Dentistry,
Birmingham, Alabama

With 258 figures, including 476 drawings and photographs

THE C. V. MOSBY COMPANY
Saint Louis   1964

Dedicated to my beloved wife

RUTH

*for her ever-present help
and encouragement*

Preface to second edition

Acceptance of the first edition of this textbook has been most gratifying and reflects a growth of interest in the subject of partial denture prosthodontics. There is no doubt that this phase of prosthetic dentistry is being taught more comprehensively than ever before. As a result the dentist is better qualified to render a more competent service to his patients. At the same time, he is better qualified to take the initiative in planning treatment and in directing the laboratory technician in the various phases of partial denture construction.

Unfortunately, the young graduate frequently follows an established pattern for partial denture treatment in which the design and construction of the prosthetic restoration are delegated entirely to the commercial dental laboratory. Too often a patient's record shows one appointment for impressions and the next appointment for the delivery of the completed restoration. A visit to the commercial dental laboratories shows that all too often the survey and design of the restoration is left to the technician. Although the teaching of prosthodontics has greatly improved in recent years, this knowledge is not always clinically applied to the best interest of all concerned. I would therefore make a plea to each graduating dentist that he assume his rightful responsibility to his profession, his laboratory, and his patient in keeping with the knowledge he has acquired as a student.

In the revision of this text, comments of reviewers, readers, and students were noted, and every attempt has been made to incorporate their suggestions. Some material has been deleted and new material has been added. Similarly, some illustrations have been improved upon and others have been replaced. However, the total amount of material remains about the same.

The chapter on terminology has been supplemented but little changed.

The publication of *Current Clinical Dental Terminology** may make such a chapter unnecessary in future editions. For the present, however, it is necessary that the terminology employed in the text be clearly defined and readily available for reference when needed.

The selected references have been brought up to date. Very few references from the first edition have been deleted. This was never meant to be a textbook bibliography alone, but rather a topical reference list to supplement the material contained in the textbook. It is hoped that the teacher of prosthetic dentistry will continue to find the references helpful in assigning supplemental reading material to his students.

The philosophies of partial denture treatment contained in the preface to the first edition remain unchanged. One reviewer of the first edition commented that this preface "might well be taken as a personal creed by dentists, dental students and dental technicians." This it was intended to be, and so it remains for subsequent editions.

W. L. McC.

---

*Boucher, Carl O. (editor): Current Clinical Dental Terminology, St. Louis, 1963, The C. V. Mosby Co.

Preface to first edition

Although I welcomed the invitation to author a textbook on the subject of partial denture construction, I realized from the outset that such a book would follow closely in the wake of several excellent textbooks on this subject. I therefore approached the task with a sense of great responsibility. However, I would not have accepted the challenge had I not felt sincerely that I could add something to what had already been written and thus produce a text in this field which is sorely needed and which provides the dental student, the dental practitioner, and the dental laboratory technician with the information necessary to produce a partial denture that is in itself a definitive restorative entity. It is my sincere hope that this textbook will be used not only by teachers of prosthetic dentistry but also by practicing dentists and dental technicians, and that in this book the dentist and dental technician may find a common meeting ground for better solution of the problems associated with the partially edentulous patient.

I am deeply grateful for the opportunities that I have had to combine private practice with teaching and for the knowledge that has evolved from this experience. Although I have attempted to present various philosophies and techniques in order that the reader may select that which to him seems most applicable, it is inevitable that certain preferences will be obvious. These are based upon convictions evolved through experience both in private practice and in the teaching of clinical prosthodontics. It is only logical, then, that I should therefore state my own personal beliefs, which are as follows:

1. I believe that the practice of prosthetic dentistry must forever remain in the hands of the dentist and that he must therefore be totally competent to render this service. In the fabrication of a partial denture restoration, the dentist

must be competent to render a comprehensive diagnosis of the partially edentulous mouth and, utilizing all of the mechanical aids necessary, plan every detail of treatment. He must either personally accomplish whatever mouth preparations are necessary or delegate to his colleagues such specialized services as surgical, periodontal, and endodontic treatment. In any case, primary responsibility for adequate mouth preparations remains his alone. He must undertake whatever impression procedures are necessary and must be primarily responsible for the accuracy of any casts of the mouth upon which work is to be fabricated. He must provide the laboratory technician with an adequate prescription in the form of diagrams and written instructions and with a master cast which has been completely surveyed with a specific design outlined upon it. He must be solely responsible for the accuracy and adequacy of any jaw relation records and must specify all materials and, in many instances, the exact method by which occlusion is to be established on the finished restoration. Finally, he must be competent to judge the excellence of the finished restoration or recognize its inadequacies and must assume the responsibility for demanding a degree of excellence from the technician that will continually raise rather than lower the standards of dental laboratory service.

2. I believe that the dental laboratory technician has a responsibility to his profession to demand a quality of leadership from the dentist which he can respect and follow without question. The responsibility for providing adequate prosthetic dentistry service to the patient must be shared by both dentist and technician, and each has not only a right to expect that the other do his part competently but also an obligation to demand a quality of service from the other that will not jeopardize the finished product. The technician therefore would do dentistry a great service if he would reject inadequate material from the dentist and respectfully suggest whatever improvements are necessary for him to produce an acceptable piece of work. As long as the technician accepts inadequate material from the dentist and the dentist is willing to place an inadequate product in the patient's mouth, the quality of removable prosthetic appliances will continue to be, as it all too frequently is, a far poorer service than the dentist and technician together are capable of rendering.

I believe also that dental laboratories should always be willing to adopt newer techniques and philosophies developed by the dental profession and being taught to dental graduates. Too often the commercial dental laboratory insists upon using stereotyped techniques that suit its production methods and actively attempts to discourage the recent graduate from putting into practice modern methods and techniques that were painstakingly taught to him in dental school by instructors whose knowledge of the subject far exceeds that of the laboratory technician who depreciates it.

3. I believe that any free-end partial denture must have the best possible support from the underlying edentulous ridge and that the design of the abutment retainers must apply a minimum of torque to the adjacent abutment teeth. I believe that some kind of secondary impression is necessary to obtain adequate support for the denture base, both through tissue placement and from the broadest possible coverage compatible with biologic requirements and limitations.

4. I believe in the functional, or dynamic, registration of occlusal relationships rather than in relying upon intraoral adjustment of an established centric occlusion or upon the ability of an instrument to simulate articulatory movements. I believe that the occlusion on a partial denture, be it fixed or removable, should be made to harmonize with the existing adjusted natural occlusion, and that this can best be accomplished by the registration of functional occlusal paths. For this to be done adequately, occlusion on the partial denture must be established upon either the final denture base(s) or upon an accurate substitute for the final base(s). The practice of attempting to submit jaw relation records to the technician prior to the fabrication of the denture framework is therefore, with few exceptions, strongly condemned.

5. I believe that a partial denture, when properly designed, carefully made, and serviced when needed, can be an entirely satisfactory restoration and can serve as a means of preserving remaining oral structures as well as restoring missing dentition. Unless a partial denture is made with adequate abutment support, with optimal base support, and with harmonious and functional occlusion, it should be clear to all concerned that such a denture should be considered only a temporary, treatment, or interim denture rather than a restoration representative of the best that modern prosthetic dentistry has to offer.

W. L. McC.

Contents

Chapter 4

Classification of partially edentulous arches, 73

Chapter 5

Surveying, 82

Chapter 6

Principles of partial denture design, 113

Chapter 7

Component parts of the partial denture: major and minor connectors, 128

Chapter 8

Occlusal rests, 151

Chapter 9

Direct retainers, 165

Chapter 14

Impression materials and procedures for partial dentures, 277

Chapter 15

Support for the free-end denture base, 300

Chapter 16

Occlusal relationships for partial dentures, 338

Chapter 17

Laboratory procedures, 370

Partial denture
construction

Chapter 1

Terminology

The subject of prosthodontic terminology has been neglected until only recently, with the result that much confusion has been allowed to exist because of conflicting terms. Thanks to the efforts of the Academy of Denture Prosthetics and its Nomenclature Committee, a *Glossary of Prosthodontic Terms* has been made available to the profession.* The efforts of the Nomenclature Committee is a continuing one in an endeavor to provide an authentic and acceptable glossary of prosthodontic terminology.

More recently, the American Dental Association, Bureau of Library and Indexing service, has published a Vocabulary of Dentistry and Oral Science.† This is the first dental vocabulary to be published since 1936 and is the result of three workshops sponsored by the American Dental Association ("Concepts of Occlusion" in 1952, "Supplementing the Dental Dictionary" in 1953, and "Troublesome Terms" in 1954) and of Denton's efforts toward compiling a comprehensive review of dental nomenclature.

Many conflicting or indefinite terms in common usage in prosthodontics require definition and clarification. Many of these are used synonomously, others incorrectly. While the following is not meant to be a complete glossary of partial denture terminology, some definitions will be given, based upon available reference material.

A *prosthesis* is the replacement of an absent part of the human body by some artificial part, such as an eye, a leg, or a denture. *Prosthetics*, then, is the art of science of supplying missing parts of the human body.

When applied to dentistry, the term prosthetics becomes *prosthodontics* and

---

*This glossary first appeared in the March, 1956, issue of The Journal of Prosthetic Dentistry (published by The C. V. Mosby Company, St. Louis, Mo.). The latest reprint, published in 1963, may be obtained from Dr. Louis S. Block, Chairman, Editorial Council of The Journal of Prosthetic Dentistry, 3939 Old Brownboro Rd., Louisville 7, Ky.

†Denton, G. B.: The Vocabulary of Dentistry and Oral Science, Chicago, 1958, American Dental Association.

denotes that branch of dental art or science that treats specifically with the replacements of missing dental and oral tissues. The term prosthodontics is somewhat preferable to the term *prosthetic dentistry*. The latter is defined by the American Dental Association as "The science or art of providing suitable substitutes for the coronal portions of teeth, or for one or more lost or missing natural teeth and their associated parts, in order that impaired function, appearance, comfort, and health of the patient may be restored." This definition is broad and may be applied to operative dentistry as well as to the restoration of individual teeth by means of cast inlays and crowns.

The replacement of missing teeth may be accomplished by a fixed, or cemented, prosthesis or by a removable prosthesis. The former may be in two pieces, with a locking joint between, or all in one piece. The latter may be attached to the abutment teeth by either intracoronal or extracoronal retainers. In any case, the prosthesis is spoken of as a *bridge* or a *bridge prosthesis*. Functionally, they all have one thing in common—they are supported entirely by abutment teeth.

A *complete denture prosthesis* is entirely supported by the tissues (mucous membrane, connective tissues, and underlying bone) upon which it rests. A *partial denture prosthesis* is neither entirely tissue supported nor entirely tooth supported. It is a prosthetic restoration which replaces missing teeth and other parts in a partially edentulous arch, but it derives its principal support from the tissues underlying its base and to a lesser degree from some of the remaining teeth that are used as abutments. The true partial denture is therefore unique in that it derives its support from both the teeth and the tissues of the residual ridge. A true partial denture will always have one or more free-end bases. There is some confusion in the use of the term *partial denture* in that some authors use the term to include all tooth-borne replacements of missing teeth in a partially edentulous arch. In such usage a cemented bridge is referred to as a *fixed partial denture* and a removable prosthesis is called a *removable partial denture*.

There are sufficient points of difference between the removable bridge and the partial denture to justify a distinction between the two types of removable restorations. Principles of design and the techniques employed in construction may be completely dissimilar. The points of difference are as follows:

1. The manner in which the prosthesis is supported.
2. The impression methods required for each.
3. The types of direct retainers best suited for each.
4. The base material best suited for each.
5. The need for indirect retention.

Although the term *removable partial denture* will be used broadly throughout this book to apply to both the tooth-supported and the tooth- and tissue-supported restoration, a distinction will be made between the bilateral removable bridge prosthesis and the true partial denture prosthesis.

The term *appliance* is correctly applied only to a device worn by the patient in the course of treatment, such as splints, orthodontic appliances, and space maintainers. A denture, an obturator, a bridge, or a crown is properly called a *prosthesis*. The terms *prosthesis, restoration,* and *denture* will generally be used synonymously in this book to avoid tiresome repetition of the single word *prosthesis.*

A *treatment denture* is a dental prosthesis used for the purpose of treating or conditioning the tissues which are called upon to support and retain a denture base.

A *provisional denture* is a dental prosthesis used for the purpose of conditioning the patient to the acceptance of an artificial substitute for missing natural teeth.

A *transitional denture* is a dental prosthesis that can be added to or replaced following changes in the oral tissues.

A *temporary or interim denture* is a dental prosthesis used for the purpose of spanning an interval of time for reasons of esthetics, mastication, occlusal support, or convenience until more complete dental treatment can be provided.

Use of the term *acrylic* as a noun will be avoided. Instead, it will be used only as an adjective, such as *acrylic resin.* The word *plastic* may be used either as an adjective or a noun, in the latter sense referring to any of various substances that harden and retain their shape after being molded. The term *resin* will be used as a broad term for substances named according to their chemical composition, physical structure, and means for activation or curing, such as *acrylic resin.*

The term *base* will be used to designate that part of a denture, either of metal or of a resin material, which supports the supplied teeth and/or receives support either from the abutment teeth or the residual ridge, or both. The term *saddle* is considered objectionable terminology when used to designate a denture base.

The tissues underlying the denture base, which have been called the *subjacent* tissues, will be spoken of as the *residual ridge* or *edentulous ridge,* referring to the residual alveolar bone with its soft tissue covering. The exact character of this soft tissue covering may vary and includes the mucous membrane and the underlying fibrous connective tissue.

Resurfacing of a denture base with new material to make it fit the underlying tissues more accurately will be spoken of as *relining.* The term *rebasing* refers to a process that goes beyond relining and involves the refitting of a denture by the replacement of the denture base with new material without changing the occlusal relations of the teeth.

Perhaps no other terms in prosthetic dentistry have been associated with more controversy than the terms *centric relation, centric position,* and *centric occlusion.* The definitions given in the *Glossary of Prosthodontic Terms* are as follows:

"*centric relation:* The most retruded relation of the mandible to the maxillae when the condyles are in the most posterior unstrained position in the glenoid fossae from which lateral movement can be made, at any given degree of jaw separation."

"*centric position:* The position of the mandible when the jaws are in centric relation."

Centric occlusion is given two definitions in the *Glossary of Prosthodontic*

Terms, as follows: (1) "the relation of opposing occlusal surfaces which provides the maximum planned contact and/or intercuspation," and (2) "the occlusion of the teeth when the mandible is in centric relation to the maxillae."

Moulton had this to say about centric occlusion:

> The initial point of contact of teeth during a mandibular closure into the terminal hinge position is fundamental to diagnosis and treatment planning for dentulous patients. This tooth relationship is termed centric occlusion.
>
> The definition of the terminal hinge position locates the condyles in their most retruded position in the glenoid fossae. This concept allows attention to be focused on a tooth relationship while the condyles have a specific correlation in the fossae. Therefore, in centric occlusion there may be an ideal cusp arrangement in this mandible-to-maxillae relationship; or possibly only one cusp of one mandibular tooth may occlude with a cusp of a maxillary tooth.
>
> This first tooth contact, regardless of the cusp relationship, is centric occlusion. After this initial contact, the mandible often shifts to bring more teeth into occlusion. This is eccentric occlusion. In closing into eccentric occlusion, the mandible follows the dictates of the neuromuscular system. The proprioceptive impulses received from receptors in the periodontal membrane cause a reaction which attempts to produce a closure that avoids the traumatic effect of deflective occlusal contacts.*

Thus it would seem that the second definition is preferable to the first, despite its long and continued usage.

In artificial dentition on complete dentures centric occlusion should be made to coincide with centric relation for that patient. In adjusting natural occlusion, the objective is to establish harmony between centric relation and centric occlusion. In dentition on partial dentures, the objective is to make the artificial occlusion coincide and be in harmony with the remaining natural occlusion. Ideally, the natural occlusion must first have been adjusted to maximum contact at centric relation, and be free of eccentric interference, before establishing a similar occlusion on the partial denture.

In describing the various component parts of the partial denture, conflicting terminology must be recognized and the preferred terms defined. A *retainer* is defined as "any form of attachment applied directly to an abutment tooth used for the fixation of a prosthetic restoration." Thus, the attachment may be intracoronal or extracoronal and may be used as a means of retaining either a removable or a fixed restoration. A solder joint may also be considered to be an attachment. The term *internal attachment* will be used in preference to the terms *precision attachment, frictional attachment,* and others to describe any mechanical retaining device that depends upon frictional resistance between parallel walls of male and female (or key and keyway) parts. The term precision attachment is discarded because its usage implies that all other types or retainers are less precise in their design and fabrication.

The term *clasp* will be used in conjunction with the words "retainer," "arm," or "assembly" whenever possible. The clasp assembly will consist of a *retentive clasp arm* and a *reciprocal* or *stabilizing clasp arm,* plus any minor connectors

---

*From Moulton, G. H.: The Importance of Centric Occlusion in Diagnosis and Treatment Planning, J. Pros. Den. **10:**921-926, 1960, and occlusal rests from which they originate or with which they are associated. The term *bar clasp arm* will be used in preference to the use of Roach's name to designate this type of extracoronal retainer and is defined as a clasp arm that originates from the base or framework, traverses soft tissue, and approaches the tooth undercut area from a gingival direction. In contrast, the term *circumferential clasp arm* will be used to designate a clasp arm that originates above the height of contour, traverses a portion of the suprabulge portion of the tooth, and approaches the tooth undercut from an occlusal direction. Both types of clasp arms terminate in a retentive undercut lying gingival to the height of contour and both provide retention by the resistance of metal to deformation rather than frictional resistance of parallel walls.

A *continuous clasp* is a component of the partial denture framework which augments the major connector(s) and lies on the lingual or facial surface of several teeth. It is most frequently used on the middle third of the lingual slope of lower anterior teeth. In such case it is called a *secondary lingual bar* in preference to the use of Kennedy's name to designate this usage of the continuous clasp. If connected to the lingual bar major connector with a thin, contoured apron, the apron is designated as a *lingual apron* or *lingual plate*.

For lack of better terminology, any thin, broad palatal coverage used as a palatal major connector is called a *palatal plate* or, if of lesser width, a *palatal strap*. The term *anatomic replica* will be used in preference to the patented term Tru-Rugae to designate cast metal palates which duplicate the topography of that portion of the patient's mouth. This is in keeping with a desire to use descriptive terminology whenever possible.

The term *occlusal rest* will be used to designate any component of the partial denture which is so placed on an abutment tooth, preferably in a seat prepared to receive it, that it limits movement of the denture in a gingival direction. Although the occlusal surface of a premolar or molar tooth offers the most ideal location for an occlusal rest, it may be placed on a canine or an incisor tooth as a *cingulum rest*, an *incisal rest,* an *incisal hook,* or an *embrasure hook.* All of these are considered to be occlusal rests since they function to prevent movement toward the tissue and assist in providing occlusal support for the prosthesis.

The terms *canine* (tooth) and *premolar* (tooth) will be used to designate those teeth commonly called cuspid and bicuspid teeth. Denton gives the chief arguments for the use of the word *canine* as "(1) it is the term used in other sciences, and (2) other terms in standard usage can be understood only in relation to *canine* tooth; for example canine eminence, canine fossa, etc." For the use of the term *premolar* he gives the following arguments: "(1) the term bicuspid is not descriptive of all teeth in that class, and (2) the acceptance of premolar makes uniform the terminology of dentistry and comparative dental anatomy."

In describing an impression and resulting cast of the supporting form of the edentulous ridge, the terms *functional impression* and *functional ridge form* will be used in the absence of a more descriptive terminology. These terms have become accepted as meaning the form of the edentulous ridge when it is supporting a denture base. It is artificially created by the use of a fluid wax impression material which displaces those tissues that can be readily displaced and that would be incapable of rendering support to the denture base. Firm areas are not displaced due to the flow characteristics of the impression material. Thus, the tissues are recorded more nearly in the form that they will assume when supporting a functional load. In contrast, the static form of the edentulous ridge as recorded in a soft impression material such as hydrocolloid, rubber-base material, or metallic oxide impression paste is spoken of as the anatomic ridge form. This is the surface form of the edentulous ridge when at rest or when not supporting a functional load.

The terms *functional occlusion* and *functional occlusal registration* are sufficiently descriptive and are used to designate a dynamic registration of opposing dentition as opposed to the recording of a static relationship of one jaw to another. While centric position is found somewhere in a functional occlusal registration, eccentric positions are also recorded, and the created occlusion is made to harmonize with all gliding and chewing movements the patient is capable of making.

The term *odontexesis* is described by Denton as being more descriptive of "tooth scraping" than the commonly used term prophylaxis. The latter is an example of a general term being reduced in meaning to refer to a specific dental treatment. As to the term *scaling* for the removal of calcareous deposits from the teeth, Denton says, "this term is not only more colloquial than professional, but lacks in descriptiveness when used alone."

The word *cast* may be used as a verb (to cast) or as an adjective (cast framework or cast metal base). It is used most frequently in this text as a noun to designate a positive reproduction of a maxillary or mandibular dental arch made from an impression of that arch. Such an objective is further designated according to the purpose for which it is made, such as *study cast, master cast,* or *investment cast.* An investment cast may also be spoken of as a *refractory cast,* since it is compounded to withstand higher temperatures without disintegrating and, incidentally, to perform certain functions relative to the burnout and expansion of the mold. A *refractory investment* is an investment material that can withstand the high temperatures of casting or soldering. Plaster of Paris or artificial stone may also be considered *investment* if it is used to invest any part of a dental restoration for the purpose of processing it.

A *wax pattern* is converted to a *casting* by the elimination of the pattern by heat, leaving a mold into which the molten metal is thrown by centrifugal force or other means. The term *casting* is therefore used most frequently as a noun, meaning "a thing shaped by being poured into a mold to harden." It is used primarily to designate the cast metal framework of a partial denture but may also be used to describe a molded denture base which is also actually cast into a mold.

The term *cast* in dentistry should always imply that it is an *accurate* reproduction of the tissues being studied or upon which a restoration may be fabricated. Any cast that is admittedly inaccurate is unpardonable and unacceptable in modern dentistry because of the excellence of impression and cast materials available today.

The term *cast* is preferable to the term *model,* which should only be used to designate a reproduction for display or demonstration purposes. A model of a dental arch or any portion thereof may be made of durable and attractive material. It need not be an accurate reproduction but should be a reasonable facsimile of the original. It is frequently made of tooth- and tissue-colored resin.

The term *mold* is also incorrect when applied to a reproduction of a dental arch or portion thereof. It is a term used to indicate either the cavity into which a casting is made or the shape of an artificial tooth.

Dental stones are used to make an artificial stone reproduction from an impression and occasionally they are used as an investment or for mounting purposes. All dental stones are gypsum products. Use of the word stone in dentistry should be applied only to those gypsum materials that are used for their hardness, accuracy, and/or abrasion resistance.

Some controversy exists over the use of the terms *x-ray, radiograph,* and *roentgenogram* in dentistry. The American Academy of Oral Roentgenology has indicated its preference for the use of the term roentgenogram, at the same time admitting that it may leave much to be desired as a descriptive terminology. Examination of several recent textbooks on dental subjects finds usage divided between all three terms. However, in deference to the terminology preferred by the American Acadmy of Oral Roentgenology, the terms *roentgenogram, roentgenographic survey,* and *roentgenographic interpretation* are used herein.

Many others terms used in prosthetic dentistry might be defined in this chapter, but such an undertaking is worthy of the efforts of those who have recently directed their thoughts to that end. The Nomenclature Committee of the Academy of Denture Prosthetics is to be commended for their efforts in compiling a glossary which may be used for future guidance in prosthodontic terminology. Familiarity with accepted prosthodontic terminology should be acquired by the dental student, for a vocabulary once acquired is always difficult to change.

The clasp partial denture

The clasp-type partial denture, utilizing the extracoronal direct retainer, is probably utilized a hundred times more frequently than the intracoronal, or internal attachment, partial denture. While the clasp partial denture has numerous disadvantages, for reasons of economy and time involved, it will probably continue to be used because it is capable of providing a physiologically sound service to the greatest number of patients needing partial denture restorations in keeping with their ability to pay for such service. Some of the possible disadvantages of a clasp partial denture are as follows:

1. Caries may develop beneath clasp components, especially if the abutments are not protected with cast restorations and the patient fails to keep the prosthesis and the abutments clean.

2. Strain is too often placed on the abutment teeth by improper clasp designs.

3. Clasps are often unesthetic, particularly when placed on visible tooth surfaces.

Despite these disadvantages, the use of removable prostheses may be preferred where there are tooth-bounded edentulous spaces of greater magnitude than can safely be restored with fixed prostheses or where cross-arch stabilization and wider distribution of stress loading is desirable. The removable partial denture retained by internal attachments eliminates some of the disadvantages of clasps, but it has other disadvantages, one of which is too great a cost for a large percentage of patients needing partial dentures. Fixed bridges should always be used whenever indicated.

When the alignment of the abutment teeth is favorable, the clinical crown is of sufficient length, the pulp size is diminished by tooth maturity, and the economic status of the patient permits, an internal attachment prosthesis is unquestionably preferable for esthetic reasons. In most instances, if the internal attachment denture is designed properly, this is its only advantage, for abutment protection and bracing components should be used with both internal and external retainers. However, economics permitting, esthetics alone may justify the use of a claspless denture.

I do not believe in the routine use of hinges or other types of stress breakers for free-end partial dentures, much less in conjunction with internal attachments. It is not because they are ineffective but because they are more frequently misused and substituted for adequate support for the partial denture base. Particularly in the mandibular arch, in the absence of the cross-arch stabilization inherent in a rigid denture design, a stress-broken distal extension frequently subjects the edentulous ridge to excessive trauma from horizontal forces.

Because it must be used in conjunction with some form of stress breaker, the internal attachment is not indicated when one or more free-end edentulous spaces exist. In the true partial denture, a rigid design is preferred, and therefore some type of extracoronal retainer must be used. Of these, the clasp retainer is still the most frequently used, and it seems likely that its use will continue until a more widely acceptable retainer is devised.

THREE PHASES OF PARTIAL DENTURE SERVICE

Partial denture service may logically be divided into three phases. Included in the first phase are *treatment planning, design of the partial denture framework, and the execution of mouth preparations.* The second phase is the *obtaining of adequate support for the free-end base.* The third and final phase is the *establishment of harmonious occlusal relationships with the opposing and remaining natural teeth.*

Treatment Planning and Design. Following a complete oral examination, including interpretation of radiographs and a survey of study casts, a treatment plan is evolved that is based upon the support available for the partial denture. Distal extension situations, where no posterior abutments remain and any free-end bases must derive their support from the underlying residual ridge, require an entirely different partial denture design than one where total abutment support is available. This is apparent from visual examination, but roentgenographic interpretation and the surveying of abutments must take into consideration the greater torque and tipping leverages of the distal extension partial denture.

Basically, the same principles apply to the unilateral free-end denture as to the bilateral free-end denture. On the other hand, entirely different principles of design apply to a prosthesis that is totally tooth suported. The latter is actually a tooth-borne removable bridge rather than a true partial denture. Each type must be designed according to the manner of support.

The dental surveyor is necessary in any dental office where partial dentures are being constructed. There is no more reason to justify its omission from a dentist's armamentarium than to ignore the need for roentgenographic equipment or the mouth mirror and explorer used for diagnostic purposes.

There are several moderately priced surveyors on the market which will adequately accomplish the diagnostic procedures necessary for designing the partial denture. And yet, in a large number of dental offices today, this most important phase of dental diagnosis must be delegated to the commercial dental laboratory because of the absence of a single necessary piece of equipment. This is a deplorable and degrading situation which makes no more sense than relying upon the technician to interpret roentgenograms and render a diagnosis therefrom.

Following treatment planning, mouth preparations may be performed with a definite goal in mind. Through the aid of study casts upon which the tentative design of the partial denture has been outlined and the mouth changes have been indicated in colored pencil, abutment restorations and abutment modifications can be accomplished which will provide for adequate support and retention of the partial denture.

Proximal tooth surfaces should be made parallel to provide guiding planes during insertion and removal of the prosthesis. Occlusal rest seats should be established that will direct occlusal forces toward the long axis of the supporting teeth, so that neither the tooth nor the denture will be displaced under occlusal loading. This dictates that the floor of the rest preparation be made to incline toward the center of the tooth and be spoon-shaped, with marginal ridge lowered to permit sufficient bulk without occlusal interference.

Retentive areas must be identified or created, which will provide for equal and uniform retention on all abutment teeth, sufficient only to resist reasonable dislodging forces. Reciprocal tooth surfaces upon which bracing clasp arms may be placed must also be identified or created.

Following mouth preparations, the impression for the master cast should be made and poured immediately. The master cast must then be surveyed to see if some slight changes in the path of insertion are indicated to accommodate for minor discrepancies in mouth preparations.

The final design of the denture framework should be outlined in pencil on the master cast, including the location of clasp arms in relation to the height of contour of the abutment teeth. It must be remembered that the location of clasp arms will be determined by the height of contour of the abutment teeth and that this exists for a given path of insertion only; hence the need for proximal guiding planes and accurate blockout of proximal tooth surfaces. The position of the cast in relation to the surveyor must be recorded so that the technician may similarly place the cast on his surveyor to parallel the blockout material. This is easily done by scoring the base of the cast on three sides parallel to the path of insertion, but this must be done before the cast is removed from the surveyor.

It is necessary that a specific design be carefully planned in advance of mouth preparations and that these mouth preparations be carried out with care, as outlined on the study cast. Specific and exact mouth preparations, including abutment restorations, will then dictate the final form of the denture framework to be outlined on the master cast. This should be penciled on the master cast after surveying so that there will be no doubt in the mind of the technician as to the exact design of the partial denture framework he is to construct.

Surveying the master cast, scoring the base of the cast to record its position on the surveyor, and drawing a definite outline on the master cast are still not enough. It is impossible to draw upon the master cast all of the details of the denture design. This should be done by labeling a colored pencil drawing upon a chart, which provides the technician with an outline of the partial denture framework and allows for marginal instructions for the technician to follow in fabricating the denture. From this information, it is possible for the technician to return a casting to the dentist superimposed upon the outline as drawn on the master cast. From any lesser instructions the technician cannot be criticized for returning a more stereotyped partial denture design.

The responsibility for the design of the partial denture framework should be the dentist's from the beginning to the finish; therefore, he is responsible for providing the technician with all the information needed. It is the responsibility of the technician to follow the written instructions given him by the dentist, but at the same time it is his prerogative to demand that these instructions be such that he can follow them without question.

Up to this point the treatment planning and design of the partial denture, the preparation of abutments, and the actual design of the denture framework and retainers may be adequately accomplished through close cooperation between dentist and technician. Given adequate jaw relation records, the technician can then complete the partial denture if it is of the tooth-supported type or if the dentist is satisfied to have free-end bases finished to the anatomic form of the edentulous ridge. This is the form that was recorded by the original impression from which the master cast was made. However, adequate support for free-end bases and the need for exact occlusal records make it necessary that the denture framework be returned to the dentist for further records before completion of the prosthesis.

Adequate Support for Free-End Bases. As was stated earlier, there are three phases in the construction of a partial denture. The second of these is adequate support for free-end bases and therefore does not apply to tooth-borne removable partial dentures. In the latter, support comes entirely from the abutment teeth through the use of occlusal rests.

For the free-end partial denture, however, a base made to fit the anatomic ridge form does not provide adequate support under occlusal loading. Neither does it provide for maximum peripheral extension nor accurate peripheral detail. Therefore, some type of correction impression is necessary. This may be accomplished by several means, all of which satisfy the requirements for support of any free-end partial denture base.

Foremost is the requirement that the tissues should be recorded or related under some loading so that the base may be made to fit the form of the ridge when under function, thereby providing support and assuring a maintenance of that support for the longest possible time. This requirement makes the free-end partial denture unique in that the support from the tissues underlying the free-end base must be made as equal to and compatible with the tooth support as possible.

A complete denture is entirely tissue supported and the entire denture can move tissueward under function. In contrast, any movement of a partial denture base is inevitably a rotational movement, which results in loss of occlusal balance and the application of forces to the abutment teeth. Therefore, every effort must be made to provide the best possible support for the free-end base in order to minimize these forces.

No single impression technique can adequately record the anatomic form of the teeth and adjacent structures and at the same time record the supporting form of the edentulous ridge. Therefore, some method must be used which will record these tissues either in their supporting *form* or in a supporting *relationship* to the rest of the denture. This may be accomplished by one of several methods. One is to reline the finished denture to provide adequate support. Another is to make a combination impression by finger loading a previously made anatomic impression at the time it is related to the rest of the arch in an over-all elastic impression. The latter method does not attempt to record a different surface form of the ridge but, instead, records the relationship of the ridge to the rigid parts of the denture in the same manner that it will be related to the rest of the arch when an occlusal load is applied. This method presumes that there will be some rebound of the tissues when an occlusal load is released.

A third method records the supporting form of the ridge with a secondary impression through the use of a mouth-temperature wax. An impression wax must be used which is capable of displacing and leveling out tissues, thereby making the supporting tissues more compact over a larger area and providing adequate support through uniformity of the supporting surface. A mouth-temperature wax must be used which will flow sufficiently to prevent overdisplacement of tissues and yet, given sufficient time, will permit a recovery of any tissues that have been overloaded. At the same time, soft tissues are made more compact and better able to render support to the partial denture base.

Although there are minor variations in this technique, the one most commonly used is the making of the wax impression in a resin base attached to the denture framework. Anatomic ridges are cut away and discarded and that portion of the master cast repoured to conform to the new wax impression. This provides a corrected master cast upon which the denture base will be processed.

When a free-end partial denture is to be made with a metal base, the master cast is usually corrected prior to making the denture casting. In this case, a resin tray technique is used, utilizing three or more occlusal stops to position the resin tray in the mouth and then back onto the master cast with the same degree of accuracy as the returning of a cast denture framework to the master cast. Thus, the master cast may be corrected prior to the making of the denture casting.

If the above procedure is not followed, the metal bases must be cast separately after the master cast has been corrected, and then the denture must be assembled by soldering or by attaching the parts with resin. The latter method offers an advantage in that the denture can be disassembled at any future time and new metal bases made without having to remake the original framework.

Establishment of Occlusal Relations. Whether the partial denture is tooth-borne or has one or more free-end bases, the recording of occlusal relationships comprises the final step in the construction of a partial denture. For the tooth-borne partial denture, ridge form is of little significance since it is not called upon to support the prosthesis. For the free-end base, however, jaw relation records should be made only after obtaining the best possible support for the denture base. This necessitates the making of a base or bases which will provide the same support as the finished denture. Therefore, jaw relation records cannot be recorded until after the denture framework has been returned to the dentist and a secondary impression has been taken. Either a new resin base or a corrected base must then be used to record jaw relation records.

Occlusal records for a partial denture may be made by several methods. The one most frequently used is the recording of a static relationship with the opposing teeth. This method presumes that allowance will be made for denture settling and that occlusal harmony will be established on the finished denture by occlusal adjustment in the mouth.

A second method, which is a graphic one, may be used to record centric jaw relation, but only where the opposing teeth and the remaining natural teeth are or can be made noninterfering. This is because a graphic record is usually made on one plane and does not allow for cuspal inclinations. Therefore, this method is usually used only where a partial denture is being made to an opposing complete denture.

A third method is the registration of functional paths. This records the opposing teeth in function and allows the occlusion on the partial denture to be made to conform to the cuspal influence of the remaining natural teeth. When there are natural teeth remaining in contact, they will influence jaw movements by cuspal guidance rather than by condylar guidance as in the completely edentulous mouth. Registration of functional paths permits seating of the denture under a functional relationship with the opposing teeth and in cuspal harmony with the remaining natural teeth.

Such a wax record is converted to a stone template and the denture teeth are modified to occlude with the template, thereby eliminating any lateral interference on the finished denture. When one considers the influence of cuspal contacts throughout the remainder of the arch, it becomes quite clear that some method of functional registration must be used or else the dentist must assume the entire responsibility for perfecting the occlusion on the partial denture in the mouth.

REASONS FOR FAILURE OF THE CLASP PARTIAL DENTURE

Experience with the clasp-type partial denture made by methods herein outlined has proved its merit and justifies its continued use. The occasional objection to the visibility of retentive clasps can be minimized through the use of wrought-wire clasp arms. There are few contraindications for use of the clasp partial denture when properly designed. Practically all of the objections to the clasp partial denture can be disposed of by pointing to deficiencies in its design and fabrication. These can be listed as follows:

1. Inadequate diagnosis and treatment planning.
2. Failure to use the surveyor during diagnosis and treatment planning.
3. Inadequate mouth preparations, usually due to insufficient planning of the design of the partial denture.
4. Failure to provide the technician with a specific design and the necessary information for following out this design.

5. Failure of the technician to follow the design and instructions outlined. (This is due either to disagreement as to the wisdom of the dentist's design or resistance on the part of the dental laboratory to follow other than stereotyped designs which may be mass produced. Either of these causes can and must be either eliminated or rectified through closer cooperation between the dentist and the technician.)

6. Incorrect use of clasp designs and improper use of cast clasps that have too little flexibility, too broad tooth coverage, and too little consideration for esthetics.

7. Failure to provide for adequate tissue support for free-end denture bases.

8. Failure to provide for posterior occlusal forms which are in harmony with the cuspal relationships of the remaining natural teeth.

A partial denture which is so designed and fabricated that it avoids the errors and deficiencies listed above is one that proves the clasp-type partial denture can be made functional, esthetically pleasing, and long lasting, without damage to the supporting structures. The proof of the merit of the clasp partial denture lies in the knowledge that (1) it permits partial denture service for the largest number of patients, as the need for this service increases with advances in other phases of dentistry, made economically possible by the avoidance of elaborate mechanical devices and high laboratory costs; (2) it provides partial dentures that are comfortable and efficient over a long period of time, with adequate support and maintenance of occlusal contact relations; (3) it provides for healthy abutments, free of caries and periodontal disease; and (4) it makes possible a partial denture service that is definitive and not merely an interim service.

Partial dentures thus made contribute to a concept of prosthetic dentistry which has as its goal the preservation of as many teeth as possible, the restoration of partially edentulous mouths, and an ultimate elimination of the need for complete dentures.

Chapter 3

Diagnosis and treatment planning

Diagnosis and treatment planning for oral rehabilitation must take into consideration some or all of the following procedures: the restoration of individual teeth with fillings, cast inlays, or crowns; the restoration of occlusal relationships; the replacement of missing teeth by fixed restorations; and the replacement of other missing teeth by means of removable partial dentures.

The treatment plan for the partial denture, which is frequently the final step in an extensive and lengthy sequence of treatment, should precede earlier treatment so that abutment teeth and other areas in the mouth may be properly prepared to support and retain the partial denture. This means that a study cast for the purpose of designing and planning partial denture treatment must be made at the time of the original diagnosis. The design that is drawn on the study cast, along with a detailed chart of mouth conditions and proposed treatment, is the master plan for the mouth preparations and the partial denture to follow.

Failures of partial dentures, other than structural defects, can usually be attributed to inadequate diagnosis, failure to properly evaluate the conditions present, and failure to prepare the mouth properly prior to construction of the master cast. The importance of the examination, the consideration of favorable and unfavorable aspects, and the importance of planning the elimination of unfavorable influences cannot be stressed too strongly.

VISUAL EXAMINATION

Visual examination will reveal many of the signs of dental disease. Consideration of *caries susceptibility* is of primary importance. The number of fillings present, signs of recurrent caries, and evidence of decalcification should be noted. Generally, the very young and the older partial denture patient are poor risks so far as the use of unprotected abutments is concerned. Only those patients in the so-called prime of life, presenting with good oral hygiene, may be considered good abutment risks without resorting to such prophylactic measures as the crowning and splinting of abutment teeth.

Evidence of periodontal disease, inflammation of gingival areas, and the degree of gingival recession should be noted at the time of initial examination. In addition, the depths of periodontal pockets should be determined by instrumentation and the degree of mobility of the teeth by digital examination. Although evidence of periodontal disease is detectable visually, the *extent* of damage to the supporting structures by periodontal disease must be determined by roentgenographic interpretation.

The number of teeth remaining and the location of the edentulous areas will have a definite bearing upon the proportionate amount of support which the partial denture will receive from the teeth and the edentulous ridges.

During the oral examination, not only must each arch be considered separately but also its occlusal relationship with the opposing arch. A situation that looks simple when the teeth are apart may be complicated when the teeth are in occlusion. For example, an extreme vertical overlap may complicate the attachment of anterior teeth to a maxillary denture. Extrusion of a tooth or teeth into an opposing edentulous area may complicate the replacement of teeth in the edentulous area, or it may create cuspal interference which will complicate the location and design of clasp retainers and occlusal rests. Where occlusal interference cannot be adequately determined by visual examination, the interposition of wax strips of varying thickness between the teeth may assist in determining the amount of interference or clearance present. Such findings will subsequently be further evaluated by a study of occluded study casts.

Need for Reshaping Remaining Teeth. Many failures of partial dentures can be attributed to the fact that the teeth were not reshaped properly to receive clasp arms and occlusal rests before the impression for the master cast was made. Of particular importance is the paralleling of proximal tooth surfaces to act as guiding planes, the preparation of adequate occlusal rest areas, and the reduction of unfavorable tooth contours. To neglect to plan such mouth preparations in advance is inexcusable.

The design of clasps is dependent upon the location of the retentive and supporting areas in relation to a definite path of insertion and removal. Failure to reshape unfavorably inclined tooth surfaces and, if necessary, place inlays and crowns with suitable contours not only complicates the design and location of clasp retainers but also frequently leads to failure of the partial denture due to poor clasp design.

A malaligned tooth or one inclined unfavorably may make it necessary to so place certain parts of the clasp that they interfere with the opposing teeth. Proximal tooth surfaces which are not parallel will not only fail to provide needed guiding planes during insertion and removal but will also make necessary excessive blockout. This inevitably results in the connectors being placed so far out of contact with tooth surfaces that undesirable food traps are created. In order to pass lingually inclined lower teeth, clearance for a lingual bar major connector may have to be so great that a food trap will result when the appliance is fully seated, and the bar will be so located that it will interfere with tongue comfort and function. These are only some of the objectionable consequences of inadequate mouth preparations.

Reduction of Unfavorable Tooth Contours. Slight reduction of unfavorable tooth contours will greatly facilitate the design of the partial denture framework. The need for modification of tooth contours must be established during the diagnosis and treatment planning phase of partial denture construction.

The amount of reduction of tooth contours should be kept to a minimum, and all modified tooth surfaces should be repolished after reduction. If it is not possible to produce the contour desired without perforating the enamel cap, inlays or crowns must be used. The age of the patient, caries activity evidenced elsewhere in the mouth, and the apparent oral hygiene habits must all be taken into consideration when deciding between reducing the enamel or modifying tooth contours with protective restorations.

Some of the areas frequently needing correction are the lingual surfaces of mandibular premolars, the mesial and lingual surfaces of mandibular molars, the distobuccal line angle of maxillary premolars, and the mesiobuccal line angle of maxillary molars. The actual degree of inclination of teeth in relation to the path of insertion and the location of retentive and supporting areas are not readily interpretable during visual examination. These are established during a comprehensive survey of the study cast with a cast surveyor, which should follow the visual examination.

DENTAL CAST SURVEYOR

The cast surveyor (Fig. 1) is a simple enough instrument but is most essential to planning partial denture treatment. Its main working parts are the vertical arm and the adjustable table that holds the cast in a fixed relation to the vertical arm. This represents the path of insertion that the partial denture will ultimately take in the mouth.

The adjustable table may be tilted in relation to the vertical arm of the surveyor until a path can be found which best satisfies all of the factors involved. A cast in a horizontal relationship to the vertical arm represents a vertical path of insertion; a cast in a tilted relationship represents a path of insertion toward the side of the cast that is tilted upward. The vertical arm, when brought in contact with a tooth surface, will indicate the areas available for retention and those available for support, as well as the existence of tooth and other tissue interference to the path of insertion.

If conditions are found that are not favorable for the particular path of insertion being considered, the conditions produced by a different path of insertion should be studied. The cast is merely tilted in relation to the vertical arm until the most suitable path is found. Mouth preparations are then planned with a definite path of insertion in mind.

The path of insertion must also take into consideration the presence of tissue undercuts which will interfere with the placement of major connectors, the location of vertical minor connectors, the origin of bar clasp arms, and the denture bases.

Recording the Path of Insertion. Once the path of insertion for all factors involved has been ascertained, the base of the cast can be scored to record the relation of the cast to the surveyor for future reference (Fig. 2, *A* and *B*). A guide line may then be scribed on the surfaces of the abutment teeth by means

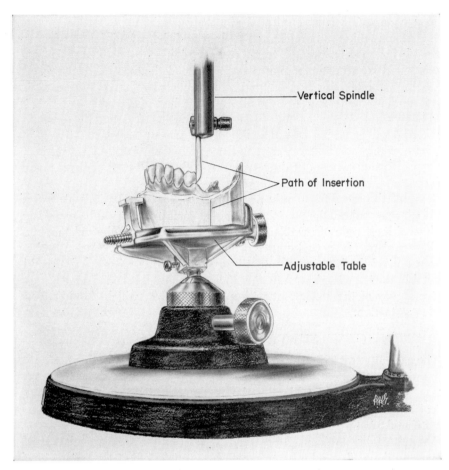

Vertical Spindle

Path of Insertion

Adjustable Table

Fig. 1. The most essential parts of a dental surveyor (Ney Parallelometer), showing the vertical arm in relation to the cast attached to the adjustable table.

of a graphite marker replacing the surveyor blade (Fig. 2, *C*). This guide line will graphically locate the division between retentive and supportive areas, as well as areas of interference. Modification of tooth contours and clasp designs may then be planned with accuracy and mouth preparations planned accordingly. The cast surveyor is an indispensable instrument in surveying the cast of the mouth prior to preparing the mouth to receive a partial denture. Only by its use can the dentist ascertain the mechanical factors upon which the success or failure of the partial denture will depend.

ORAL EXAMINATION

A complete oral examination should precede any mouth rehabilitation procedures. An oral examination should be complete—not limited to only one arch. It should include, in addition to a visual examination of the teeth and surrounding tissues with mouth mirror and explorer, a complete intraoral roentgenographic survey, a vitality test of critical teeth, and an examination of occluded study casts.

Fig. 2. A and **B,** The path of insertion having been determined, the base of the cast is scored to record its relation to the surveyor for future repositioning. **C,** The height of contour is then delineated by substituting a carbon rod for the surveyor blade.

During the examination, the objective to be kept foremost in mind should be the consideration of the possibilities for maintaining the remaining oral structures in a state of health for the longest period of time. In addition to the elimination of infection, the primary objectives should be the prevention of tooth migration and the elimination or correction of traumatic influences. Secondarily should be the consideration as to how best to restore lost function within the limits of tissue tolerance of the patient. Thirdly, and not before, should the decision be made as to how best to maintain or improve upon the appearance of the mouth. As the first two objectives are satisfied, so will the requirement of a comfortable and esthetically pleasing restoration be also satisfied.

Objectives of Prosthodontic Restoration. The objectives of any prosthodontic restoration may be stated thus: (1) the elimination of disease, (2) the preservation of the health and relationship of the teeth and the health of the remaining oral tissues, and (3) the restoration in part of lost teeth and function in an esthetically pleasing manner.

Patients with missing teeth may specifically request their replacement, especially where anterior teeth are missing and they are concerned only with the cosmetic implications. On the other hand, they may seek diagnosis and advice, the result of which is frequently the recommendation that the missing teeth be replaced with either fixed or removable restorations. In any case, the patient is usually concerned only with the replacement of the missing teeth. The dentist's primary obligation to the patient is to emphasize the importance of restoring the total mouth to a state of health and of preserving the remaining teeth and surrounding tissues. Incident to this is the functional and esthetically acceptable replacement of missing teeth in a harmonious relation with the remaining teeth and surrounding structures.

In many instances, restoration of lost function must be modified and minimized to avoid overloading the supporting structures. The prevention of tooth migration, healthful stimulation of oral tissues, and the preservation of the remaining teeth are of greater importance. The amount that lost masticatory function can be restored depends upon the tissue tolerance of the individual, as influenced by his age, his general health, and the health of the oral tissues.

Sequence for Oral Examination. An oral examination should be accomplished in the following sequence:

1. *A thorough and complete oral prophylaxis (odontexesis).* An adequate examination can best be accomplished with the teeth free of accumulated calculus and debris. Also, an accurate study cast reproduction of the dental arches can be obtained only if the teeth are clean; otherwise the teeth reproduced on the study casts are not a true representation of tooth and gingival contours. Cursory examination may precede odontexesis, but a thorough oral examination should be deferred until the teeth have been thoroughly cleaned and true surfaces uncovered.

2. *The placement of temporary or treatment fillings.* This is advisable not only to relieve discomfort arising from tooth defects but also to determine as early as possible the extent of caries and to arrest further caries activity until definitive treatment can be instituted. By restoring tooth contours with temporary restorations, the impression will not be torn in removal from the mouth, and a more accurate study cast may be obtained.

3. *A complete intraoral roentgenographic survey* (Fig. 3). The objectives of a roentgenographic examination are (a) to locate areas of infection and other pathosis that may be present, (b) to reveal the presence of root fragments, foreign objects, bone spicules, and irregular ridge formations, (c) to reveal the presence and extent of hidden caries and the relation of carious lesions to the pulp, (d) to permit evaluation of existing restorations as to evidence of recurrent caries, marginal leakage, and overhanging gingival margins. (e) to reveal the presence of pulp canal fillings and to permit their evaluation as to future prognosis (the design of the partial denture may hinge upon the decision to retain or extract a nonvital tooth), (f) to permit an evaluation of periodontal conditions present and to establish the need and possibilities for treatment, and (g) to evaluate the remaining alveolar support of abutment teeth—the number and supporting length of their roots, the amount of alveolar bone loss suffered through pathogenic processes, and the amount of alveolar support remaining.

Fig. 3. A complete intraoral roentgenographic survey of the remaining teeth and adjacent edentulous areas reveals much information vital to effective diagnosis and treatment planning. The response of bone to previous stress is of particular value in establishing the prognosis of teeth that are to be used as abutments.

4. *Vitality tests of remaining teeth,* particularly those to be used as abutments and those having deep restorations or deep carious lesions. This may be done either by thermal or by electronic means, whichever the operator has learned best to interpret.

5. *The exploration of teeth and investing structures* by instrumentation and by visual means. This should include a determination of tooth mobility, an examination of ridge form and anatomic irregularities, and the clinical examination of occlusal relationships. At this time, the presence of tori and other bony protuberances should be noted and their clinical significance evaluated. Also, history and diagnosis charts should be filled out at this time, as well as a simple working chart for future reference (Figs. 4 and 5). The latter does not become part of the patient's permanent record but records the nature and sequence of treatment which the dentist can use as a check list during treatment. A breakdown of the fee may be recorded on the back of this chart for easy reference should adjustments or substitutions become necessary by changes in the diagnosis as the work progresses.

6. *Impressions for accurate study casts,* preferably articulated on a suitable instrument. The importance of accurate study casts and their use will be discussed later in this chapter.

The fee for examination, which should include the cost of the roentgenographic survey and the examination of articulated study casts, should be established prior to the examination and should not be related to the cost of treatment. It should be understood that the charge for examination is based upon the time involved and the service rendered and that the material value of the roentgenographs and study casts is incidental to the effectiveness of the examination.

The examination record should always be available in the office for future consultation. Should consultation with another dentist be requested, modern respect for the hazards of unnecessary radiation justifies the dentist loaning the roentgenograms for this purpose. Preferably, however, double film packs should be used, so that one copy may be retained in the dentist's files.

PARTIAL DENTURE DIAGNOSIS AND TREATMENT RECORD

Patient:_____Reg. No._____

Student:_____Date:_____

Pertinent Radiographic Findings:_____

	UPPER	LOWER
Kennedy Classification		
Initial	Class_____, Mod._____	Class_____, Mod._____
Final	Class_____, Mod._____	Class_____, Mod._____
Abutment Teeth		
Teeth to be Extracted and Reason		
Surgical Preparation of Ridges		
Abutment Restorations (Tooth No. & Type Restorations)		
Final Mouth Preparations:		
Guiding Planes		
Reduction of Tooth Contours		
Occlusal Rests		
Date above completed		
Impression Materials Used:		
For Master Cast		
For Correction of Supporting Ridges		
Denture Base Materials		
Tooth Selection		
Occlusal Registration; Methods Used		
Drawing of Partial Denture Design: Metal framework in blue, Resin bases or attachments in red, Wrought retentive clasp arms in red.	MAXILLARY OCCLUSAL VIEW	MANDIBULAR OCCLUSAL VIEW
Insertion Date:		
Post-insertion Notes:		

Fig. 4. A diagnosis and treatment record chart for recording the treatment plan and pertinent data.

Fig. 5. A simple working chart. Fillings, crowns, and bridges to be made may be marked on the chart and checked off as completed during mouth preparations. Some may prefer to chart from an external viewpoint. In such case, the left and right sides of the chart are reversed.

ROENTGENOGRAPHIC INTERPRETATION

Many of the reasons for roentgenographic interpretation during oral examination are outlined herein and are considered in greater detail in other texts. The aspects of such interpretation which are the most pertinent to partial denture construction are those relative to the prognosis of remaining teeth that may be used as abutments.

The quality of the alveolar support of an abutment tooth is of primary importance, because the tooth will be called upon to withstand greater stress loads when supporting a dental prosthesis. Abutment teeth providing total abutment support to the prosthesis, be it either fixed or removable, will have to withstand a greater vertical load than before and, to some extent, greater horizontal forces. The latter may be minimized by establishing a harmonious occlusion and by distributing the horizontal forces among several teeth through the use of rigid connectors. Bilateral stabilization against horizontal forces is one of the attributes of a properly designed tooth-borne removable prosthesis. In many instances, abutment teeth are aided more than weakened by the presence of a bilaterally rigid partial denture.

In contrast, abutment teeth adjacent to free-end bases are subjected not only to vertical and horizontal forces but to torque forces as well, due to the movement of the tissue-supported base. Vertical support and stabilization against horizontal movement through rigid connectors are just as important as with a tooth-borne prosthesis, and the partial denture must be designed accordingly. But, in addition, the abutment tooth adjacent to the free end will be subjected to torque in proportion to the design of the retainers, the tissue support received by the base, and the total occlusal load applied. With this in mind, each abutment tooth must be carefully evaluated as to the alveolar support present and the past reaction of that bone to occlusal stress.

The Value of Interpreting Bone Density. The quality and quantity of bone in any part of the body is often evaluated by roentgenographic means. A detailed treatise dealing with the bone support of the abutment tooth should include many considerations not possible to include in this text because of space limitations. The reader should realize that subclinical variations in bone may exist but may not be observed because of the limitations inherent in technical methods and equipment.

Of importance to the prosthodontist when evaluating the quality and quantity of the alveolar bone are the height and the quality of the remaining bone. In estimating bone height, care must be taken to avoid interpretive errors resulting from angulation factors. Technically, when making an exposure, the central ray should be directed at right angles to both the tooth and the film. The most commonly used roentgenographic technique, i.e., the short-cone technique, does not follow this principle; instead, the ray is directed through the root of the tooth at a predetermined angle. This technique invariably causes the buccal bone to be projected higher on the crown than the lingual or palatal bone. Therefore, when interpreting bone height, it is imperative to follow the line of the lamina dura from the apex toward the crown of the tooth until the opacity of the lamina materially decreases. At this point of opacity change, a less dense bone extends farther toward the tooth crown. This additional amount of bone represents false bone height. Thus, the true height of the bone is ordinarily where the lamina shows a marked decrease in opacity. At this point the trabecular pattern of bone superimposed upon the tooth root is lost. That portion of the root between the cementoenamel junction and the true bone height has the appearance of being bare or devoid of covering.

Roentgenographic evaluation of bone quality is hazardous but is often necessary. It is essential to emphasize that changes in bone calcification up to 25 per cent often cannot be recognized by ordinary roentgenographic means. Optimum bone qualities are ordinarily expressed by normal-sized interdental trabecular spaces which usually tend to decrease slightly in size as examination of the bone proceeds from the root apex toward the coronal portion. The normal interproximal crest is ordinarily shown by a relatively thin white line crossing from the lamina dura of one tooth to the lamina dura of the adjacent tooth. Considerable variation in the size of trabecular spaces may exist within the limits of normal, and the roentgenographic appearance of crestal alveolar bone may vary considerably, depending upon its shape and the direction which the x-ray takes as it passes through the bone.

Normal bone usually responds favorably to ordinary stresses. Abnormal stresses, however, may create a reduction in the size of the trabecular pattern, particularly in that area of bone directly adjacent to the lamina dura of the affected tooth. This decrease in size of the trabecular pattern (i.e., *so-called bone condensation*) is often thought of as a favorable bone response, indicative of an improvement in bone quality. This is not necessarily an accurate interpretation. Such bone changes usually indicate stresses which should be relieved, for should the resistance of the patient decrease, the bone may exhibit a progressively less favorable response in future roentgenograms.

An increased thickness of the periodontal space near the neck of the tooth or over its entire dimension ordinarily suggests varying degrees of tooth mobility. This should be evaluated clinically. Roentgenographic evidence coupled with clinical findings may suggest to the prosthodontist the inadvisability of utilizing such a tooth as an abutment. Furthermore, an irregular intercrestal bone surface should make the prosthodontist suspicious of active bone deterioration.

It is essential that the prosthodontist realize that roentgenographic evidence shows the *result* of changes which have taken place and may not necessarily represent the present condition. For example, periodontal disease may have progressed beyond the stage visibly demonstrated in the roentgenograms. As was pointed out earlier, roentgenographic changes are not observed until approximately 25 per cent of the calcific content has been depleted. On the other hand, bone condensations probably do represent the present situation.

Roentgenographic findings should serve the prosthodontist as an adjunct to his clinical observations. Too often the roentgenographic appearance alone is used in arriving at a diagnosis. Roentgenographic interpretation will also serve an important function if used periodically *after* the prosthesis has been inserted. Future bone changes *of any type* suggest traumatic interference from some source. The nature of such interference should be determined and corrective measures taken.

Index Areas. Index areas are those areas of alveolar support which disclose the reaction of bone to additional stress. Favorable reaction to such stress may be taken as an indication of future reaction to an added stress load. Teeth that have been subjected to abnormal loading due to the loss of adjacent teeth or have withstood tipping forces in addition to occlusal loading may be better risks as abutment teeth than those which have not been called upon to carry an extra occlusal load (Fig. 6). If occlusal harmony can be improved and unfavorable forces minimized by the reshaping of occlusal surfaces and the favorable distribution of occlusal loading, such teeth may be expected to carry the prosthesis without difficulty. At the same time, other teeth, although not at present carrying an extra load, may be expected to react favorably because of the favorable reaction of alveolar bone to abnormal loading elsewhere in the same arch.

Such index areas are those around teeth that have been subjected to abnormal occlusal loading, those that have been subjected to diagonal occlusal loading due to tooth migration, and those that have reacted to additional loading, such as around existing bridge abutments. The reaction of the bone to additional stresses in these areas may be either positive or negative, with evidence of a supporting trabecular pattern, a heavy cortical layer and a dense lamina

Fig. 6. The reaction of bone adjacent to teeth that have been subjected to abnormal stress serves as an indication of the probable reaction of that bone when such teeth are used as abutments for fixed or removable restorations. Such areas are called *index areas*.

dura, or the reverse response. With the former, the patient is said to have a *positive bone factor,* meaning the ability to build additional support where needed. With the latter, he is said to have a *negative bone factor,* meaning inability to respond favorably to stress.

Alveolar Lamina Dura. The alveolar lamina dura is also considered when making a roentgenographic interpretation of abutment teeth. The lamina dura is the thin layer of hard cortical bone that normally lines the sockets of all teeth. It affords attachment for the fibers of the periodontal membrane, and, like all cortical bone, its function is to withstand mechanical strain. In a roentgenogram, the lamina dura shows as a *radiopaque* white line around the radiolucent dark line that represents the periodontal membrane.

When a tooth is in the process of being tipped, the center of rotation is not at the apex of the root but in the apical third. Resorption occurs where there is pressure, and apposition occurs where there is tension. Therefore, during the active tipping process, the lamina dura is uneven, with evidence of both pressure and tension on the same side of the root. For example, in a mesially tipping lower molar, the lamina dura will be thinner on the coronal mesial and apical distal aspects, and thicker on the apical mesial and coronal distal aspects, due to the fact that the axis of rotation is not at the root apex but above it. When the tooth has been tipped into an edentulous space by some change in the occlusion and becomes set in its new position, the effects of leverage are discontinued. The lamina dura on the side to which the tooth is sloping becomes uniformly heavier, which is nature's reinforcement against abnormal stresses. The bone trabeculations are arranged at right angles to the heavier lamina dura.

Thus, it is possible to say that, for a given individual, nature is able to build support where it is needed and on this basis to predict future reaction elsewhere in the arch to additional loading of teeth used as abutments. However, since bone is approximately 30 per cent organic, and this mostly protein, and since the body is not able to store a protein reserve in large amounts, any change in body health may be reflected in the patient's ability to maintain this support permanently. When systemic disease is associated with faulty protein metabolism and the ability to repair is diminished, bone is resorbed and the lamina dura is disturbed. The loading of any abutment tooth must therefore be kept to a minimum inasmuch as the patient's future health status and the eventualities of aging are unpredictable.

STUDY CASTS

A study cast should be an *accurate* reproduction of the teeth and adjacent tissues. In a partially edentulous arch, this must include the edentulous spaces, since these also must be evaluated in determining the type of denture base to be used and the extent of support available for its support.

A study cast is usually made of dental stone because of its greater strength and the fact that it is less easily abraded. Generally, the improved dental stones, such as Duroc and Vel-Mix, are not used for study casts because of their cost. Their greater resistance to abrasion does, however, justify their use for master casts. Therefore, the study cast can be easily differentiated from the master cast in the laboratory by the identifying color of each, the study cast being buff and the master cast a light greenish yellow or pink.

The impression for the study cast is usually made with an alginate hydrocolloid in either a perforated or rim-lock partial denture impression tray. The type and size of the arch will determine the type and size of the tray to be used. The tray should be sufficiently oversize to assure an optimal thickness of impression material to avoid distortion or tearing upon removal from the mouth. Ordinarily the tray need not be built up or extended, except where a high vault is present. In such case, utility wax may be used to extend the height of the tray in this area. The technique for the making of impressions will be covered in more detail in Chapter 14.

Purposes for Which the Study Casts Are Used. Study casts serve a number of purposes as an aid to diagnosis and treatment planning. Some of these are as follows:

1. To supplement the oral examination by permitting a view of the occlusion from the lingual as well as from the buccal aspect. Analysis of the existing occlusion is made possible when opposing casts are occluded, as well as a study of the possibilities for improvement either by occlusal adjustment or occlusal reconstruction, or both. The degree of overclosure, the amount of interocclusal

space needed, and the possibilities of interference to the location of occlusal rests may also be determined.

2. To permit a topographic survey of the dental arch that is to be restored by means of a partial denture. The cast of the arch in question may be surveyed individually with a cast surveyor to determine the parallelism or lack of parallelism of tooth surfaces involved and to establish its influence on the design of the partial denture. The principal considerations in studying the parallelism of tooth and tissue surfaces of the dental arch are (a) proximal tooth surfaces which can be made parallel to serve as guiding planes, (b) retentive and nonretentive areas of the abutment teeth, and (c) areas of interference to insertion and removal. From such a survey, a path of insertion may be selected which will satisfy requirements of parallelism and retention to the best mechanical, functional, and esthetic advantage. Mouth preparations may then be planned accordingly.

3. To permit a logical and comprehensive presentation to the patient of his present and future restorative needs, as well as the hazards of future neglect. Occluded and individual study casts can be used to point out to the patient (a) evidence of tooth migration and the existing results of such migration, (b) the effects of further tooth migration, (c) loss of occlusal support and its consequences, (d) the hazards of traumatic occlusal contacts, and (e) the cariogenic and periodontal implications of further neglect.

Treatment planning may actually be accomplished with the patient present, so that economic considerations may also be discussed. Such use of study casts permits a justification of the proposed fee through the patient's understanding of the problems involved and the treatment needed. Inasmuch as mouth rehabilitation procedures are frequently protracted, there must be complete accord between dentist and patient before beginning extensive treatment, and financial arrangements must be consummated during the planning phase.

4. Individual impression trays may be fabricated upon the study casts, or the study cast may be used in selecting and fitting a stock impression tray for the final impression. If wax blockout is to be used in the fabrication of individual trays, a duplicate cast made from an alginate impression of the study cast should be used for this purpose. The study cast is too valuable for future reference to risk damage resulting from the making of an impression tray. On the other hand, if only a wet asbestos blockout is used, the study cast may be used without fear of damage.

Since essential areas will be known in advance of making the final impression, the tray may be selected or made with these in mind. Such areas as recorded in the final impression may then be examined critically for possible artifacts.

5. Study casts may be used as a constant reference as the work progresses. Penciled marks indicating the type of restorations, areas of tooth surfaces to be modified, location of occlusal rests, and the design of the partial denture framework, as well as the path of insertion and removal, may all be recorded on the study cast for future reference (Fig. 7). These steps may then be checked off the work sheet as they are completed.

Areas of abutment teeth to be modified may first be changed on the study

Path
of
Insertion

Fig. 7. The proposed mouth changes and the design of the partial denture framework are indicated in pencil on the study cast in relation to a previously determined path of insertion.

cast by trimming the stone cast with the surveyor blade. A record is thus made of the location and degree of modification to be done in the mouth. This must be done in relation to a definite path of insertion. Any mouth preparations to be accomplished with new cast restorations require that wax patterns be shaped in accordance with a previously determined path of insertion. Even so, the shaping of abutment teeth on the study cast serves as a guide to the form of the abutment pattern. This is particularly true if the contouring of wax patterns is to be delegated to the technician, as it must be in any busy practice.

6. Study casts should become a permanent part of the patient's record, because a record of conditions existing before treatment are just as important as preoperative roentgenograms.

Mounting Study Casts. Although study casts may be occluded by hand, occlusal analysis is much better accomplished when they are mounted on some kind of articulator. A simple hinge device may be used if a study of centric occlusion is all that is desired. By definition, an articulator is "a mechanical device that represents the temporomandibular joints and jaw members, to which maxillary and mandibular casts may be attached." Since the dominant influence on mandibular movement in a partially edentulous mouth is the cusps of the remaining teeth, an anatomic reproduction of condylar paths is probably neither necessary nor obtainable. Still, movement of the casts in relation to one another as influenced by the cusps of the remaining teeth, when mounted at a reasonably accurate radius from the axis of condylar rotation, permits a reasonably valid analysis of occlusal relationships. This is much better than a simple hinge mounting.

It is probably still better that the casts be mounted in relation to the axis-orbital plane to permit better interpretation of the plane of occlusion in relation to the horizontal plane. While it is true that an axis-orbital mounting has no functional value on a non-arcon instrument, since that plane ceases to exist when opposing casts are separated, the value of such a mounting lies in the orientation of the casts in occlusion. (An *arcon* articulator is one in which the condyles are attached to the lower member as they are in nature, the term being a derivation coined by Bergström from the words *ar*ticulation and *con*dyle [Fig. 8]. All of the more widely used articulators, such as the Hanau, Dentatus,

Fig. 8. A, The Bergström arcon articulator showing the condyle attached to the lower arm of the articulator and the condyle path to the upper arm. **B,** The Bergström face-bow attached to the articulator prior to mounting the upper cast. (Courtesy Dr. H. O. Beck.)

and improved Gysi, have the condyles attached to the upper member and are therefore non-*arcon* instruments.)

Mounting the Upper Cast to the Axis-Orbital Plane. The face-bow is a relatively simple device used to obtain a transfer record for the purpose of orienting a maxillary cast on an articulating instrument. Originally, the face-bow was used only to transfer a *radius* from condyle reference points so that a given point on the cast would be the same distance from the condyles as on the patient. The addition of an adjustable infraorbital pointer to the face-bow and the addition of an orbital plane indicator to the articulator makes possible also the transfer of the *elevation* of the cast in relation to the axis-orbital plane. This permits the maxillary cast to be correctly oriented in the articulator space comparable to the relationship of the maxilla to the Frankfort horizontal on the patient. In order to accommodate a maxillary cast so oriented and still have room for the mandibular cast, the posts of the conventional articulator must be lengthened. The older Hanau model H articulator will not usually permit a face-bow transfer using an infraorbital pointer.

A face-bow may be used to transfer a comparable radius from arbitrary reference points, or it may be so designed that the transfer can be made from hinge-axis points. The latter type of transfer requires that a hinge bow attached to the mandible be used initially to determine the hinge-axis points, to which the face-bow is then adjusted for the purpose of making the hinge-axis transfer.

A face-bow transfer of the maxillary cast oriented to the axis-orbital plane to a suitable articulator is an uncomplicated procedure. Hanau models S-M, S-M-X, and H-2, and the Dentatus model ARH will accept this transfer, since these models have the longer posts and orbital plane indicator necessary to such a transfer (Figs. 13 and 14). Both the Hanau face-bow model S-M and the Dentatus face-bow type AEB incorporate the infraorbital pointer which permits transfer of the infraorbital plane to the articulator. Neither of these is a hinge-axis bow but is used instead at an arbitrary point.

Fig. 9. Location of an arbitrary axis 11 to 13 mm. anterior to the upper one third of the tragus of the ear from a line extending from the upper margin of the external auditory meatus to the outer canthus of the eye. The lowest point on the inferior orbital margin is marked as the third point of reference for establishing the axis-orbital plane.

Fig. 10. The face-bow is positioned on the face so that calibrations on the shaft on either side read the same as they rest lightly on the two dots located anterior to the external auditory meatus. The infraorbital pointer is adjusted to rest lightly on the infraorbital point previously marked on the face.

Fig. 11. A, Model H-2 Hanau articulator with S-M face-bow attached. Note the orientation of the face-bow to the orbital plane indicator, supported by the adjustable screw on the face-bow. **B,** New Hanau University articulator, model 130-2, a basic model of the new Hanau articulator series. Due to its several improved features, this model may supplant the model H-2, but techniques will remain unchanged. (Courtesy Hanau Engineering Co., Buffalo, N. Y.)

The location of this arbitrary point or axis has long been the subject of some controversy. Gysi and others have placed it 11 to 13 mm. anterior to the upper one third of the tragus of the ear on a line extending from the upper margin of the external auditory meatus to the outer canthus of the eye (Fig. 9). Others have placed it 13 mm. anterior to the posterior margin of the center of the tragus of the ear on a line extending to the corner of the eye. Bergström has located the arbitrary axis 10 mm. anterior to the center of a spherical insert for the external auditory meatus and 7 mm. below the Frankfort horizontal plane.

In a series of experiments reported by Beck it was shown that the arbitrary axis suggested by Bergström falls consistently closer to the kinematic axis than the other two. It is, of course, desirable that an arbitrary axis be placed as close as possible to the kinematic axis. While most authorities agree that any of the three will permit a transfer of the maxillary cast with reasonable accuracy, it would seem that the Bergström point compares most favorably with the kinematic axis.

The lowest point on the inferior orbital margin is taken as the third point of reference for establishing the axis-orbital plane. Some authorities use the point on the lower margin of the bony orbit in line with the center of the pupil of the eye. For the sake of consistency, the right infraorbital point is usually used and the face-bow assembled in this relationship. All three points (right and left

Fig. 12. Cast support attached to the lower arm of the Hanau H-2 articulator. This device is used to support a maxillary cast at the determined elevation while it is being plastered to the upper arm of the articulator. The orbital pointer and orbital plane indicator may then be removed to facilitate mounting the maxillary cast. (Courtesy Hanau Engineering Co., Buffalo, N. Y.)

Fig. 13. The Hanau face-bow model S-M attached to the articulator prior to mounting the maxillary cast. Note the elevation of the face-bow with the orbital plane indicator.

axis and infraorbital point) are marked on the face with an ink dot before making the transfer.

The face-bow bite fork is covered with a roll of softened baseplate wax and formed to the teeth of the upper arch. If the study cast has been made previously, the wax may be adapted to it. The bite fork should be attached with the offset to the left. This is done to avoid interference with the infraorbital pointer which will be located on the right.

The bite fork is then placed in position in the mouth and the patient asked to close the lower teeth into the wax to stabilize it in position. This wax imprint is not used for mounting the lower cast.

With the bite fork in position, the face-bow is slipped over its shaft and positioned so that the calibrations on the shaft on either side read the same as they rest lightly on the two dots located anterior to the exterior auditory meatuses. The calibrated shafts are then locked in this bilaterally equal position. The face-bow may have to be removed to accomplish this. It is then returned to position and locked to the bite fork while being held with equal contact over the dots on either side of the face. This accomplishes the *radius* aspect of the face-bow transfer.

With the infraorbital pointer on the extreme right side of the face-bow, it is angled toward the infraorbital point previously identified with an ink dot. It is then locked into position with its tip lightly touching the skin at the dot

(Fig. 10). This establishes the *elevation* of the face-bow in relation to the axis-orbital plane. Extreme care must be taken to avoid any slip which might damage the patient's eye.

With all elements tightened securely, the patient is asked to open the mouth, and the entire assembly is removed intact, rinsed with cold water, and set aside. The face-bow records not only the radius from the condyles to the incisal contacts of the upper central incisors but also the angular relationship of the occlusal plane to the axis-orbital plane.

The face-bow must be positioned on the articulator in the same axis-orbital relation as on the patient (Figs. 11, *A*, 13, and 14). The calibrated condyle rods of the face-bow will not ordinarily fit the condyle shafts of the articulator unless the width between the condyles just happens to be the same. With a model C face-bow the calibrations must be re-equalized when in position on the articulator. For example, they might have read 7.4 (mm.) on each side of the patient but must be adjusted to read 6.9 (mm.) on each side of the articulator. With some later model articulators having adjustable condyle rods, these may instead be adjusted to fit the face-bow. It is necessary that the face-bow be centered in either case.

The third point of reference is the orbital plane indicator, which must be swung to the right so as to be above the tip of the infraorbital pointer. The entire face-bow with maxillary cast in place must be raised until the tip of the pointer contacts the orbital plane indicator (Figs. 11, *A*, 13, and 14). The elevation

Fig. 14. The Dentatus face-bow, type AEB, attached to the Dentatus articulator prior to mounting the maxillary cast. Note the wax record attached to the bite fork and the elevation of the face-bow with the orbital pointer in contact with the orbital plane indicator.

having thus been established, for all practical purposes the orbital plane indicator and pointer may now be removed, for they may interfere with placing the mounting plaster.

The Hanau Company makes available an auxiliary device called a cast support which is used to support the maxillary cast during the plastering operation (Fig. 12). With this device the weight of the cast and mounting plaster is supported separately from the face-bow, thus preventing possible downward movement resulting from their combined weight. The cast support is raised to supporting contact with the bite fork after the face-bow height has been adjusted to the level of the orbital plane. Its use is highly recommended as an adjunct to face-bow mounting.

The keyed and lubricated maxillary cast is now attached to the upper arm of the articulator with laboratory plaster, thus completing the face-bow transfer. Any dimensional change in plaster of Paris during setting will not be enough to be of any consequence. Not only will the face-bow have permitted the upper cast to be mounted with reasonable accuracy, but it also will have served as a convenient means of supporting the cast during mounting. The ease and speed with which a face-bow transfer can be effected makes ridiculous the frequently expressed objection to its use on the basis of time involved. Rather, once mastered, its use becomes a great convenience rather than a time-consuming nuisance.

Fig. 15. Upper study cast mounted by face-bow transfer. Note that the cast has been keyed prior to mounting and may be removed for repositioning on the surveyor by means of the scratch lines on its base.

If the study casts have been made previously, and the upper cast keyed, it may now be lubricated and attached to the upper arm of the articulator (Fig. 15). It is preferable that the upper cast be mounted while the patient is still present, thus eliminating a possible reappointment should the face-bow record be unacceptable for some reason. Not too infrequently, the face-bow record has to be redone with the bite fork repositioned to avoid interference with some part of the articulator.

Jaw Relationship Records for Study Casts. In some instances, study casts may be satisfactorily occluded by cuspal interdigitation and perhaps with greater accuracy than by interposing a wax "bite." It must be remembered that *centric occlusion* is the relation of the opposing occlusal surfaces which provides the maximum cusp contact. This position rarely coincides with the *centric relation* of the mandible to the maxilla in a partially edentulous arch, due to the effects of tooth migration and the interference of opposing cusps. However, since we are attempting to mount casts in their *existing* relationship for the purposes of study, a recording of the casts in centric occlusion rather than in centric relation is used.

A second jaw relationship record at centric relation may also be desirable. After the casts have first been mounted in their existing relationship, a second mounting of the mandibular cast is made, which reveals occlusal discrepancies at centric relation. Treatment planning may then take into consideration the need for correction of the existing occlusion prior to any occlusal reconstruction.

Where teeth are missing posteriorly, some base is necessary over the edentulous ridge when recording centric occlusion. A sprinkled acrylic base is the most accurate means of supporting edentulous areas. This is easily made by sprinkling a suitable resin polymer and monomer onto the surface of the cast which has been painted with a tin-foil substitute until a base of sufficient thickness has been obtained. A wax occlusion rim is then added until contact in centric occlusion is established. This is for the purpose of supporting occlusion in the edentulous areas while the jaw relationship is recorded with some suitable recording medium.

Materials and Methods for Recording Centric Occlusion. Materials available for recording simple centric occlusion are (1) wax, (2) modeling plastic, (3) quick-setting impression plaster, and (4) metallic oxide impression paste. Of these, wax is the least satisfactory material because it may not be uniformly softened when introduced into the mouth and it does not remain rigid and dimensionally stable after removal.

Modeling plastic is a satisfactory record medium since it can be flamed and tempered until uniformly soft before placing it into the mouth. After chilling, it is sufficiently stable to permit mounting casts with accuracy. For these reasons, it is a very satisfactory medium for recording occlusal relations for either complete or partial dentures. It can also be used with opposing natural teeth.

Impression plaster has advantages of softness when introduced and rigidity when set, which makes it a very satisfactory material for recording jaw relations on denture bases. However, it is too friable and too brittle for use between opposing natural dentition.

Fig. 16. The adjustable bite frame may be used either bilaterally or unilaterally. Each gauze bib is made with a tube which is slid over the open lingual portion of the frame and attached to its buccal portion with sticky wax. For bilateral use the frame must be adjusted to the mouth or cast to avoid interference distal to the last teeth in occlusion. A metallic oxide impression paste is applied to both sides of the gauze, the frame is inserted in the mouth, and the patient's mouth is closed into a rehearsed occlusal relation until the paste hardens. This is usually, although not always, in centric occlusion, with the opposing teeth making maximum contact. After the set record is removed from the mouth, the sticky wax is released from the frame and the tube is slid off the frame. Gross excess and any sharp projections into interproximal spaces and into deep sulci are trimmed with a sharp knife before the record is placed between the occlusal casts for mounting on the articulator.

Impression paste offers many of the advantages of plaster, with less friability. Although not strong enough to be used alone, when supported by a gauze mesh it is perhaps the most satisfactory of all recording media for opposing dentition. It may also be used on occlusion rims. Therefore, it is the material of choice for recording jaw relations with accuracy, either between opposing dentition or between opposing occlusion rims, or any combination of the two.

The adjustable bite frame* was devised for use with those materials that have the combined advantage of offering no resistance when the patient closes and of being firm and stable when set. It consists of an adjustable wire frame to which gauze bibs are added for the purpose of supporting the impression paste (Fig. 16). Pastes which set rapidly to a hard state are the most satisfactory, although any metallic oxide impression paste may be used.

---

*Kerr Manufacturing Co., Detroit, Mich.

The frame is adjusted to fit the lower cast. Each gauze bib has incorporated into it a tube which may be slid over the lingual extension on each side of the arch. These bibs are so placed that a space remains distal to the gauze so that the operator can see to place the frame beyond the last tooth; otherwise the patient might close on the cross bar of the frame. The gauze is then attached to the buccal wing of the frame with sticky wax.

An impression paste is mixed according to the manufacturer's directions and is applied on both sides of the gauze bibs. The frame is then placed in the mouth while the patient closes in centric occlusion. When edentulous bases with wax occlusion rims are being used to support the occlusion in those areas, the wax must have been trimmed and adjusted previously to provide for simultaneous occlusal contact throughout. The cross bar of the frame must be placed posterior to any occlusion rims or any remaining posterior teeth.

After the paste has set, the frame is removed from the mouth and the buccal side of the gauze released where it has been secured with sticky wax. The tube on the lingual side may then be slid off the lingual extension of the frame. The frame is not needed when mounting casts with this type of bite registration, for the tube alone lends sufficient support to the registration.

The lower cast should be mounted on the lower arm of the articulator with the articulator inverted. The articulator is first locked in centric position and then the position of the vertical pin is checked or made flush with the upper arm for future reference. (The pin on the Dentatus articulator is calibrated and always projects above the arm, whereas the pin on the Hanau articulator should be flush with the upper arm.) The projection of the pin on the Dentatus articulator serves most conveniently as the third leg of a tripod for supporting the articulator while mounting the lower cast, whereas the Hanau, when inverted, must be supported by other means. A plastering stand for this purpose is available (Fig. 17).

The base of the cast should be keyed and lubricated for future removal. With the articulator inverted, the operator's thumbs should be pressed through the soft mounting plaster onto the base of the cast to reseat it into the occlusal registration. This is done to prevent a faulty mounting should the angle of closure into the mounting plaster have caused the cast to be displaced slightly. The articulator is then propped up in the inverted position until the plaster has set.

An articulator mounting thus made will have recorded the casts in the centric occlusal relation existing at the time of oral examination. The operator can then proceed to make an occlusal analysis by observing the influence of cusps in relation to one another and in relation to the proposed plan of treatment.

If desired, a second mounting of the lower cast may be made from a rest position record taken in much the same manner as the centric record but without cuspal influence. Such a record is made as follows:

The patient must be trained through exercises, such as recommended by Boos, to assume a rest position without making tooth contact. When such patient cooperation can be obtained, a rest position record may be made by interposing any soft recording material that will remain stable after removal. Here, impression plaster may be used because the greater thickness of a rest bite per-

Fig. 17. The Hanau plastering stand for use with any model H or SMX articulator is supported in an inverted position while the mandibular cast is being mounted. (Courtesy Hanau Engineering Co., Buffalo, N. Y.)

mits the use of the more friable material. Such a plaster record may be trimmed with a sharp knife after removal before placing onto the cast surfaces for mounting and may be secured there with sticky wax.

A mounting record from rest position presumably may be closed into tooth contact at or near to centric jaw relation for the purpose of locating cuspal interference. The fact that the upper cast was not mounted in relation to the hinge axis does not prevent a reasonable interpretation of cusp relationships for purposes of study.

After an occlusal analysis has been made, the casts may be removed from their mounting for the purpose of surveying them individually and for other purposes as outlined previously. The mounting record also should be retained throughout the course of treatment in the event that further study should be needed. It is advisable that the mounting be identified with the articulator used, so that it may always be placed back onto the same articulator.

Factors Involved in Occlusal Analysis. From the occlusal analysis made from mounted study casts, the dentist must decide whether it is best to accept and maintain the existing occlusion or attempt to improve upon it by means of occlusal adjustment and the restoration of occlusal surfaces. It must be kept in mind that the partial denture can only supplement the occlusion that exists at the time the prosthesis is constructed. The dominant force dictating the occlusal pattern will be the cuspal harmony or disharmony of the remaining teeth and their proprioreceptal influence on kinematic movement. At best, the supplied teeth can only be made to harmonize with the cause and effect of the existing occlusion.

Improvements in the natural occlusion must be accomplished prior to the construction of the denture, not subsequent to it. The objective of occlusal reconstruction by any means should be occlusal harmony of the restored dentition in relation to the natural forces already present or established. Therefore, one of the earliest decisions in planning reconstructive treatment must be whether to accept or reject the existing occlusion. If occlusal adjustment is indicated, cuspal analysis should always precede any corrective procedures in the mouth by selective grinding. On the other hand, if reconstruction is to be the means of correction, the manner and sequence should be outlined as part of the over-all treatment plan.

EXAMINATION DATA

As a result of the oral examination and diagnosis, certain data should be recorded, much of which is based upon decisions that are the result of the diagnosis. These are as follows:

1. *Patient's present and predictable future health status.*

2. *Periodontal conditions present* throughout the mouth in general and around abutment teeth in particular. This includes the amount of alveolar support remaining and the past and predictable future reaction to additional occlusal stress. Evidence of tooth mobility should be noted, as well as suggestions as to its cause and the corrective measures to be employed. This may involve simple correction of occlusal disharmony, or it may involve extensive periodontal treatment and, in some instances, splinting of periodontally weakened teeth.

3. *Oral hygiene habits* of the patient and the likelihood of patient cooperation in this regard, as well as the likelihood that the patient will return periodically for maintenance following reconstruction. The teeth remaining will need attention no less after placement of a partial denture and perhaps more so. Denture bases may need relining to compensate for changes in the supporting tissues. Therefore, the patient must be willing to share with the dentist the responsibility for maintaining the health of the mouth following restorative treatment.

The most decisive evidence of oral hygiene habits is the condition of the mouth prior to the initial prophylaxis. Good or bad oral hygiene is basic to the patient's nature, and although it may be influenced somewhat by patient education, the long-range view must be taken. It is reasonably fair to assume that the patient will do little better in the long-term future than he has done in the past. In making decisions as to the method of treatment based upon oral hygiene, the future in years, instead of in weeks and months, must be considered. Probably in this instance it is better not to give the patient the benefit of any doubt as to future oral hygiene habits. Rather, the benefit should come from protective measures where any doubt exists as to future oral hygiene habits.

4. *Caries activity* in the mouth, past and present, and the need for protective restorations. The decision to use full coverage is based upon the age of the patient, evidence of caries activity, and the patient's oral hygiene habits. Generally, both the very young and the patient past middle age need full coverage of all abutment teeth. Occasionally, partial veneers (three-quarter crowns) may be used where buccal or lingual surfaces are completely sound, but intracoronal restorations (inlays) are seldom indicated in any mouth with evidence of past extensive caries or precarious areas of decalcification, erosion, or exposed cementum.

5. *Need for surgery or extractions.* The same criteria apply to surgical intervention in the partially edentulous arch as in the completely edentulous arch. Mandibular tori should be removed if they will interfere with the placement of a lingual bar connector or a favorable path of insertion. Any other areas of bony prominence which will interfere with the path of insertion should also be removed. The path of insertion will be dictated primarily by the tooth guidance of the abutment teeth. Therefore, some areas may present interference to the path of insertion of the partial denture by reason of the fact that other unalterable factors, such as retention and esthetics, must take precedence in selecting that path.

Extraction of teeth may be indicated for one of three reasons.

(a) If the tooth cannot be restored to a state of health, extraction may be unavoidable. Modern advancements in the treatment of periodontal disease and in restorative procedures, including endodontic therapy, have resulted in the saving of teeth once considered untreatable. All avenues of treatment should be considered both from a prognostic and an economic standpoint before recommending extraction.

(b) A tooth may be removed if its absence will permit a more serviceable partial denture design. Teeth that are in extreme malposition, such as lingually inclined mandibular teeth, buccally inclined maxillary teeth, and mesially inclined teeth posterior to an edentulous space, may be removed if an adjacent tooth in good alignment and with good support is available for use as an abutment. Justification for extraction lies in the decision that a suitable crown cannot be fabricated which will provide satisfactory contour and support. An exception to the arbitrary removal of a malposed tooth is where by so doing a free-end partial denture base would have to be made instead of the more desirable tooth-supported base through the use of the tooth in question. If alveolar support is adequate, a posterior abutment should be retained if at all possible in preference to a tissue-supported free-end base.

Teeth that are deemed to have insufficient alveolar support may be extracted if their prognosis is poor and if other adjacent teeth may be used to better advantage as abutments. The decision to extract such a tooth should be based upon the degree of mobility and other periodontal considerations and upon the number, length, and shape of the roots contributing to its support.

(c) A tooth may be extracted if it is so unesthetically placed as to justify its removal to improve appearance. In this regard, a veneer crown should be considered in preference to removal. If removal is advisable because of unesthetic tooth position, the biomechanical problems involved in replacing anterior teeth with a removable partial denture must be weighed against the problems involved in making an esthetically acceptable fixed restoration. Admittedly, the removable replacement is frequently the more esthetic of the two, despite modern advancements in retainers and pontics. Yet, the mechanical disadvantage of the removable restoration frequently makes the fixed replacement of missing anterior teeth preferable.

6. *Need for fixed restorations for tooth-bounded spaces* rather than include them in the partial denture to the detriment of isolated abutment teeth. The advantages of splinting must be weighed against the total cost, with the weight of experience always in favor of utilizing fixed restorations for tooth-bound spaces. One of the least successful of partial denture designs is where multiple tooth-bounded areas are replaced with the partial dentures in conjunction with isolated abutment teeth and free-end extensions. Biomechanical considerations and the future health of the remaining teeth should be given preference over economic considerations where such a choice is possible.

7. *Need for occlusal correction,* either by selective grinding of tooth cusps or by occlusal restorations, or both.

8. *Need for periodontal consultation and treatment.*

9. *Need for orthodontic treatment of malposed and disarranged teeth.* Occasionally, orthodontic movement of teeth followed by retention through the use of fixed restorations makes possible a better partial denture design, mechanically and esthetically, than could otherwise be used.

10. *Need for restorations elsewhere in either arch,* including individual restorations, fixed bridges, and/or splinted abutments.

DIFFERENTIAL DIAGNOSIS: FIXED OR REMOVABLE PARTIAL DENTURES

It must be assumed that diagnosis of the partially edentulous mouth is accomplished with objectivity and without prejudice, utilizing all the diagnostic aids available to modern dentistry. It also must be assumed that total treatment or total oral rehabilitation is the ultimate objective rather than, as is too often the case, only the replacement of a few missing teeth. Errors in diagnosis and treatment occur more often as a result of too limited a consideration of the long-term needs of the patient than for any other reason.

There is some confusion in the use of the terms "fixed partial denture" and "removable partial denture." A "fixed partial denture" or a "fixed bridge" is one which is cemented to abutment teeth and is not removable by the patient. A "removable partial denture" may be either totally tooth supported or supported in part by the tissue of the residual ridge. If it is supported entirely by abutment teeth, it may logically be called a "removable bridge" even though it may be bilateral in design.

According to the terminology which I believe is the most logical, a true partial denture differs from a removable bridge prosthesis in that it has one or more free-end bases and derives its support from both the teeth and the edentulous residual ridge.

At the risk of oversimplification, I believe a rule may be stated to the effect that the replacement of missing teeth by means of fixed restorations always should be the method of preference, and the decision to use a removable restoration instead should be based on just and logical reasons for doing so. Unless a fixed bridge restoration is contraindicated for some reason, one cannot justify the use of a removable restoration for arbitrary reasons alone.

Indications for Use of Fixed Restorations

Tooth-Bounded Edentulous Regions. Generally, any unilateral edentulous space with teeth remaining at each end which can be used as abutments should be restored with a fixed bridge cemented to one or more abutment teeth at each end. The length of the span and the periodontal support of the abutment teeth will determine the number of abutments required.

Lack of parallelism of the abutment teeth need not necessarily rule out the making of a fixed bridge, because copings or locking recesses may be utilized to provide parallel sectional insertion when this is necessary. Neither should the presence of sound abutment teeth influence the decision to use a removable restoration where a fixed bridge restoration is otherwise indicated; instead, this should be looked on as an opportunity to use more conservative retainers such as inlays rather than full crowns, especially where not more than two teeth are being replaced. The age of the patient, evidence of caries activity, oral hygiene habits and the soundness of remaining tooth structure must all be considered in any decision to use less than full coverage for any abutment tooth.

Only rarely should economics be allowed to dictate the use of a unilateral removable bridge where a fixed bridge is indicated. In most instances the patient will be better served by using properly prepared abutment restorations which will provide better support and retention for the prosthesis and also better protection for the abutment teeth. The total cost of the removable bridge will thus be comparable to that of a fixed bridge when the cost of the abutment restorations is added, and little is gained economically by the use of a removable prosthesis.

One frequently hears the arguments in favor of removable unilateral bridges that the patient will not allow a sound tooth to be cut for the sake of placing abutment restorations or that the patient's health will not allow such procedures. In answer to the former, the dentist must be allowed to follow the best procedure for the welfare of his patient just as the medical surgeon prescribes the best method of treatment for his. The patient is always free to seek more than one opinion if he so desires, but if there is a conflict in the method of treatment recommended by more than one dentist, the responsibility for the choice of dental treatment becomes the patient's. In answer to the latter, it is doubtful that the patient who, for reasons of health, cannot undergo reasonable operative procedures should be encumbered with an appliance that will be less than adequate. When a removable unilateral restoration is made for such a patient, it should be considered primarily as a space maintainer and an interim appliance until more definitive treatment is possible. In the meantime, the patient should be cautioned against continuous wear of the appliance unless meticulous oral hygiene is maintained.

There are two specific contraindications for the use of unilateral fixed restorations. One is where the edentulous span is very long and the abutment teeth would not be able to withstand the trauma of horizontal and diagonal occlusal forces. The other is where abutment teeth weakened by periodontal disease would benefit from the bracing effect of cross-arch stabilization. In either situation, and frequently the two exist together, a bilateral removable restoration can be used to replace the missing teeth more effectively than unilateral fixed restorations. As with any removable restoration, properly contoured abutment retainers, either inlays or full crowns, will better insure the success of the removable partial denture.

Modification Spaces. In the Kennedy method of classification of partially edentulous arches, any edentulous space not contributing to the initial classification is spoken of as a modification of that class. A removable partial denture for a Class III arch is better supported and stabilized when a modification area on the opposite side of the arch is present. Such an edentulous area would not be restored by a fixed bridge since it is essential to the design of the removable partial denture. Additional modification spaces, however, particularly those involving single missing teeth, are better restored separately by means of fixed bridges. Not only is a lone-standing abutment thus stabilized by the splinting effect of a fixed bridge, but a possible teeter-totter effect on the partial denture is avoided. Moreover, the partial denture is made less complicated by not having to include other abutment teeth for the support and retention of an additional edentulous space or spaces.

Frequently an edentulous space which is a modification of either a Class I or Class II arch exists anterior to a lone-standing abutment tooth. This tooth would be subjected to trauma by the movements of a free-end partial denture far in excess of its ability to withstand such stresses. The components of such stresses are mesiodistal, horizontal and rotational. This makes the splinting of the lone abutment to the nearest tooth mandatory. Splinting is best accomplished in such a situation by means of a fixed bridge uniting the two teeth on either side of the edentulous space. This is almost always a specific indication for a fixed bridge. The abutment crown should be contoured so as to provide support and retention for the partial denture, and, in addition, means of supporting a stabilizing component on the anterior abutment of the fixed bridge or on the occlusal surface of the bridge pontic usually should be provided.

Anterior Modification Spaces. I believe the statement can be justified that any missing anterior teeth in a partially edentulous arch, except in a Kennedy Class IV arch where only anterior teeth are missing, are best replaced by means of a fixed bridge. There are exceptions, of course. Sometimes a better esthetic result is obtainable when the anterior replacements are supported by the partial denture, especially where abutment restorations on the adjacent natural teeth are not otherwise necessary. This is also true where excessive resorption would necessitate the placement of bridge pontics too far posteriorly for good esthetics and an acceptable relation with the opposing teeth. Also, economics may dictate the replacement of anterior teeth with the partial denture rather than by means of an anterior fixed bridge. But from both a mechanical and a biological standpoint, anterior replacements are best accomplished with fixed restorations.

When anterior teeth are replaced with a removable partial denture, support for the anterior segment is difficult to obtain unless multiple rests on several adjacent teeth are used. Incisal rests cannot be used because of the leverage induced, not to mention their objectionable display of metal. Therefore, multiple crown ledges and occlusal rests must be used to support the anterior segment. It is often better to avoid the numerous components necessary to support an anterior segment of the partial denture by resorting to the use of an anterior fixed bridge instead. The replacement of the missing posterior teeth with a partial denture is then made much less complicated and with more satisfactory results.

These considerations are even more applicable where the partial denture will have one or two posterior free ends. I would prefer always to replace missing anterior teeth separately by means of a fixed bridge even where the posterior restoration was totally supported and retained by abutment teeth. But with one or more free-end bases, some anterior-posterior rotation, or teetering, will inevitably result, to the detriment of both the abutment teeth and the residual ridge. The distal end of a tooth-borne partial denture is prevented from moving tissueward by the occlusal rests on the posterior abutment; it is prevented from rotating away from the tissues by the direct retainer on the same abutment. In contrast, a free-end partial denture base is free to move in either direction. Tissueward movement is limited by the quality of tissue support and the accuracy of fit of the denture base. Movement away from the tissues is limited to some extent by the presence of indirect retainers, and by the inherent retention of the denture base. But some teetering action is inevitable when a free-end partial denture is used to support missing anterior teeth. This can best be avoided by replacing the missing anterior teeth separately with a fixed bridge or by supporting the anterior denture base with a fixed bar soldered to adjacent abutment castings.

Nonreplacement of Missing Molars. Frequently the decision must be made whether or not to replace missing molars on one side of the arch only. To do so with a removable partial denture necessitates the making of a free-end partial denture with the major connector joining that side to retentive and stabilizing components located on the opposite, nonedentulous, side of the arch. Leverage factors are always unfavorable in such a situation, and the retainers which must be used on the non-edentulous side are frequently unsatisfactory. Several factors, therefore, will influence the decision to make a unilateral free-end partial denture.

First, the opposing teeth must be considered. If they are to be prevented from extrusion and migration, some opposing occlusion must be provided. This would influence the replacement of the missing molars far more than any improvement in masticating efficiency which might result. I can think of no instance where the replacement of missing molars on one side is necessary for reasons of mastication alone.

Second, the future of a maxillary tuberosity must be considered. Left uncovered, the edentulous tuberosity frequently will seem to drop and increase in size. Whether this is due to unilateral posterior closure with intrusion of adjacent remaining teeth or to a migration of the maxillary tuberosity is not known. However, covering the tuberosity with a partial denture base, in combination with the stimulating effect of the intermittent occlusion provided, helps to maintain the normalcy of the tuberosity. This may be of considerable importance in any future denture replacements the patient may require. In such an instance, it may be better to make a unilateral partial denture than to leave a maxillary tuberosity uncovered.

A third consideration is the condition of the opposing second molar, if present. If this tooth is missing or can logically be ignored or eliminated, then only first molar occlusion need be supplied. This is perhaps accomplished best by "throwing off" a molar pontic from two bicuspid abutments, in other words, by utilizing a cantilever fixed bridge. Occlusion need be only minimal to maintain occlusal relations between the natural first molar in the one arch and the prosthetic molar in the opposite arch. Such a pontic should be made narrow buccolingually and need not be made to occlude with more than two thirds of the opposing tooth. Frequently such a fixed bridge is the preferred method of treatment, thus avoiding the necessity of making a unilateral removable partial denture.

Indications for Removable Partial Dentures

Generally, a removable partial denture should be considered only when a fixed bridge is contraindicated for one reason or another. However, there are a number of specific indications for the use of a removable restoration.

Free-end Situations. Except where the replacement of missing second (and third) molars is either not advisable or unnecessary, or where unilateral replacement of a missing first molar can be accomplished by means of a cantilever fixed bridge, replacement of missing posterior teeth without the assistance of a posterior abutment must be accomplished with a removable partial denture. The most common partially edentulous situations are the Kennedy Class I (bilateral free-end) and Class II (unilateral free-end). With the latter, an edentulous space on the opposite side of the arch is often conveniently present to aid in the effective retention and stabilization of the partial denture. If not, embrasure clasps or intracoronal retainers usually must be used. In some instances, a questionable tooth, preferably the first molar, can be extracted to provide an edentulous space. All other edentulous areas, especially those involving missing anterior teeth or a missing tooth anterior to a lone-standing abutment, are best replaced with fixed bridges.

After Recent Extractions. The replacement of teeth after recent extractions cannot be accomplished satisfactorily with a fixed restoration. Where rebasing will be required later or where a fixed bridge will be constructed later, a removable partial denture must be used. In any situation in which ultimate replacement can be accomplished better with a fixed restoration, the partial denture should be considered only as a temporary or interim appliance. In such instances, an all-resin denture is used rather than a more elaborate partial denture, and the cost to the patient for the temporary appliance is therefore much less.

A tooth-bounded edentulous area that otherwise could be restored with a fixed bridge, but because of recent extractions some change in the residual ridge is anticipated, is also best restored with a removable partial denture. Although the relining of a tooth-supported resin denture base thus is made possible, this is usually done only to improve esthetics, oral cleanliness, or patient comfort, and rarely, if ever, to provide support to the denture. Support for such a restoration should come from the occlusal rests on the abutment teeth lying at each end of the edentulous space.

Long Span. A long span may be totally tooth-supported if the abutments and the means of transferring the support to the denture are adequate and the denture framework is rigid. There is little, if any, difference between the support afforded a removable partial denture and that afforded a fixed bridge by the adjacent abutment teeth. However, the fixed bridge does not have the advantage of bilateral stabilization that the removable partial denture may have, and, therefore, more than a single abutment at each end should be used whenever possible to compensate for the lack of bilateral stabilization.

An example where a fixed bridge may be contraindicated is an edentulous span from cuspid to lone second or third molar. Obviously, the strength of double abutments is not obtainable posteriorly, and the inclusion of the lateral incisor as an additional abutment is impractical and of little value. Therefore, a fixed bridge would have to comprise three or four pontics supported by a single abutment at each end. In the absence of cross-arch stabilization, the torque and leverage on the two abutment teeth would be excessive. Instead, a removable partial denture deriving retention, support and stabilization from abutment teeth on the opposite side of the arch is indicated as the logical means of replacing the missing teeth. As always, this is better accomplished when an edentulous space, preferably at the second bicuspid or first molar, exists on the opposite side of the arch.

Need for Effect of Bilateral Bracing. In a mouth weakened by periodontal disease a partial denture may do more for the abutment teeth than the abutment teeth can do for the partial denture. Because of the lack of cross-arch stabilization, a fixed bridge may jeopardize the future of abutment teeth involved in periodontal disease unless the splinting effect of multiple abutments is employed. Indeed, those prosthodontists and periodontists who strongly favor fixed splinting in all instances usually insist on encircling the arch with united restorations rather than relying on unilateral splinting alone. The partial denture, on the other hand, may act as a periodontal splint through its effective cross-arch bracing of teeth weakened by periodontal disease. However, this is true only when vertical tooth surfaces are available or created which may act as positive guiding planes, when occlusal rests in definite prepared areas are used, and when the abutment teeth are so contoured that uniform retention and rigid bracing components are made possible. It is unlikely that a partial denture made for a mouth that has not been subjected to careful survey and meticulous mouth preparation will provide the degree of stabilization to the arch that is possible by a carefully executed design. But when a number of abutment teeth throughout the arch are properly prepared, and more often than not this necessitates the use of carefully contoured abutment retainers, the beneficial effect of a partial denture may be far greater than the effect of a unilateral fixed bridge.

Esthetics in Anterior Region. Where the replacement of missing anterior teeth in a partially edentulous arch is the primary consideration, esthetic and cosmetic demands sometimes are better served by the use of denture teeth rather than bridge pontics. This is particularly true where a number of anterior teeth are missing, such as in a Kennedy Class IV arch, or where a better tooth arrangement and better contours and shading are possible through the use of denture teeth.

There is no need to go into the types of anterior bridge pontics one might use, and the limitations and disadvantages of each. However, where an anterior fixed bridge involving more than two missing teeth is constructed, I prefer one method over all others which provides an opportunity to use denture teeth as one would with a partial denture. In this method, resin denture teeth are selected for shade, size and contour and set on the master cast in an acceptable arrangement. A plaster index then is made of the labial surfaces of these teeth in relation to the cast, and the teeth are attached to a wax trial base. They then are tried in the mouth and any alterations made for esthetic or functional reasons.

The teeth then are returned to the cast, hollowed out lingually, and a cast bar which will also form the cingulum of each tooth is constructed with retentive loops projecting labially. After soldering to the abutment castings, the bridge is finally assembled by attaching the teeth with resin of the same shade. Such a bridge comes as close as possible to equaling the esthetic result of a partial denture with all of the advantages of a fixed bridge.

Excessive Loss of Residual Bone. The pontic of a fixed bridge must be related to the residual ridge in such a manner that the contact with the mucosa is gentle. Where excessive resorption has occurred, however, teeth supported by a denture base may be set in a more acceptable buccolingual position than is possible with a fixed bridge.

Posteriorly, loss of residual bone occurs for the most part from the buccal aspect. Although two opposing bridges made concurrently or a bridge to which an opposing complete or partial denture will be made to occlude might be acceptable with pontics resting on the resorbed ridge, the opposing denture teeth cannot then be set as far buccally as the natural dentition. Tongue and cheek contact is therefore abnormal, and function is impaired. Food impaction and masticatory inefficiency result from the failure to restore natural contours. In contrast, artificial teeth supported by a denture base can be set without regard to the crest of the residual ridge and more nearly in the position of the natural dentition. This is particularly true of a maxillary denture. All too commonly the technician has learned to set teeth "on" the residual ridge, which locates them too far lingually. When supported by a denture base, the teeth may be set in a more acceptable buccolingual position than is possible with a fixed bridge where excessive bone resorption has occurred.

Anteriorly, loss of residual bone occurs from the labial aspect. Often, the incisive papilla lies at the crest of the residual ridge. Knowing that the location of the incisive papilla does not change, and knowing that the central incisors are normally located anterior to this landmark, any other location of artificial central incisors is unnatural. An anterior fixed bridge made for such a mouth will have pontics resting on the labial aspect of this resorbed ridge that are too far lingual to provide desirable lip support. Frequently the only way the incisal edges of the pontics can be made to occlude with the opposing lower anterior teeth is to use a labial inclination that is excessive and unnatural, and both esthetics and lip support suffer thereby. Although the same applies to a removable partial denture in which the anterior teeth are abutted on the residual ridge, there are times when a labial flange must be utilized to permit the teeth to be located more nearly in their natural position. With denture-base staining technics and a wide selection of denture-base shades to choose from, this can usually be done acceptably and with much better effect than with improperly located pontics.

The same applies to the replacment of missing lower anterior teeth. All dentists have seen lower anterior bridges six or more units in length where the remaining space necessitates either leaving out one anterior tooth or using the original number of teeth but with all of them too narrow for esthetics. In either instance, the bridge is nearly in a straight line as the pontics follow the form of the resorbed ridge. Again, a removable partial denture permits the location of the replaced teeth in a favorable relation to the lip and opposing dentition regardless of the shape of the residual ridge. When such a removable prosthesis is made, however, positive support must be obtained from the adjacent abutments either in the form of definite rests or through the use of a fixed bar soldered to abutment retainers.

Unusually Sound Abutment Teeth. Too often the excuse has been offered for making a removable restoration where a fixed restoration is clearly indicated that the dentist or patient, or both, did not want to see sound teeth crowned or prepared for other types of abutment retainers. The reasons for the loss of the teeth being replaced must be considered first. If for reasons of neglect or caries, then it is likely that caries also will occur eventually in the abutment teeth and even more so because of the effect of the denture components on those teeth. If the teeth were lost because of periodontal disease, then the periodontium of the remaining teeth must be evaluated carefully and the possible advantages of splinting several abutment teeth considered. If the teeth were lost for other reasons, such as the neglect of minimal caries, and if the caries activity which preceded extraction has since become diminished or arrested, the utilization of existing tooth surfaces to support a removable restoration may be justified. If caries activity is not apparent, the oral hygiene habits of the patient are favorable, and the abutment teeth are sound with good periodontal support, unprotected abutments may be used to support and retain a removable restoration. However, such a combination of circumstances is very uncommon. When it does exist, the dentist should not hesitate to reshape and modify existing enamel surfaces to provide proximal guiding planes, occlusal rest areas, optimal retentive areas, and surfaces on which nonretentive stabilizing components may be placed. An enamel surface thus prepared and repolished is no more likely to become carious in the future than the original surface and, in many instances, less likely because of the effect of repolishing the new surface.

It is only in selected instances, then, that the making of a removable prosthetic restoration on unprotected abutments can be justified just because the abutment teeth are sound. Certainly other criteria should be used in making a decision to use unprotected abutments.

Economic Considerations. Just as the existence of sound abutments should not be the only factor deciding the choice of restorative treatment, neither should economics alone be allowed to dictate the method of treatment. Too frequently the dentist allows this to influence the type of restorative treatment recommended. A removable partial denture is then made on unprotected abutments with little or no attempts at mouth preparations, involving a minimum of chair-time and a maximum of assistance from the commercial laboratory. This practice cannot be condemned too strongly, for it is the prime factor in all impending "denturist" legislation. Prosthetic dentistry is being betrayed by those who, for selfish reasons, delegate professional responsibilities to the dental technician outside of their own office. Moreover, respect for the profession suffers in the long run, because too often all that the patient receives is a partial denture that is forever a foreign body in his mouth, with eventual loss of remaining teeth due to caries or periodontal disease. In most such instances, the patient would have been better served with no replacements at all. On the other hand, had the advantages of a complete service been explained to him, who can say that the means of financing such service could not have been found. A look at the financial status of the parents of children receiving orthodontic treatment is proof that the means will be found if the desire is great enough. Unfortunately, however, with some families this is the very reason why the parents cannot afford necessary prosthetic treatment.

When, for economic reasons or because the prognosis of the remaining teeth is poor, complete treatment is inadvisable or out of the question, and yet replacement of missing teeth is indicated, the type of restoration dictated by these considerations must be described clearly to the patient as being of a temporary or interim nature and not representative of the best that modern dentistry has to offer. In some instances, such as after recent extractions, the restoration may be replaced at some future time with more complete treatment. Such a removable prosthesis can render satisfactory service for a period of time and yet the patient must clearly understand its purpose and limitations. Depending on many factors such as oral cleanliness and other caries and periodontal control measures, a removable partial denture of this kind may indeed have a very useful life. Ordinarily, however, a prosthesis which is made to satisfy economic considerations alone is doomed to failure, and both professional esteem and the patient suffer thereby.

A free-end situation usually necessitates the making of a removable partial denture. In all other situations, factors of esthetics, periodontal health, preservation of remaining teeth, mechanical and biological factors, and the patient's economic status must all be taken into consideration. Rarely, if ever, should a removable restoration be used where a fixed replacement is clearly indicated. Some of the few exceptions to this are after recent extractions, where the prognosis of the remaining teeth is poor, or where the patient's economic position does not permit optimal treatment.*

THE CHOICE BETWEEN COMPLETE DENTURES AND PARTIAL DENTURES

In making the diagnosis preceding prosthetic service, the probable length of service which can be expected from a partial denture must always be weighed against the patient's economic status. A decision may have to be made between a partial denture and a complete denture, in either arch or both. The dentist is not in a position to know the patient's own estimate of the value of his teeth. One patient may prefer complete dentures to the traumatic experience of complete oral rehabilitation, regardless of his ability to pay. Another may be so determined to keep his own teeth that he will make great financial sacrifices to do so if given reasonable assurance of the success of oral rehabilitation.

The value of listening to the patient during the examination and the diagnostic procedures should not be disregarded nor treated lightly. During the presentation of pertinent facts, time should be allowed for the patient to express himself freely as to his desires in retaining and restoring his natural teeth. At this time, a treatment plan may be influenced or even drastically changed to conform to the expressed and implied desires of the patient.

For example, there may be a reasonable possibility of saving teeth in both arches through the use of partial dentures. With only anterior teeth remaining, a partial denture can be made to replace the posterior teeth by utilizing good abutment support and, in the maxillary arch, utilizing full palate coverage for retention and stability. If the patient expresses a desire to retain his anterior teeth "at any cost" and the remaining teeth are esthetically acceptable and func-

---

*From McCracken, William L.: Differential Diagnosis: Fixed or Removable Partial Dentures, J. A. D. A. **63:**767-775, 1961.

tionally sound, then the dentist should do his best to make successful partial dentures for both arches and thus fulfill his professional obligation to the patient.

On the other hand, if for economic or other reasons the patient feels that a complete upper denture would best satisfy his denture requirements, but for fear of difficulty in wearing a complete lower denture he would prefer restoration of that arch with a partial denture, then all factors being acceptable, his wishes should be respected and treatment planned accordingly.

Still another patient, for economic or other reasons, may prefer to have complete dentures made for both arches rather than undergo complete rehabilitation of the partially edentulous arches. It is frequently unwise to insist on the latter course with such a patient. The professional obligation to present the facts and then do the best in accordance with the patient's expressed desires still applies.

Still another patient may wish to retain the remaining teeth for an indefinite but relatively short period of time, with eventual complete dentures a foregone conclusion. In this instance the professional obligation may be to recommend interim partial dentures without extensive mouth preparations. Such dentures will aid in mastication and/or provide esthetic replacements while at the same time serve as conditioning appliances which will make the later transition to complete dentures somewhat easier. Such partial dentures should be designed and fabricated with care, but the total cost of partial denture service will be considerably less.

An expressed desire on the part of the patient to retain only six lower anterior teeth must be considered carefully before being agreed to as the planned treatment. The advantages to the patient are obvious: he may retain six esthetically acceptable teeth, he does not become totally edentulous, and he has the advantage of direct retention that would not be possible if he were completely

A   B

Fig. 18. The effect of retaining six lower anterior teeth in opposition to a maxillary complete denture. **A**, The extreme resorption of the maxillary ridge due to the trauma exerted by the remaining lower anterior teeth. **B**, A roentgenogram of the same patient, showing resorption of the maxillary ridge all the way to the anterior nasal spine.

edentulous. Retaining even the lower canine teeth would accomplish the latter two objectives. These advantages cannot be denied. Yet, the disadvantages, which are less obvious to the patient, must also be considered and explained to him. These are mechanical and functional considerations; namely, that the edentulous maxilla anteriorly is structurally not able to withstand the trauma of positive tooth contact against natural opposing teeth. The inevitable result is the loss of residual maxillary bone, loosening of the maxillary denture due to the tripping influence of the natural lower teeth, and the loss of basal foundation for the support of future prostheses (Fig. 18). The presence of inflamed hyperplastic tissue is a frequent sequel to continued loss of support and denture movement.

The prevention of this sequence of events lies in the maintenance of positive occlusal support posteriorly and the continual elimination of traumatic influence from the remaining anterior teeth. Such support is sometimes impossible to maintain without frequent relining or remaking of the lower partial denture base. On the other hand, this may cause undesirable resorption of the posterior ridges due to overloading. The results in any event are undesirable and the patient must be made aware of the hazards involved.

While some patients are able to wear a lower partial denture supported only by anterior teeth against a complete upper denture, the odds are that the consequences will be disastrous. In no other situation in treatment planning is the general health of the patient and the quality of residual alveolar bone as critical as in the above situation.

In addition to considering the age and health of the patient and his ability to build bone in response to stress, it is well to consider why the teeth being replaced were extracted. In all probability, any history of periodontal disease precludes the wearing of such combination dentures successfully. On the other hand, the loss of teeth due to caries or the premature loss of teeth that might have been saved justifies the conclusion that the residual bone is probably healthy and will be able to withstand stresses within reasonable limits. In such instances, combination dentures may be made if the patient is made aware of the need for periodic re-examination and is willing to make the transition to a complete lower denture upon the first signs of serious damage to supporting structures.

COMPUTING THE TOTAL FEE

The final treatment plan should represent the best possible course for the patient after considering all of the physical, mechanical, esthetic, and economic factors involved. Only then may the cost be computed and the total fee quoted to the patient.

The total fee will be the *total cost of all rehabilitation procedures*. This will include the cost of individual restorations and the cost of any multiple fixed restorations elsewhere in the arch. The total cost of partial denture service is the cost of the prosthesis *plus* the cost of abutment restorations *plus* the cost of maintenance. The latter will be influenced by the patient's caries attack rate, his future oral hygiene, the extent of periodontal treatment needed, and the response of supporting bone, both alveolar and residual, to the added stress of the partial denture.

Chapter 4

Classification of partially
edentulous arches

Several methods of classification of partially edentulous arches have been proposed and are in use today. This has led to much confusion and disagreement as to which method should be adopted and by which method all possible combinations can best be classified.

It has been estimated that there are over 65,000 possible combinations of teeth and edentulous spaces. It is obvious that no single method of classification can be descriptive of any but the most basic types. Therefore, a basic classification should be sufficient. It is unfortunate that no single method has been universally adopted by the profession. This fact has probably done more to prevent a comprehensive approach to the principles of partial denture design than any other single factor.

The most familiar classifications are those originally proposed by Cummer, Bailyn, and Kennedy. The Cummer classification is less widely used than the others and is based on the position of the direct retainers and the variations in the position of the indirect retainers. There can be some disagreement with Cummer's statement that "the classification occurs as a by-product of design rather than design as a by-product of classification." Cummer's classification is actually, therefore, a classification of the finished partial denture rather than of the partially edentulous arch.

METHODS OF CLASSIFICATION

Cummer's Classification. Cummer divided all partial dentures into four classes:

Class I. Diagonal. Direct retainers (two in number) diagonally opposite. The fulcrum line of the direct retainers passes diagonally across, with the location of the indirect retainer nearly at right angles to the fulcrum line, as tooth support permits.

Fig. 19. Representative examples of partially edentulous arches classified by the Bailyn, Kennedy, and Skinner methods of classification.

Class II. Diametric. Direct retainers (two in number) diametrically opposite. The fulcrum line passes diametrically across the arch, and the indirect retainer is located as nearly at right angles to the fulcrum line as possible.

Class III. Unilateral. Direct retainers (two in number) on the same side. No indirect retainers are used. *(This is actually a unilateral removable bridge rather than a true partial denture.)*

Class IV. Multilateral. Direct retainers (three or more in number) in a triangular or quadrangular relationship. No indirect retainers are used.

The Bailyn and Kennedy methods are more widely used and are classifications of the partially edentulous arch (Fig. 19). These classifications have been modified and enlarged upon by others, generally with some improvement over the original classification.

Bailyn's Classification. Bailyn's original classification as proposed in 1928 is as follows:

Class I. Available abutment teeth at each extremity of an edentulous space with not more than three teeth missing between the abutments.

Class II. Available tooth support at only one extremity of an edentulous space.

Class III. Available abutment tooth support at each extremity of an edentulous space but with more than three teeth missing between the abutments.

These classes are still further divided into (a) edentulous spaces lying anterior to the first premolar tooth and (b) edentulous spaces lying posterior to the canine tooth.

Bailyn proposed that each class be considered as a guide to the design of the partial denture. This should be the primary objective in classifying any partially edentulous arch. However, one may differ with the arbitrary position that although a span replacing three teeth or less may be tooth borne, a span of greater than three teeth should be considered to be tissue supported. Rather, the quality of abutment support available, the magnitude of the occlusal area involved, the harmony of occlusion obtainable, and the quality of the residual ridge must all be taken into consideration in deciding the proportionate amount of support the teeth and tissues are capable of providing.

Although some tooth-bounded edentulous spaces are too great and some abutment teeth too weak to permit a long edentulous span to be entirely tooth supported, every effort should be made to avoid the necessity for tissue support alone. The splinting of weak abutment teeth, absolute rigidity of the denture frame, reduction in the number and width of teeth supplied, and occlusal harmony within toleration limits will all contribute to the success of a tooth-borne prosthesis. Any such tooth-bounded edentulous area may therefore be considered to have abutments which are potentially capable of supporting the prosthesis, and mouth preparations and design should be treated accordingly.

Beckett and Wilson's Classification. Recognizing some need for further classification of the Bailyn classification, Beckett and, more recently, Wilson have proposed the following classification:

Class I. Teeth are available at each end of the edentulous space which are fully qualified to support the partial denture by means of occlusal rests. The mucosa may be covered but it is not used for support in any way whatsoever.

Class II. (a) A tooth is present at only one end of the edentulous area. Some support for the partial denture is given by the abutment tooth and some is given by the mucosa and underlying bone.

(b) A tooth is present at only one end of the edentulous area, but the support for the denture base comes entirely from the mucosa and underlying bone.

Class III. Teeth are present at each end of the edentulous space, but they are not as well qualified to provide occlusal support as are the abutment teeth at each end of a Class I area.

Wilson further elaborates on this latter classification by stating that a mandibular Class III is treated as a Class I, whereas a maxillary Class III may be treated as either a Class I or a Class II, depending on the extent and location of the edentulous span. It is admitted that the Class III type is difficult to determine but is generally agreed that a Class I or tooth-borne design is preferable if adequate abutment support can be obtained.

As in any method of classification, a weak or malposed posterior abutment may best be removed before fabricating the denture, if the prognosis is poor and a free-end base will serve better. Although this decision must be based upon a careful evaluation of the abutment tooth in question, it is often desirable to retain the tooth as an abutment originally but to provide for a partial denture design which will permit later conversion to a free-end base if it becomes necessary (Fig. 20). Such a denture would have to be designed to function as a Class II (a) should the posterior abutment support be lost.

Skinner's Classification (Fig. 19). Skinner has proposed a classification that he claims is based upon the relations of the anatomic-physiologic factors of the maxillary and mandibular arches. In this classification he attempts to relate the remaining abutment teeth to the alveolar supporting area. According to Skinner, a logical working classification of partially edentulous arches should be expressive both to the dentist from a physiologic standpoint and to the technician from a technical standpoint.

Skinner further states that "the total value of any partial denture is based upon the coordination of the abutment teeth and the alveolar ridge support to the maximum degree. Therefore, a classification should be based upon the morphology and physiology of each dental arch. These factors in turn should be the guiding values as to the design and the arrangement of the various connectors to be related to the alveolar ridge support. Such a classification would be very

Fig. 20. A lower partial denture framework designed for later conversion to a free-end base if it becomes necessary due to the loss of the posterior abutments. Combination clasps on the premolars and dual indirect retention would then be effective when the denture was converted to a bilateral free-end partial denture. The design of the retention for the resin bases is such that adequate retention will remain after the posterior clasp assemblies are cut off following the loss of the posterior teeth.

beneficial in determining the particular type of connector to be used, and in determining the correlation required in selecting the type of broken stress as applied to that relationship of function between the abutment teeth and the supporting alveolar ridge."[*]

The Skinner classification is as follows:

Class I. That group of partial dentures characterized by anatomic relationship of the remaining abutment teeth in which they are related both anterior and posterior to the denture base area. These groups of partial dentures are found in both the maxillary arch and the mandibular arch. They may occur unilaterally or bilaterally. Of the total classification this group constitutes about 14 per cent of the cases involving either arch.

Class II. That group of partial dentures which are characterized by a morphologic pattern of the remaining abutment teeth in which all of the teeth are posterior to the denture base area which functions as a partial denture unit. This principle is found in the maxillary arch and also in the mandibular arch. The condition can be either unilateral or bilateral in character. This group constitutes approximately 8.5 per cent of the whole.

Class III. That group of partial dentures which are characterized by the anatomic relationship in which all of the abutment teeth remaining are related anterior to the denture base area which functions as a partial denture base. This principle holds true of the maxillary arch and also of the mandibular arch. The condition exists unilaterally or bilaterally in either arch. This group constitutes about 72 per cent of all partial dentures.

Class IV. That group of partial dentures which are characterized by anatomic relationships in which the denture base areas are both anterior and posterior to the remaining teeth. Observe in this instance that the abutment teeth are in the center or between the functional denture bases. These relations are found in the maxillary arch and in the mandibular arch. Again, these cases can be either unilateral or bilateral in character. This group is approximately 3 per cent of the whole.

Class V. That group of partial dentures characterized by a specific relationship in which all of the remaining abutment teeth are unilateral to the denture base area. This group is about 2.5 per cent of the total classification.

Kennedy's Classification (Fig. 19). The Kennedy method of classification was originally proposed by Dr. Edward Kennedy in 1925. Like the Bailyn classification, and also the Skinner classification, it attempts to classify the partially edentulous arch in a manner that will suggest, if not govern, the partial denture design for a given situation. Contrary to Cummer, it seems more logical for the design to be a by-product of the classification, inasmuch as the key to the design lies in the type of support the partial denture is to receive from the oral tissues.

Kennedy divided all partially edentulous arches into four main types. Edentulous areas, in addition to those determining the main types, were designated as *modification spaces.*

---

[*]From Skinner, C. N.: A Classification of Removable Partial Dentures Based Upon the Principles of Anatomy and Physiology, J. Pros. Den. **9:**240, 1959.

The Kennedy classification is as follows:

Class I. Bilateral edentulous areas located posterior to the remaining natural teeth.

Class II. A unilateral edentulous area located posterior to the remaining natural teeth.

Class III. A unilateral edentulous area with natural teeth remaining both anterior and posterior to it.

Class IV. A single, but bilateral (crossing the midline), edentulous area located anterior to the remaining natural teeth.

One of the principal advantages of the Kennedy method is that it permits immediate visualization of the partially edentulous arch. Those schooled in its use and in the principles of partial denture design which are based upon it may immediately compartmentalize their thinking as to the basic partial denture design that will be used. It permits a logical approach to the problems of design. It makes possible the application of sound principles of partial denture design and is therefore the most logical method of classification.

Applegate's Rules for Applying the Kennedy Classification. The Kennedy classification would be difficult to apply to every situation without certain rules for application. Applegate has provided the following eight rules governing the application of the Kennedy method:

Rule 1. Classification should follow rather than precede any extractions of teeth that might alter the original classification.

Rule 2. If the third molar is missing and not to be replaced, *it is not considered in the classification.*

Rule 3. If a third molar is present and is to be used as an abutment, *it is considered in the classification.*

Rule 4. If a second molar is missing and is not to be replaced, *it is not considered in the classification* (for example, if the opposing second molar is likewise missing and is not to be replaced).

Rule 5. The *most posterior edentulous area* (or areas) always determines the classification.

Rule 6. Additional edentulous areas other than those determining the classification are spoken of as *modifications* and are designated by their number.

Rule 7. The *extent* of the modification is not considered, only the *number* of additional edentulous areas.

Rule 8. There can be no modification areas in Class IV arches. (Other edentulous area lying posterior to the "single bilateral area crossing the midline" would instead determine the classification.)

More recently, Applegate has proposed two additional classes to the original four of Kennedy.* Class V, according to Applegate, differs from Class III only in that a very weak anterior boundary tooth located at one end of a long edentulous span is not utilized as an abutment. Instead, a free-end base extend-

---

*From Applegate, O. C.: The Rationale of Partial Denture Choice, J. Pros. Den. **10:**891-907, 1960.

ing anteriorly is used to support the artificial occlusion in much the same manner as a distal free-end base. Most of the principles of design common to treating a Class II arch are applied similarly to this Class V situation. In a Class V design a posterior abutment on the opposite side of the arch is used for indirect retention rather than an anteriorly placed indirect retainer as in Class II. The Class V situation is most commonly found in the maxillary arch, and the weak anterior boundary tooth is usually a lateral incisor. (Fig. 21.) Applegate points out, however, that if multiple splinting of anterior abutments can successfully be employed, the design should follow that of a typical bilateral Class III.

In Class VI, Applegate describes the unilaterally edentulous situation which can be successfully treated with a tooth-supported unilateral removable prosthesis. However, he rightly states, "In such instances the fixed prosthesis is the restoration of choice." Thus it is recognized that the Kennedy system of classification can logically be applied to any partially edentulous arch, even though in Classes III, IV, and VI the choice of treatment may be by means of a fixed prosthetic restoration.

Other Methods of Classification. Still other methods of classification have been proposed and are in limited use. For the most part, however, attempts to improve upon or replace existing classifications have met with little acceptance.

One suggested change in the order of the Kennedy classification is an attempt to correlate the Class I and Class II partially edentulous arches with the number of edentulous areas involved. Thus, Class I would be a unilateral edentu-

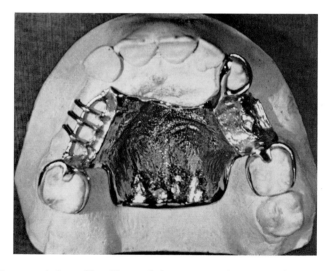

Fig. 21. Cast framework for a Class V partial denture according to Applegate. Since the lateral incisor is deemed too weak to serve as an abutment the partial denture is designed as a unilateral free-end type, extending anteriorly instead of posteriorly. The fulcrum line extends from the patient's right molar to the canine, and the occlusal rest on the left molar abutment serves as an indirect retainer.

lous area posterior to the remaining teeth, and Class II would be a bilateral edentulous area posterior to the remaining teeth.

While it is true that there is some confusion in the mind of the student initially as to why Class I should refer to two edentulous areas and Class II should refer to one, the principles of design make this position logical. Either by design or by accident, presumably the former, Kennedy placed the Class II unilateral free-end between the Class I bilateral free-end and the Class III tooth-bounded classification. Any change in this order would be illogical for the following reasons. The Class I partial denture is designed as a tooth- *and* tissue-supported denture. Three of the features necessary for the success of such a denture are adequate support for the free-end base, flexible direct retention, and some provision for indirect retention. The Class III partial denture is designed as a tooth-borne removable bridge, without need for indirect retention, without base support from the ridge tissues, and with direct retention, the only function of which is to retain the prosthesis. An entirely different design is therefore common to each class due to the difference in support.

The Class II partial denture, however, especially where tooth-borne modifications are present, must embody features of both. Having a tissue-supported free end, it must be designed similarly to a Class I, but frequently there is a tooth-supported, or Class III, component elsewhere in the arch. Thus, the Class II partial denture rightly falls between the Class I and the Class III, for it embodies design features common to both. In keeping with the principle that design is based upon the classification, the application of such principles of design is simplified by retaining the original classification of Kennedy.

Another proposed alteration of the Kennedy method is to add the letters "A" and "P" to designate modifications. Thus, an additional edentulous space is identified specifically as being anterior or posterior. It is doubtful that this change in the original classification adds little, if any, clarification to it. However, if it is used only to supplement the original classification rather than to replace it, there can be little objection to the use of the "A" and "P" designations. It cannot be applied to the Class IV arch, however, since Class IV can have no modifications.

REQUIREMENTS OF AN ACCEPTABLE METHOD OF CLASSIFICATION

The classification of a partially edentulous arch should satisfy the following requirements.

1. It should permit immediate visualization of the type of partially edentulous arch being considered.

2. It should permit immediate differentiation between the removable bridge and the partial denture; that is, between tooth support and tooth-tissue support.

3. It should serve as a guide to the type of design to be used.

4. It should be universally acceptable.

5. It should have stood the test of years of successful application.

Any method of classification that will satisfy these requirements is acceptable, but in the interest of a more comprehensive understanding of the principles of partial denture design, it seems that the universal adoption of the Kennedy method is desirable.

Chapter **5**

Surveying

A dental surveyor has been defined as an instrument used for determining the relative parallelism of two or more surfaces of the teeth or other parts of the cast of a dental arch.

Any one of the several moderately priced surveyors on the market will adequately accomplish the procedures necessary in the design and construction of a partial denture. In addition, these surveyors may be used to parallel precision rests and intracoronal retainers. With handpiece holder added, they may also be used to fabricate precision rests and to parallel guiding plane surfaces of abutment restorations.

DESCRIPTION OF A DENTAL SURVEYOR

Perhaps the most widely used surveyors are the Ney (Fig. 22) and the Jelenko (Fig. 23) surveyors. Both of these are precision-made instruments but differ principally in that the Jelenko arm swivels whereas the Ney arm is fixed. The technique for surveying and trimming blockout is therefore somewhat different. Other surveyors also differ in this respect, and the operator may prefer one over another for this reason.

The principal parts of the Ney surveyor are as follows:

1. A platform upon which the base is moved.
2. A vertical arm which supports the superstructure.
3. A horizontal arm from which the surveying tool suspends.
4. A table to which the cast or model is attached.
5. A base upon which the table swivels.
6. A paralleling tool or guide line marker. This tool contacts the convex surface to be studied in a tangential manner. The relative parallelism of one surface to another may thus be determined. By substituting a carbon marker, the height of contour may then be delineated on the surfaces of the abutment teeth and also areas of interference requiring reduction or blockout.
7. Mandrel for holding special tools (Fig. 25).

Fig. 22. The Ney surveyor is perhaps the most widely used of all dental surveyors and is preferred as a teaching instrument for dental school use because of its simplicity and durability. In several dental schools the students are required to own such a surveyor. By becoming familiar with and dependent upon its use, they are more likely to continue using the surveyor in practice as a necessary piece of equipment toward more adequate diagnosis, effective treatment planning, and the performance of many other aspects of prosthodontic treatment. (Courtesy the J. M. Ney Co., Hartford, Conn.)

The principal parts of the Jelenko surveyor are essentially the same as the Ney surveyor except that by loosening the nut at the top of the vertical arm, the horizontal arm may be made to swivel. The objective of this feature, originally designed by Dr. Noble Wills, is to permit freedom of movement of the arm in a horizontal plane rather than to depend entirely upon the horizontal movement of the cast. To some, this is confusing because two horizontal movements must thus by coordinated. For those who prefer to move the cast only in a horizontal relationship to a fixed vertical arm, the nut may be tightened and the horizontal arm used in a fixed position.

Another difference in the two surveyors is that the vertical arm on the Ney surveyor is retained by friction within a fixed bearing. The shaft may be moved up or down within this bearing but remains in any vertical position until again

Fig. 23. The Jelenko surveyor. Note the spring-mounted paralleling tool and the swivel at the top of the vertical arm. The horizontal arm may be fixed in any position by tightening the nut at the top of the vertical arm. (Courtesy J. F. Jelenko & Co., Inc., New York, N. Y.)

moved. The shaft may be fixed in any vertical position desired by tightening a set screw. In contrast, the vertical arm of the Jelenko surveyor is spring mounted and returns to the top position when released. It must be held down against spring tension while in use, which to some is a disadvantage. The spring may be removed, but the friction of the two bearings supporting the arm does not hold it in position as securely as a bearing designed for that purpose. These minor differences in the two surveyors lead to personal preference on the part of the operator but do not detract from the effectiveness of either surveyor when properly used.

Since the shaft on the Ney surveyor is stable in any vertical position, yet may be moved vertically with ease, it lends itself well for use as a drill press when a handpiece holder is added (Fig. 26). The handpiece may thus be used to cut recesses in gold restorations with precision by using burs or carborundum points of various sizes in a dental handpiece.

A number of other surveyors have been designed and are in use today (Figs. 27, 28, and 29). Many of these are more elaborate and costly and therefore are used primarily by larger laboratories where volume justifies the more costly equipment. Their main advantage lies in the incorporation of some kind of gauge for locating the desired undercut to be used with plastic patterns of standard dimensions. When used properly, they permit the technician to be more precise in selecting the amount of retention for a given clasp design, in proportion to the characteristics of the particular casting alloy being used. Since most laboratories use one chrome alloy all of the time, standardization of clasp retention is made possible through the use of retention gauges. It must be presumed, of course, that

Fig. 24. The new Williams surveyor which features a Gimbal stage table that is adjustable to any desired anterior, posterior, or lateral tilt. The degree of inclination can be recorded for re-positioning of the cast at any time. A distinct advantage of this table over the universal tilt table is that the center of rotation always remains constant. The superstructure of this surveyor consists of a jointed arm and spring-supported survey rod, all components of which can be locked in a fixed position if desired. This surveyor is perhaps best suited for the placement of internal attachments, rather than for cast analyzing and other purposes. (Courtesy Williams Gold Refining Co., Buffalo, N. Y.)

the precision possible with such a surveyor is utilized to its fullest advantage by the technician or else little is gained through the use of the more elaborate instrument.

Recently, an electronic surveyor was developed at the School of Aviation Medicine, Randolph Air Force Base, by Colonel Donald C. Hudson, Director, Research Dentistry Division (Fig. 30). The object of this surveyor is not so much the evaluation of the cast, which can be done just as well on a conventional surveyor, but the marking of the height of contour and a selected amount of under-cut by electronic means once the relation of the cast to the vertical arm of the surveyor (i.e., the path of insertion) has been established.

The marking of a stone cast is accomplished by chemical change at the surface due to passage of a weak electric current through the damp cast material

Ney undercut gauges

A

.01

.02

.03

B Jelenko undercut
gauge

C Ney carbon marker
and sheath

D Jelenko carbon marker

Path of Insertion

Blockout wax

2° taper tool

6° taper tool   E

Ney wax
trimmer

F

Ney surveyor
blade

G

Fig. 25. Various tools which may be used with a dental surveyor. **A,** Ney undercut gauges. **B,** Jelenko undercut gauge. **C,** Ney carbon marker with metal reinforcement sleeve. **D,** Jelenko carbon marker. **E,** Tapered tools, 2- and 6-degree, for trimming blockout where some non-parallelism is desired. **F,** Ney wax trimmer for paralleling blockout. **G,** A surveying blade being used for trimming blockout.

to the point of contact with the metal surveying tool. An indicator sensitive to pH changes (0.5 per cent phenolphthalein in alcohol) produces the marking.

Current is supplied from two flashlight batteries in the case at the rear of the upright post and is controlled through a foot-operated switch. The movable arm of the surveying instrument is insulated from the post by means of a nonconducting bushing.

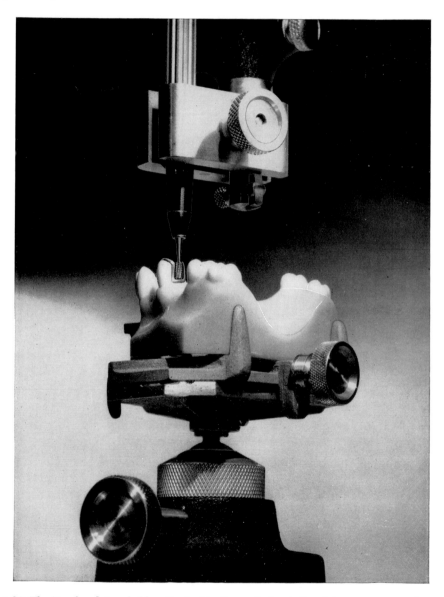

Fig. 26. The Ney handpiece holder attached to the vertical spindle of the surveyor may be used as a drill press to cut precision rests and recesses in wax patterns and/or gold castings and to establish lingual surfaces above a ledge, which are parallel to the path of insertion in abutment restorations. (Courtesy the J. M. Ney Co., Hartford, Conn.)

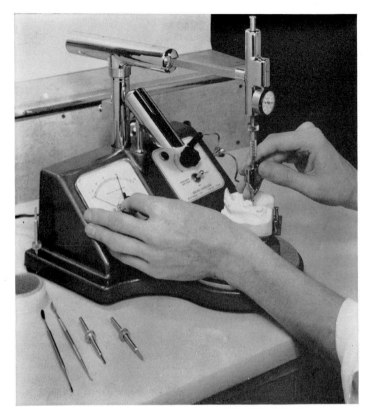

Fig. 27. The Austenal Micro-Analyzer. Undercuts are measured electrically in millimeters in relation to selected Flexseal pre-formed clasp patterns which are used as the standards of measurement. The Micro-Analyzer also aids in determining the path of insertion, marking the height of contour and relieving or blocking out undesirable undercuts. It is equipped with a vertical gauge calibrated in hundredths of a millimeter up to .51. A sweep dial indicator shows the desired amount of undercut, and a flashing light tells when the exact depth has been reached. (Courtesy Austenal, Inc., Chicago, Ill.)

Upon closure of the switch, current flows through the post and platform, through the table holding the cast and through the cast, to the surveying tool, returning through the horizontal arm to complete the circuit. The tool is negative to the cast, attracting Ca^{++} ions to the surface at the point of contact, where recombination with moisture produces a pH change and this in turn produces a color change in the indicator.

No marking occurs unless the switch is closed to permit current flow, but upon closing the switch, the height of the contour is marked on the cast at the point of contact. Thus, the location of the height of contour is accurately established without resorting to the use of a graphite marker which is frequently too broad and is easily smeared.

The precise location of an undercut on a tooth to be clasped may also be marked by replacing the surveying tool with a Ney undercut gauge. Undercut gauges of .010, .015, .020, and .030 inch are used and are selected according to

Fig. 28. The Ticonium Stress-o-graph. The left arm contains a spring-mounted paralleling tool for performing the usual surveying and relieving operations. The right arm holds a micrometer gauge and marking pen with a vernier travel screw. The gauge is divided into hundredths of an inch up to .05 inch. A case-hardened, nickel-silver marking pen is used to make a fine ink line with a slow-drying ink. The gauge is used to measure the degree of tooth undercut sloping away from the height of contour. It is recommended that a clasp tip never be placed farther into the tooth undercut than the suprabulge measurement from height of contour to occlusal marginal ridge. The following reason is given: "Because the suprabulge angle of a tooth acts as a wedge, it will pass over the height of contour and close back into contact with the tooth undercut. If the clasp tip is arbitrarily placed in an undercut angle that is greater than the suprabulge angle, undue pressure can be placed on the tooth as the clasp passes over the height of contour. The result is damage to the periodontium and danger of overloading the fatigue limit of a clasp. Also, when a clasp is placed too far into an undercut, it will not be opened by the suprabulge angle of the tooth and will require relieving on the inside before it will seat on the stone cast without chipping the teeth, thus weakening the clasp arm."* (Courtesy Ticonium Division, Consolidated Metal Products Corp., Albany, N. Y.)

---

*From Ticonium Technique Manual, Consolidated Metal Products Corp., Albany, N. Y.

Fig. 29. The Saddle-Lock Retentoscope, designed to be used with the Saddle-Lock principle of concealed clasp retention. In addition to a paralleling tool and a separate heated tool for paralleling blockout, a calibrated dial gauge accurately measures and marks with a carbon rod the location of the desired amount of undercut. The table may be raised and lowered in relation to a fixed vertical arm until the desired undercut area is located. (Courtesy Saddle-Lock, Inc., Brooklyn, N. Y.)

the length, size, diameter, and material of the clasp arm to be used. The selected undercut gauge is used to determine the amount of undercut that will be engaged by the tip of the clasp arm. This spot is marked on the cast electronically when the projection of the undercut gauge is allowed to contact the tooth below the height of contour simultaneous with contact of its shaft against the height of contour. This point or line represents the gingival edge of the clasp tip that will engage the undercut. (Fig. 31.)

The red mark made by the electronic surveyor has been described as a *captive* mark that gradually disappears as the cast becomes dry. However, this mark can easily be overlayed with a crayon-type pencil before the captive mark disappears, rendering it permanent for future reference.

Fig. 30. Electronic surveyor developed at the School of Aviation Medicine, Randolph Air Force Base, Texas. A weak current passing through the paralleling tool onto the treated cast surface marks the height of contour and location of undercut areas electronically. (U. S. Air Force Photo, School of Aviation Medicine, Randolph Air Force Base, Texas.)

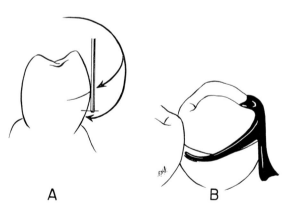

A   B

Fig. 31. An undercut on an abutment tooth may be located electronically through the use of an undercut gauge attached to the electronic surveyor. Simultaneous contact of the undercut gauge with the height of contour and the selected amount of tooth undercut is marked on the cast electronically as shown in **A.** As shown in **B,** this point or line is used to locate the gingival edge of the clasp tip that will engage the undercut.

PURPOSES FOR WHICH THE SURVEYOR IS USED

Some of the purposes for which a surveyor may be used are surveying the study cast, contouring wax patterns, surveying the master cast, placing the intracoronal retainers, and placing precision rests.

Surveying the Study Cast. Surveying the study cast is essential to effective diagnosis and treatment planning. The objectives are as follows:

1. To determine the most acceptable path of insertion that will eliminate or minimize interference to insertion and removal (Fig. 32). *The path of insertion is the direction in which a restoration moves from the point of initial contact of its rigid parts with the supporting teeth to the terminal resting position, with occlusal rest seated and the denture base in contact with the tissues.* The *path of removal* is exactly the reverse, being the direction of restoration movement from its terminal resting position to the last contact of its rigid parts with the supporting teeth. When the restoration is properly designed to have positive guiding planes, the patient may insert and remove the restoration with ease in one direction only, due to the guiding influence of tooth surfaces made parallel to that path of insertion.

2. To identify proximal tooth surfaces that are or can be made parallel so as to act as guiding planes during insertion and removal.

3. To locate and measure areas of the teeth that may be used for retention.

4. To determine whether or not tooth and bony areas of interference will need to be eliminated either by extraction or by selecting a different path of insertion.

5. To determine the most suitable path of insertion which will permit the placement of retainers and artificial teeth to the best esthetic advantage.

6. To permit an accurate charting of the mouth preparations to be made. This includes the disking of proximal tooth surfaces to provide guiding planes and the reduction of excessive tooth contours to eliminate interference and to permit a

Path of Insertion

Fig. 32. The tilt of the cast on the adjustable table of the surveyor in relation to the vertical arm establishes the path of insertion and removal that the partial denture will take. All mouth preparations must be made to conform to a previously determined path of insertion, which has been recorded by scoring the base of the cast.

more acceptable location of reciprocal and retentive clasp arms. By marking these areas on the study cast with red pencil, and then trimming them on the stone cast with the surveyor blade, the angulation and extent of tooth reduction may be established prior to preparing the teeth in the mouth. With the study cast on the surveyor at the time of mouth preparations, disking and reduction of tooth contours may thus be accomplished with acceptable accuracy.

7. To delineate the height of contour on abutment teeth and to locate areas of undesirable tooth undercut which are to be avoided, eliminated, or blocked out. This will include areas of the teeth to be contacted by rigid connectors, the location of nonretentive reciprocal and stabilizing arms, and the location of retentive clasp terminals.

8. To record the cast position in relation to the selected path of insertion for future reference. This may be done by locating three dots or parallel lines on the cast, thus establishing the horizontal plane in relation to the vertical arm of the surveyor (Fig. 2).

Contouring Wax Patterns. The surveyor blade is used as a wax carver during this phase of mouth preparation so that the proposed path of insertion may be maintained throughout the preparation of cast restorations for abutment teeth.

All proximal surfaces of wax patterns should be made parallel to the previously determined path of insertion. Similarly, all other tooth contours that will be contacted by rigid connectors should be made parallel whenever possible. The surfaces of restorations upon which reciprocal and stabilizing components will be placed should be so contoured to permit their location well below occlusal surfaces and upon nonretentive areas. Those surfaces of the restoration which are to provide retention for clasp arms should be contoured so that retentive clasps may be placed in the cervical one third of the crown and to the best esthetic advantage. Generally, a small amount of undercut (.015 inch or less) is sufficient for retentive purposes.

Placement of Intracoronal Retainers (Internal Attachments). In this application, the surveyor is used as follows:

1. To select a path of insertion in relation to the long axes of the abutment teeth which will avoid areas of interference elsewhere in the arch.

2. To cut recesses in the stone teeth on the study cast for the purpose of estimating the proximity of the recess to the pulp (in conjunction with roentgenographic information as to pulp size and location). Also, to facilitate the fabrication of metal or resin jigs to guide the preparations of the recesses in the mouth.

3. To carve recesses in wax patterns, or to place internal attachment trays in wax patterns, or to cut recesses in the gold casting with the handpiece holder, whichever method is preferred.

4. To place the keyway portion of the attachment in the casting prior to investing and soldering, each located parallel to the other similar attachments elsewhere in the arch.

Placement of Precision Rests. The surveyor may be used as a drill press, with a dental handpiece attached to the vertical arm by means of a handpiece holder. Precision rests may be carved on the wax pattern and further refined with the handpiece after casting, or the entire rest may be cut in the cast restoration with the handpiece. It is best that the outline form of the rest be carved first in wax and merely refined on the casting with the handpiece.

A precision rest differs from an internal attachment in that some portion of the cast prosthesis is waxed and cast to fit into the rest instead of a matched key and keyway attachment being used. The former is usually nonretentive but provides a definite seat for a removable restoration or a cantilever rest for a broken-stress fixed bridge. When used with fixed bridges, nonparallel abutment pieces may thus be inserted separately.

The precision rest in partial denture construction provides a positive occlusal support that is more favorably located in relation to the rotational axis of the abutment tooth than the conventional spoon-shaped occlusal rest. It also provides horizontal stabilization through the parallelism of the vertical walls, thereby serving the same purpose as bracing arms placed extracoronally. Due to the movement of a free-end base, more torque may be applied to the abutment tooth by this type of rest, and for this reason its use in conjunction with a free-end partial denture is contraindicated. The ball-and-socket or spoon-shaped occlusal rest should be used in all free-end partial denture designs. The use of the precision rest should be limited to tooth-borne removable appliances, except where it is used in conjunction with some kind of stress breaker between the abutment pieces and the movable base. The use of stress breakers will be considered in Chapter 11.

Precision rests may be made in the form of a nonretentive box, a retentive box fashioned after the internal attachment, or a semiretentive box. In the latter, the walls are usually parallel and nonretentive, but a recess in the floor of the box prevents proximal movement of the male portion. These are cut with dental burs of various sizes and shapes. Tapered or cylindrical fissure burs are used to form the vertical walls, and small round burs are used to cut recesses in the floor of the rest.

Machining Cast Restorations. With handpiece holder attached (Fig. 26), vertical surfaces of cast restorations may be refined by machining with a suitable cylindrical carborundum point. Proximal surfaces of crowns and inlays, which will serve as guiding planes, and vertical surfaces above crown ledges may be improved by machining, but only if the relationship of one crown to another is correct. Unless the seating of removable dies is very accurate and held in place with additional stone or plaster, cast restorations should first be tried in the mouth and then transferred by means of a plaster index impression to a reinforced stone cast for machining purposes. The new cast is then positioned on the surveyor, conforming to the path of insertion of the partial denture, and vertical surfaces are machined with a true-running cylindrical carborundum point.

While machined parallelism may be considered ideal and beyond the realm of everyday application, its merits more than justify the additional steps required to accomplish it. Where such parallelism is accomplished and reproduced in a master cast, it is essential that subsequent laboratory steps be directed toward the utilization of these parallel guiding plane surfaces.

Surveying the Master Cast. Since surveying the master cast follows mouth preparations, the path of insertion, location of retentive areas, and the location of remaining interference must be known before proceeding with the final design of the denture framework. The objectives are as follows:

1. To select the most suitable path of insertion following mouth preparations which satisfy the requirements of *guiding planes, retention, noninterference, and esthetics.*

2. To permit measurement of retentive areas and to identify the location of clasp terminals in proportion to the flexibility of the clasp arm being used. Flexibility will depend upon many factors: (a) the alloy used for the clasp, (b) the design and type of the clasp, (c) whether its form is round or half-round, (d) whether it is of cast or wrought material, and (e) the length of the clasp arm from its point of origin to its terminal end. Retention will then depend upon (a) the flexibility of the clasp arm, (b) the magnitude of the tooth undercut, and (c) the depth the clasp terminal is placed into this undercut.

3. To locate areas of undesirable remaining undercut which will be crossed by rigid parts of the appliance during insertion and removal. These must be eliminated by blockout.

4. To trim blockout material parallel to the path of insertion prior to duplication.

USE OF THE SURVEYOR

The partial denture must be so designed that it can be easily inserted and removed by the patient, will be retained against reasonable dislodging forces, and will have the best possible appearance. It is necessary that the study cast be surveyed with these principles in mind. Mouth preparation should therefore be planned in accordance with certain factors that will influence the path of insertion and removal.

FACTORS THAT WILL DETERMINE THE PATH OF INSERTION AND REMOVAL

The factors that will determine the path of insertion and removal are guiding planes, retentive areas, interference, and esthetics.

Guiding Planes. Proximal tooth surfaces that bear a parallel relationship to one another must either be found or be created to act as *guiding planes* during insertion and removal. Guiding planes may be compared to the valve guides in an engine and act to assure a definite path of insertion as the rigid parts of the prosthesis contact parallel tooth surfaces.

Guiding planes are necessary to ensure the passage of the rigid parts of the prosthesis past existing areas of interference. Thus, the denture can be easily inserted and removed by the patient without strain upon the teeth contacted or upon the denture itself and without damage to the underlying soft tissues.

Guiding planes are also necessary to assure predictable clasp retention. For a clasp to be retentive, its retentive arm must be forced to flex. Hence, guiding planes are necessary to give a positive direction to the movement of the appliance to and from its terminal position.

Retentive Areas. Retentive areas must exist for a given path of insertion which will be contacted by retentive clasp arms that will be forced to flex over a convex surface during insertion and removal. Satisfactory clasp retention is no more than the resistance of metal to deformation. For a clasp to be retentive, its path of escapement must be other than parallel to the path of removal of the appliance itself; otherwise it would not be forced to flex and thereby generate the resistance known as retention. Clasp retention is therefore dependent upon the existence of a definite path of insertion and removal.

Retention at each principal abutment should be balanced in relation to the tooth on the opposite side of the arch, that is, equal and opposite in magnitude and relative location. It should be sufficient only to resist reasonable dislodging forces. In other words, it should be the minimum acceptable for adequate retention against reasonable dislodging forces.

Balanced retention may be obtained by one of two means. One is to change the path of insertion so as to increase or decrease the angle of cervical convergence of opposing retentive surfaces of abutment teeth. The other is to alter the flexibility of the clasp arm by changing its design, its size and length, and/or the material of which it is made.

Interference. The prosthesis must be so designed that it may be inserted and removed without encountering tooth or tissue *interference*. A path of insertion may be selected which encounters interference only if that interference can be eliminated during mouth preparations, or on the master cast by means of a reasonable amount of blockout. Interference may be eliminated during mouth preparations by surgery, extraction, disking of interfering tooth surfaces, or altering tooth contours with cast restorations.

Generally, interference which *cannot* be eliminated for one reason or another will take precedence over the factors of retention and guiding planes. Sometimes certain areas can be made noninterfering only by selecting a different path of insertion at the expense of existing retentive areas and guiding planes. These must then be modified with restorations that are in harmony with the path dictated by the existing interference. On the other hand, if areas of interference *can* be eliminated by various reasonable means, this should always be done. By so doing, the contour of existing abutments may frequently be utilized with little or no alteration.

Esthetics. By one path of insertion, the most esthetic placement of artificial teeth is made possible and less clasp metal and/or less base material may be displayed.

The location of retentive areas may influence the path of insertion selected, and therefore retentive areas should always be selected with the most esthetic placement of clasps in mind. Where restorations are to be made for other reasons, they should be so contoured to permit the least display of clasp metal. Generally, less metal will be displayed if the retentive clasp is placed at a more distogingival area of tooth surface, made possible either by the path of insertion selected or by the contour of cast restorations.

Esthetics may also dictate the choice of path selected when missing anterior teeth must be replaced with the partial denture. In such cases, a more vertical path of insertion is necessary so that neither the artificial teeth nor the adjacent natural teeth will have to be modified excessively (Fig. 33). In this instance,

Fig. 33. Where anterior teeth must be replaced with a partial denture, a vertical path of insertion may be necessary to avoid excessively altering the adjacent abutment teeth and/or the supplied teeth.

esthetics may take precedence over all other factors. This necessitates the elimination of interference and the preparation of abutment teeth to provide guiding planes and retention *in harmony with* that path of insertion dictated by esthetic factors.

Esthetics should ordinarily not be the primary factor in partial denture design. Therefore, the replacement of missing anterior teeth should be accomplished by means of fixed restorations whenever possible rather than permit their replacement to influence the mechanical and functional effectiveness of the partial denture. Since the primary considerations should always be the preservation of the remaining oral tissues, esthetics should never be allowed to jeopardize the success of the partial denture.

STEP-BY-STEP PROCEDURE IN SURVEYING A STUDY CAST

Attach the cast to the adjustable surveyor table by means of the clamp provided. Position the adjustable table so that the occlusal surface of the teeth are approximately parallel to the platform (Fig. 34). (This is only a tentative, but practical, way to start considering the factors that influence the path of insertion and removal.)

Guiding Planes. Determine the relative parallelism of proximal tooth surfaces by contacting proximal tooth surfaces with the surveyor blade. Alter the cast position anteroposteriorly until the proximal surfaces are in a parallel relation to one another or near enough that they can be made parallel by disking. This will determine the *anteroposterior tilt* of the cast in relation to the vertical arm of the surveyor (Fig. 35). (Although the surveyor table is universally adjustable, it should be thought of as having only two axes, thus allowing only anteroposterior and lateral movement.)

Fig. 34. The recommended method for manipulating the dental surveyor. The heel of the right hand is braced on the horizontal arm of the surveyor and the fingers are used as illustrated to raise and lower the vertical shaft in its spindle. The left hand holding the cast on the adjustable table slides horizontally on the platform in relation to the vertical arm. The right hand must be used also to loosen and tighten the tilting mechanism as a suitable anteroposterior and lateral tilt of the cast in relation to the surveyor is being determined.

In making a choice between having contact with a proximal surface at the cervical area only or contact at the marginal ridge only, the latter is preferred because a plane may then be established by disking (Fig. 36). It is obvious that when only gingival contact exists, a cast restoration is the only means of establishing a guiding plane. Therefore, if a tilt is accepted which does not provide proximal contact, the proximal surface must be established with some kind of restoration. In making a choice between having a good guiding plane on one proximal surface and none on another as against having a good plane on one and disking the other, the latter is preferred and the need for disking is so indicated on the study cast with red pencil. This holds true only when cast restorations are not otherwise necessary.

Where all of the proximal surfaces are to be restored anyway, then an arbitrary tilt may be established and all restorations made with parallel proximal surfaces. Where all but one proximal surface is to be restored for other reasons, that one will usually dictate the anteroposterior tilt.

The end result of selecting a suitable anteroposterior tilt should be *to provide the greatest area of parallel proximal surfaces that may act as guiding planes.*

Retentive Areas. By contacting buccal and lingual surfaces of abutment teeth with the surveyor blade, the amount of retention existing below their height of convexity may be determined. This is best accomplished by directing a small source of light toward the cast from the side away from the operator. The *angle of cervical convergence* is best observed as a triangle of light between the surveyor blade and the tooth surface being studied.

Alter the cast position by tilting the cast laterally until equal retentive areas exist on the principal abutment teeth. If only two abutment teeth are involved, as

Fig. 35. Relative parallelism of proximal tooth surfaces will determine the anteroposterior tilt of the cast in relation to the vertical arm of the surveyor.

A   B

Fig. 36. **A,** In selecting the most desirable anteroposterior tilt of the cast in relation to the surveyor blade, a choice must be made between the positions illustrated in **A** and in **B.** In **A** the distal surface of the left premolar abutment would have to be extended by means of a cast restoration. In **B** the right premolar could be disked slightly to provide an acceptably parallel guiding plane. Unless cast restorations are necessary for other reasons, the tilt shown in **B** is always preferred.

in a Kennedy Class I partially edentulous arch, they are both principal abutments. Or, if four abutment teeth are involved, as in a Kennedy Class III, modification 1, arch, they are all principal abutments, and retention should be equalized on all four. But if three abutment teeth are involved, as in a Kennedy Class II, modification 1, arch, the posterior abutment on the tooth-borne side and the abutment on the free-end side are considered to be the principal abutments and retention is equalized accordingly. The third abutment may be considered to be secondary and less retention expected from it than from the other two. An exception is when the posterior abutment on the tooth-borne side has a poor prognosis and the denture is designed to ultimately be a Class I with bilateral free ends. In such a case, the two stronger abutments are considered to be principal abutments.

In tilting the cast laterally to establish uniformity of retention, it is necessary that the table be rotated about an imaginary longitudinal axis without disturbing the anteroposterior tilt previously established. The resulting position is one that provides or makes possible parallel guiding planes and provides for acceptable and uniform retention on the abutment teeth. Note that we have not, as yet, taken into consideration possible interference to this tentative path of insertion.

Interference. If a mandibular cast is being surveyed, check the lingual surfaces which will be crossed by a lingual bar major connector during insertion and removal. Bony prominences and lingually inclined premolar teeth are the most common causes of interference to a lingual bar connector.

If the interference is bilateral, surgery and/or disking of lingual tooth surfaces may be unavoidable. If it is only unilateral, a change in the lateral tilt may be necessary to avoid an area of tooth or tissue interference. In changing the path of insertion to avoid interference, previously established guiding planes and uniformity of retention may be lost. The decision must then be made whether to remove the existing interference by whatever means necessary or to resort to restorations on the abutment teeth, thereby changing the proximal and retentive areas to conform to the new path of insertion.

In like manner, bony undercuts which will offer interference to the insertion of denture bases must be studied and the decision made to remove them surgically, change the path of insertion at the expense of guiding planes and retention, or design denture bases so as to avoid such undercut areas. The latter may be done by eliminating buccal and labial flanges and distolingual extension of denture bases. It should be remembered that the maximum area available for support of the denture base should be utilized whenever possible. Generally, however, undercut areas are not supporting areas, and as long as sufficient horizontal stabilization is available elsewhere, the absence of a flange in an undercut area will not jeopardize the stability of the denture.

Interference to major connectors rarely exists in the maxillary arch. Areas of interference are usually found on buccally inclined posterior teeth and those bony areas on the buccal aspect of edentulous spaces. As with the mandibular cast, the decision must be made whether to eliminate them, change the path of insertion at the expense of guiding planes and retention, or design the connectors and bases so as to avoid them.

Other areas of possible interference to be studied are those surfaces of abutment teeth that will support or be crossed by minor connectors and clasp arms. While interference to vertical minor connectors may be blocked out, doing so may cause discomfort to the patient's tongue and the creation of objectionable spaces for the trapping of food. Also, it is desirable that tooth surfaces contacted by vertical connectors be utilized as auxiliary guiding planes whenever possible. Too much relief is perhaps better than too little because of the possibility of irritation to soft tissues, but it is always better that the relief be placed intentionally rather than as a blockout of interference. If possible, a minor connector should pass vertically along a tooth surface that is either parallel to the path of insertion (which is considered ideal) or tapers occlusally. If tooth undercuts exist which would necessitate the use of an objectionable amount of blockout, they may be eliminated or minimized by slight changes in the path of insertion or eliminated during mouth preparations. The need for such alteration should be so indicated on the study cast in red pencil following final acceptance of a path of insertion.

Tooth surfaces upon which reciprocal and stabilizing clasp arms will be placed should be studied to see if sufficient areas exist above the height of convexity for the placement of these components. The addition of a clasp arm to the occlusal third of an abutment tooth adds to its occlusal dimension and therefore to the occlusal loading of that tooth. Much of this is unavoidable. Still, nonretentive and stabilizing clasp arms are best located in the middle third of the crown rather than upon the occlusal third.

Areas of interference to more ideal placement of clasp arms can usually be eliminated by reshaping tooth surfaces during mouth preparations, and this is so indicated on the study cast. Gross areas of interference to the placement of clasps may necessitate minor changes in the path of insertion or changes in the clasp design. For example, a bar clasp arm originating mesially from the major connector to provide bracing might be substituted for a distally originating circumferential arm.

Areas of interference frequently overlooked are the distal line angles of premolar abutment teeth and the mesial line angles of molar abutments. These areas frequently offer interference to the origin of circumferential clasp arms. If not detected at the time of initial survey, they are not included in the plan for mouth preparations. Where such an undercut exists, three alternatives may be considered:

1. It may be blocked out the same as any other area of interference. This is by far the least satisfactory method, because the origin of the clasp must then stand away from the tooth in proportion to the amount of blockout used. While this is perhaps less objectionable than its being placed occlusally, it may be objectionable to the tongue and the cheek and may create an objectionable food trap.

2. It may be circumvented by approaching the retentive area from a gingival direction with a bar clasp arm. This is frequently a satisfactory solution to the problem if other contraindications to the use of a bar clasp arm are not present, such as a severe tissue undercut or a retentive area that is too high on the tooth.

3. It may be eliminated by reducing the tooth contour during mouth preparation. This permits the use of a circumferential clasp arm originating well below the occlusal surface in a satisfactory manner. If the tooth is to be modified during mouth preparations, it should be so indicated on the study cast with red pencil.

Where the retentive area is located objectionably high on the abutment tooth or the undercut is too severe, interference may also exist on tooth surfaces that are to support retentive clasps. Such areas of extreme or high convexity must be considered as areas of interference and should be reduced accordingly. There areas are likewise indicated on the study cast for reduction during mouth preparations.

Esthetics. The path of insertion thus established must yet be considered from the standpoint of esthetics, both as to the placement of clasps and the arrangement of substitute teeth.

Clasp designs may usually be selected which will provide satisfactory esthetics for any given path of insertion. In some instances, gingivally placed bar clasp arms may be used to advantage; in others, circumferential clasp arms located cervically may be used. This is especially true where other abutment teeth located more posteriorly may bear the major responsibility for retention. In still other instances, a tapered wrought-wire retentive clasp arm may be placed to better esthetic advantage than a cast clasp arm. The placement of clasp arms for esthetic reasons does not ordinarily justify altering the path of insertion at the expense of mechanical factors. It should, however, be considered concurrently with other factors, and if a choice between two paths of equal merit permits a more esthetic placement of clasp arms by one path than the other, that path should be given preference.

Where anterior replacements are involved, the choice of path is limited to a more vertical one for reasons previously stated. In this instance alone must esthetics be given primary consideration even at the expense of altering the path of insertion and making all other factors conform. This factor should be kept in mind when considering the other three factors, so that compromises can be made at the time other factors are being considered.

FINAL PATH OF INSERTION

The final path of insertion will be the anteroposterior and lateral position of the cast in relation to the vertical arm of the surveyor that best satisfies all four factors, i.e., *guiding planes, retention, interference,* and *esthetics.*

All proposed mouth changes should be indicated on the study cast in red pencil, with the exception of restorations to be done. These may also be indicated on an accompanying chart if desired. Extractions and surgery are given priority to allow for healing. The remaining red marks represent the actual modifications of the remaining teeth to be done, which consists of the disking of proximal surfaces, the reduction of buccal and lingual surfaces, and, last, the preparation of occlusal rests. Except where they are placed in the wax pattern for a cast restoration, the preparation of occlusal rests should always be deferred until all other mouth preparations have been completed.

The actual location of occlusal rests will be determined by the proposed design of the denture framework. Therefore, the tentative design should be sketched on the study cast in pencil after the path of insertion has been decided upon. This is done not only to locate occlusal rest areas but also to record graphically the plan of treatment prior to mouth preparations. In the intervening time between patient visits, other partial denture cases may have been considered. The dentist should have the plan of treatment before him at each succeeding appointment to avoid confusion and to refresh his memory as to what is to be done and in what sequence.

The plan for treatment should include (1) the study cast with the mouth preparations and the denture design marked upon it, (2) a chart showing the proposed design and the planned treatment for each abutment, (3) a working chart showing the total treatment involved which will permit a quick review and a check-off of each step as the work progresses, and (4) a record of the fee quoted for each phase of treatment which can be checked off as it is recorded on the patient's permanent record.

Red pencil marks on the study cast are used to indicate the location of areas to be disked or otherwise modified, as well as the location of occlusal rests. While it is not necessary that rest areas be prepared on the study cast, it is advisable for the beginning student to have done so before proceeding to cut into the abutment teeth. This applies equally also to crown and inlay preparations on abutment teeth. It is advisable, however, for even the most experienced operator to have trimmed the stone teeth with the surveyor blade wherever tooth reduction is to be done. This identifies not only the *amount* to be removed in a given area but also the *plane* in which the tooth is to be cut. For example, a proximal surface may need to be disked in only the upper third or the middle third to establish a guiding plane that will be parallel to the path of insertion. This is not usually parallel to the long axis of the tooth, and if the disk is laid against the side of the tooth, the existing surface angle will be maintained rather than establishing a new plane that is parallel to the path of insertion.

The surveyor blade representing the path of insertion may be used to advantage to trim the surface of the abutment tooth whenever a red mark appears. The resulting surface represents the amount of tooth to be removed in the mouth and indicates the angle at which the handpiece must be held. The cut surface on the stone tooth is not again marked with red pencil but is *outlined* in red pencil to positively locate the area to be disked.

RECORDING THE RELATION OF THE CAST
TO THE SURVEYOR

Some method of recording the relation of the cast to the vertical arm of the surveyor must be used so that it may be returned to the surveyor for future reference, especially during mouth preparations. The same applies to the need for returning any working cast to the surveyor for the purpose of shaping wax patterns, or trimming blockout on the master cast, or locating clasp arms in relation to undercut areas.

Obviously, the trimmed base will vary with each cast, so recording the position of the surveyor table is of no value. If it were, calibrations could be incorporated on the surveyor table, which would allow the same position to be re-established. Instead, the position of each cast must be established separately and any positional record applies only to that cast.

Of several methods, two seem to be the most convenient and accurate. One method is to locate three dots on the surface of the cast, thus establishing a horizontal plane in relation to the vertical arm of the surveyor. On returning the cast to the surveyor, it may be tilted until the tip of the surveyor blade again contacts the three dots in the same plane. This will reproduce the original cast position and therefore the original path of insertion. This is known as *tripoding* the cast.

A second method, and the one which I prefer, is to score two sides and the dorsal aspect of the base of the cast with a sharp instrument held against the surveyor blade (Fig. 2). By tilting the cast until all three lines are again parallel to the surveyor blade, the original cast position can be re-established. Fortunately, the scratch lines will be reproduced in any duplication thereby, permitting any duplicate cast to be related to the surveyor in a similar manner. While a study cast and a master cast cannot be made interchangeable, a refractory cast or a fitting cast, being duplicates of the master cast, can be repositioned on the surveyor at any time. The technician must be cautioned not to trim the sides of the cast on the model trimmer and thereby lose the reference marks for re-positioning.

SURVEYING THE MASTER CAST

The master cast must be surveyed as a new cast, but the prepared proximal guiding plane surfaces will indicate the correct anteroposterior tilt. Some compromises may be necessary, but the amount of guiding plane surface remaining after blockout should be the maximum for each tooth. Areas above the point of contact with the surveyor blade are not considered to be part of the guiding plane area and neither are gingival undercut areas which will be blocked out.

The lateral tilt will be that position which provides equal retentive areas on all principal abutments in relation to the planned clasp design. Factors of flexibility and the need for extra flexibility on free-end abutments must be considered in deciding what will provide equal retention on all abutment teeth. For example, cast circumferential or cast bar retention on the tooth-borne side of a Class II design will be balanced against the 18-gauge wrought-wire retention on the free-end abutment only if the more rigid cast clasp engages a lesser undercut than the wrought-wire clasp arm. Therefore, the degree of undercut alone does not assure equal retention unless clasp arms of equal length, diameter, form, and material are used.

Gross interference will have been eliminated during mouth preparation. Therefore, for a given path of insertion providing guiding planes and balanced retention, any remaining interference must be eliminated with blockout. If mouth preparations have been adequately planned and executed, the undercuts remaining to be blocked out should be minimal.

The base of the cast is now scored or tripoded as described previously. The surveyor blade may then be replaced with a carbon marker and the height of convexity of each abutment tooth delineated. Similarly, any areas of interference to the rigid parts of the framework during insertion and removal should be indicated with the carbon marker to locate areas to be blocked out or relieved.

The final design may now be drawn upon the master cast with a fine crayon pencil, preferably one that will not come off during duplication. Graphite is usually lifted in duplication, but some crayon pencil marks will withstand duplication without blurring or transfer.* Sizing or spraying the master cast to protect such pencil marks is usually not advisable unless done with extreme care to avoid obliterating the surface detail.

MEASURING RETENTION

The surveyor is used with the master cast for two purposes: (1) to delineate the height of convexity of the abutment teeth for the purpose of locating clasp arms and to identify both the location and magnitude of retentive undercuts and (2) to trim blockout of any remaining interference to the insertion and removal of the denture. The areas so involved are those that will be crossed by rigid parts of the denture framework.

Prior to locating retentive clasp terminals in the penciled design, undercut areas may be measured if the operator feels that greater accuracy is possible by doing so. This is particularly true where plastic patterns are to be placed on blockout ledges. The experienced operator, however, may prefer to rely on his judgment and experience in locating clasp terminals. This may actually be better than measuring blockout, unless a very precise technique is followed.

Undercuts may be measured with the use of either an undercut gauge, such as those provided with the Ney and Jelenko surveyors, or by a dial gauge, such as is incorporated in the Saddle-Lock Retentoscope, the Ticonium Stress-o-graph, or the Austenal Micro-Analyzer. Whether an undercut gauge or a dial gauge is used, the amount of undercut is measured in hundredths of an inch, the gauges allowing measurements up to .03 inch. Theoretically, the amount of undercut used may vary with the clasp to be used up to a full .03 inch. Actually, however, many undercuts of less than .01 inch are adequate for cast retention, an amount that cannot be measured with practical accuracy, whereas wrought-wire retention may safely utilize up to .02 inch without inducing undesirable torque on the abutment tooth. The use of .03 inch is rarely, if ever, justified with any clasp. When greater retention is required, such as where abutment teeth remain on only one side of the arch, multiple abutments should be used rather than an increase of the retention on any one tooth.

When a source of light is directed toward the tooth being surveyed, a triangle of light is visible. This triangle is bounded by the surface of the abutment tooth

---

*Such as the Dixon Thinex pencil (No. 379 black).

Fig. 37. A tooth undercut is best viewed against a good source of light passing through a triangle which is bounded by the surface of the abutment tooth, the surveyor blade, and the gingival tissues.

on one side and the blade of the surveyor on the other, the apex being the point of contact at the height of convexity and the base of the triangle being the gingival tissues (Fig. 37). Retention will be determined by (1) the magnitude of the angle of cervical convergence below the point of convexity, (2) the depth at which clasp terminal is placed in the angle, and (3) the flexibility of the clasp arm. The intelligent application of various clasp designs and their relative flexibility is of far greater importance than the ability to measure an undercut with precise accuracy.

BLOCKING OUT THE MASTER CAST

Following the establishment of the path of insertion and the locating of undercut areas on the master cast, any undercut areas that will be crossed by rigid parts of the denture (which is every part of the denture framework but the retentive clasp terminals) must be eliminated by blockout.

In the broader sense, the term *blockout* includes not only the areas crossed by the denture framework during insertion and removal but also (1) those areas not involved that are blocked out for convenience, (2) ledges upon which clasp patterns are to be placed, (3) relief beneath connectors to avoid tissue impingement, and (4) relief to provide for later attachment of the denture base to the framework.

Ledges or shelves for locating clasp forms may or may not be used. However, this should not be confused with the actual blocking out of undercut areas which would offer interference to the insertion of the denture framework. Only the latter is made on the surveyor, with the surveyor blade being used as a paralleling device.

Blockout material may be purchased, or it may be made up according to the following formula:

> Melt and mix together:
> 4½ sheets of baseplate wax
> 4½ sticks of temporary gutta percha stopping
> 3   sticks of sticky wax
> ½ tsp. kaolin
> Add ½ tube lipstick for color.

Some of the ready-made blockout materials contain a mixture of wax and clay. Pink baseplate wax may also be used satisfactorily as a blockout material. It is easily applied and is easily trimmed with the surveyor blade. Trimming is facilitated by slightly warming the surveyor blade. While it is true that baseplate wax will melt more readily than a wax-clay mixture if the temperature of the duplicating material is too high, it should be presumed that the duplicating material will not be used at such an elevated temperature. If the temperature of the duplicating material is high enough to damage a wax blockout, other distortions resulting in an inaccurate duplication will also be likely.

Paralleled blockout is necessary beneath guiding plane surfaces and over all undercut areas that will be crossed by minor connectors and the originating parts of clasp arms. Other areas that are to be blocked out for convenience and to avoid difficulties in duplication should be blocked out with an oil-base modeling clay (artist's modeling clay). A modeling clay that is water-soluble should not be used where duplication procedures are involved. Such areas are the labial surfaces and labial undercuts not involved in the denture design and sublingual and distolingual areas beyond the limits of the denture design. These are blocked

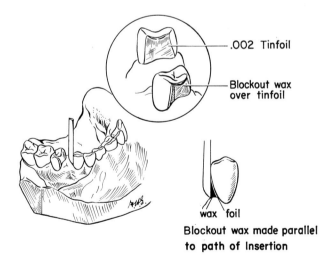

.002 Tinfoil

Blockout wax
over tinfoil

wax foil

**Blockout wax made parallel
to path of Insertion**

Fig. 38. All guiding plane areas must be parallel to the path of insertion, and all other areas that will be contacted by rigid parts of the denture framework must at least be free of undercut if not parallel. These areas are first covered with .002 tin foil, and then any overlying blockout is trimmed parallel to the path of insertion with the surveyor blade.

out arbitrarily with clay, but since they have no relation to the path of insertion, they do not require the use of the surveyor.

Areas to be crossed by rigid connectors, on the other hand, should be trimmed with the surveyor blade parallel to the path of insertion (Fig. 38). This imposes a considerable responsibility upon the technician. Should he fail to trim the blockout sufficiently to expose guiding plane surfaces, the effect of these guiding planes, so carefully established by the dentist, will be nullified. If, on the other hand, the technician is overzealous in paralleling the blockout, the stone cast may be abraded by heavy contact with the surveyor blade. While the resulting cast framework would seat back onto the master cast without interference, interference to insertion in the mouth would result. This would necessitate relieving the casting at the chair, which is not only an embarrassing and time-consuming operation but also one which may have the effect of obliterating guiding plane surfaces.

Fortunately, the hazard can be avoided by the simple expedient of placing a .002-inch thickness of tin foil over all areas where blockout is to be trimmed.

Such areas are first identified and then tin foil is adapted and cemented to

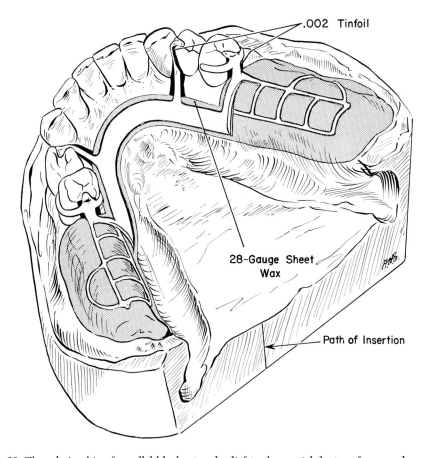

Fig. 39. The relationship of parallel blockout and relief to the partial denture framework.

place, covering slightly more than the area to be blocked out. The tin foil may be extended onto marginal ridge areas but must not extend into occlusal rest areas. *Care must be taken not to allow the cement to flow beyond the tin foil, especially into occlusal rest areas.* If so, it must be removed with a solvent before duplication or a false surface on the investment cast will result.

The placing of tin foil beneath trimmed blockout serves two purposes. One is that the master cast is thus protected against abrasion during the paralleling of blockout. Should the surface of the tin foil be penetrated at any point, the defect is immediately discernible and can be corrected. Another is that a .002-inch relief is provided, which serves as a margin for error in the casting under all rigid connectors contacting tooth surfaces. Since occlusal rest areas are not so relieved, the terminal rest position of the denture framework is not affected.

RELIEVING THE MASTER CAST

Tissue undercuts which must be blocked out are paralleled in much the same manner as tooth undercuts. The difference between *blockout* and *relief* must be clearly understood. For example, tissue undercuts which would offer interference to the seating of a lingual bar connector are blocked out with blockout wax and trimmed parallel to the path of insertion. This does not in itself afford relief to avoid tissue impingement. In addition to such blockout, a

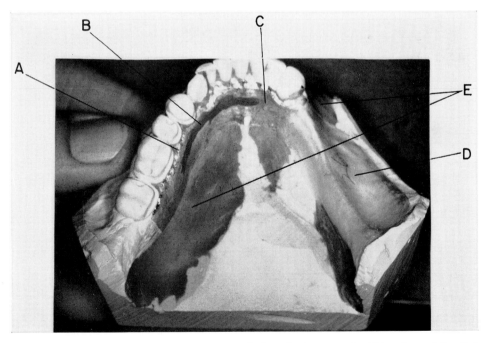

Fig. 40. Relief and blockout of a master cast before duplication. **A,** .002-inch tin-foil relief over the free gingivae and the adjacent lingual slope. **B,** Clay blockout of lingual undercut. **C,** 26- or 28-gauge sheet wax relief, a little wider than the lingual bar which will be placed over it. **D,** 26- or 28-gauge sheet wax relief over edentulous area. **E,** Arbitrary clay blockout of areas not involved in the denture design.

Table 1. Differentiations Between Paralleled Blockout, Shaped Blockout, Arbitrary Blockout, and Relief

Site	Material	Thickness
Paralleled Blockout		
Proximal tooth surfaces to be used as guiding planes	Blockout material or pink baseplate wax over .002-inch tin foil	Only undercut remaining gingival to contact of surveyor blade with tin-foiled tooth surface
Beneath all minor connectors	Blockout material or pink baseplate wax over .002-inch tin foil	Only undercut remaining gingival to contact of surveyor blade with tin-foiled tooth surface
Tissue undercuts to be crossed by rigid connectors	Blockout material or pink baseplate wax over .002-inch tin foil	Only undercut remaining below contact of surveyor blade with surface of cast
Tissue undercuts to be crossed by origin of bar clasps	Blockout material or pink baseplate wax over .002-inch tin foil	Only undercut remaining below contact of surveyor blade with tin-foiled surface of cast
Tissue undercuts to be crossed by flanges of metal bases	Oil-base clay	Only undercut remaining below contact of surveyor blade with surface of cast
Shaped Blockout		
On buccal and lingual surfaces to locate plastic patterns for clasp arms	Blockout material	Ledges for location of nonretentive reciprocal clasp arms to follow height of convexity so that they may be placed as low as possible without becoming retentive
		Ledges for location of retentive clasp arms to be placed as low as tooth contour permits; point of origin of clasp to be above height of convexity, crossing survey line about halfway, and to include an undercut area previously selected in keeping with flexibility of type of clasp being used.

Arbitrary Blockout

All gingival crevices	Baseplate wax or oil-base clay	Enough to eliminate gingival crevice
Deep interproximal spaces to be covered by minor connectors or lingual plates and aprons	Oil-base clay	Only sufficient to block out acute angle between teeth; small end of No. 7 wax spatula may be used to trim away excess clay, leaving sufficient interproximal blockout
Gross tissue undercuts situated below areas involved in design of denture framework	Oil-base clay	Leveled arbitrarily with spatula and fingers
Tissue undercuts distal to cast framework	Oil-base clay	Smoothed arbitrarily with spatula or knife
Labial and buccal tooth and tissue undercuts not involved in denture design	Oil-base clay	Filled and tapered to within upper third of crowns of teeth with spatula and fingers

Relief

Beneath lingual bar connectors	Adhesive wax sealed to cast; should be wider than width of major connector to be placed upon it	28-gauge minimum; 26-gauge where more desired; two thicknesses 28-gauge maximum
Beneath minor connectors	Tin foil adapted and cemented to cast	.002 inch minimum, .004 inch maximum
Over gingival areas to be crossed by vertical connectors	Tin foil adapted and cemented to cast	.002 inch minimum, .004 inch maximum
Beneath bar clasps arms, from their point of origin to or beyond the blockout of gingival crevice	Tin foil adapted and cemented to cast	.002 inch minimum, .004 inch maximum
Areas where cast bases or connectors will contact thin tissue coverings, such as hard areas so frequently found on lingual of mandibular ridge	Tin foil adapted and cemented to cast	.002 inch minimum, .004 inch maximum
Beneath extensions onto ridge areas for attachment of resin bases	Adhesive wax, sealed to cast well beyond area involved	28-gauge usually sufficient, especially where a wax secondary impression will follow making of cast framework

relief of varying thickness must be used, depending upon the location of the connector and the predictable effect of denture settling. Generally, this is a minimum of 28-gauge thickness beneath a lingual bar connector and .002 inch beneath minor connectors and the origin of bar clasp arms (Fig. 39). The former is usually sheet wax adapted and sealed to the master cast, whereas the latter is usually tin foil adapted and cemented to the master cast. Low-fusing casting wax, such as Kerr's green casting wax, should not be used for this purpose, for it is too easily thinned during adapting and may be affected by the temperature of the duplicating material. Pink casting wax may be used, but it is difficult to adapt uniformly. A pressure-sensitive adhesive-coated casting wax is preferable because it adapts readily and adheres to the cast surface. Any wax, even the adhesive type, should be sealed all around its borders with a hot spatula to prevent its lifting when the cast is moistened prior to or during duplication.

Additional relief may be advisable in certain instances, such as (1) where the lingual slope of the tissues beneath a lingual bar connector is gradual, since there is more danger of the inferior border of a lingual bar settling into the tissues than where the slope is more nearly vertical, and (2) where the supporting abutment teeth have been out of function for some time and intrusion of those teeth may be anticipated due to the fact that they are again being called upon to support an occlusal load. Such intrusion may result in the denture settling more than in cases where abutment teeth have remained in occlusion. In either case, the amount of relief should be increased accordingly, generally by doubling the usual relief.

Still other areas requiring relief are the gingival crossings and gingival crevices. All gingival areas should be protected from possible impingement due to settling of the denture framework, and all gingival crevices should be bridged by the denture framework. Wax or clay may be used to block out gingival crevices, over which one or two thicknesses of .002-inch tin-foil relief may be placed for additional relief (Fig. 40).

PARALLELED BLOCKOUT, SHAPED BLOCKOUT, ARBITRARY BLOCKOUT, AND RELIEF

Table 1 differentiates between *paralleled blockout, shaped blockout, arbitrary blockout,* and *relief*. The same factors apply to both the maxillary and mandibular arches, except that relief is ordinarily not used beneath palatal major connectors as it is with mandibular lingual bar connectors.

Chapter 6

Principles of partial
denture design

DIFFERENTIATION BETWEEN TWO MAIN TYPES

Strictly speaking, a partial denture is a prosthetic restoration which derives its support principally from the tissues underlying its base and only to a minor degree from some of the remaining natural teeth that we use as abutments (Fig. 41). Any partial denture having a unilateral or bilateral free-end base is, then, a true *partial denture*.

Where there are natural teeth that may be used as abutments, remaining both anterior and posterior to the edentulous area, we still speak of such a prosthetic restoration as a partial denture. Again, strictly speaking, such a restoration actually is a *removable bridge,* even though it is bilateral in design. This is true because the restoration derives its support from two or more remaining teeth through the placement of occlusal rests on those abutment teeth. The tissues underlying the base of this removable bridge type of partial denture do not contribute appreciably to the support of the denture. (Fig. 42.)

Thus, it is clear that two distinctly different types of partial dentures exist. Certain points of difference exist between the Class I and Class II types of partial dentures on the one hand and the Class III, or removable-bridge type of partial denture, on the other. The first consideration is the *manner in which each is supported*. The Class I type and the free-end side of the Class II type derive their support primarily from the tissues underlying the base and only to a minor degree from the abutment teeth, whereas the Class III type derives all of its support from the abutment teeth lying at each end of the edentulous space.

Second, for reasons directly related to the manner of support, the *method of impression registration* required for each type will vary.

Third, the *need for some kind of indirect retention* exists in the free-end type of partial denture, whereas in the tooth-borne, Class III type, there is no free-end base which can lift away from the supporting tissues due to the action of sticky foods and movements of the tissues of the mouth against peripheries

Fig. 41. A Kennedy Class I partially edentulous arch. The major support for the denture bases must come from the residual ridges, tooth support from occlusal rests being effective only at the anterior portion of each base. (From McCracken, W. L.: Mouth Preparation for Partial Dentures, J. Pros. Den. **6**:39-52, 1956.)

Fig. 42. A Kennedy Class III, modification 1, partially edentulous arch which provides total tooth support for the prosthesis. A removable partial denture made for this arch is totally supported by properly prepared occlusal rest seats on the four abutment teeth. (From Mc-Cracken, W. L.: Mouth Preparation for Partial Dentures, J. Pros. Den. **6**:39-52, 1956.)

of the denture. This is because each end of each saddle is secured by a direct retainer on an abutment tooth. Therefore, the tooth-borne partial denture does not rotate about a fulcrum as does the free-end partial denture.

Fourth, the manner in which the free-end type of partial denture is supported often necessitates the *use of a base material that can be relined* to compensate for tissue changes. Acrylic or some other resin is usually used as a base material for free-end saddles. The Class III partial denture, on the other hand, being entirely tooth-supported, does not require rebasing except when it is advisable to eliminate an unhygienic, unesthetic, or uncomfortable condition resulting from loss of tissue contact. Metal bases, therefore, are more frequently used in tooth-borne restorations, since rebasing is not likely to be necessary.

Differences in Support. The true partial denture, since it derives its major support from the elastic, fibrous connective tissue covering of the residual ridge, is dependent upon the quality of that support for its stability under functional loading. Some areas of this residual ridge are firm, with limited displaceability, whereas other areas are very displaceable, depending upon the thickness and structural character of the tissues overlying the residual alveolar bone. The movement of the base under function determines the occlusal efficiency of the partial denture and also the degree to which the abutment teeth are subjected to torque and tipping stresses.

Impression Registration. An impression registration for the construction of a partial denture must fulfill two requirements:

1. The anatomic form and relationship of the remaining teeth in the dental arch, as well as the surrounding soft tissues, must be recorded accurately so that the denture will not exert any pressure on those structures and its retentive and stabilizing components may be properly placed. Some impression material which can be removed from undercut areas without permanent distortion must be used to fulfill this requirement. The elastic impression materials, such as agar or alginate hydrocolloid, mercaptan rubber base (Thiokol), and silicone impression materials are therefore used for this purpose.

2. The supporting form of the soft tissues underlying the free-end base of the partial denture should be recorded so that firm areas are not overloaded and softer areas are made more compact and more capable of supporting their share of the total work load. Only in this way can maximum support of the partial denture base be obtained. An impression material which is capable of displacing tissue sufficiently to register the supporting form of the ridge will fulfill this second requirement. One of the fluid mouth-temperature waxes, such as Kerr's Korecta wax No. 4, is usually used for this purpose.

No single impression material can satisfactorily fulfill both of the above requirements. To compromise by recording only the anatomic form of both teeth and supporting tissues can result only in inadequate support for the free-end base of the partial denture.

Differences in Clasp Design. A fifth point of difference between the two main types of partial denture lies in their *requirements for direct retention*.

Direct retainers may be classified as being either intracoronal or extracoronal in type. The clasp-type partial denture, utilizing the extracoronal direct retainer, is probably utilized a hundred times more frequently than the intracoronal, or internal attachment, partial denture. This is not necessarily an indication of increasing preference for the clasp denture, nor is it a reflection upon the excellence of the internal attachment denture. The fact remains, however, that although the internal attachment was devised more than forty-five years ago, for economic and other reasons, the clasp denture is the more widely used. The clasp denture permits the rendering of a physiologically sound partial denture service to the greatest number of patients in keeping with the ability of the majority of patients to pay for such service.

The tooth-borne partial denture, being totally supported by abutment teeth, is retained and stabilized by a clasp at each end of each edentulous space. The only requirement of such clasps is that they flex sufficiently during insertion and removal of the denture to pass over the height of contour of the teeth in approaching or escaping from an undercut area. While in its terminal position on the tooth a retentive clasp should be passive and should not be called upon to flex except when engaging the undercut area of the tooth for the purpose of resisting a vertical dislodging force.

Cast retentive arms are usually used for this purpose. These may be either of the circumferential (or Akers) type, arising from the body of the clasp and approaching the undercut from an occlusal direction, or of the bar (or Roach) type, arising from the base of the denture and approaching the undercut area from a gingival direction. A modification of the latter type is the infrabulge clasp (DeVan). Each of these two types of cast clasps has its advantages and disadvantages.

The direct retainer adjacent to a free-end base must perform still another function, in addition to that of resisting vertical displacement. Because of the lack of tooth support distally, the denture base will move tissueward under function proportionate to the quality of the supporting tissues, the accuracy of the impression registration, the accuracy of the denture base, and the total occlusal load applied. Because of this tissueward movement, those elements of the clasp that lie in an undercut area must be able to flex sufficiently to dissipate stresses which would otherwise be directly transmitted to the abutment tooth as leverage.

The cast clasp cannot effectively act to dissipate this stress for two reasons. First, the material itself can have only a limited flexibility, or else other parts of the casting which must be rigid, such as lingual and palatal bars, would also tend to be flexible. The material used being the same, the only variable factor is the bulk and diameter used in each component part. Second, and probably more important, the cast clasp is of necessity made half-round in shape. Since edgewise flexing is negligible, the clasp can flex in only one direction and therefore cannot effectively dissipate, by flexing, the torque stresses placed upon it. For this reason, some torque is inevitably transmitted to the abutment tooth, which is magnified by the length of the lever arm.

Immediately there comes to mind the stress breakers which are often incorporated into the partial denture design for this very reason. There are those who strongly feel that a stress breaker is the best means of preventing leverage from being transmitted to the abutment teeth. It is just as strongly felt by others that a wrought-wire retentive arm more effectively accomplishes this purpose with greater simplicity and ease of application. It cannot be denied that a retentive clasp arm made of wrought wire can flex more readily in all directions than the cast half-round clasp arm and thereby more effectively dissipate those stresses that would otherwise be transmitted to the abutment tooth. The advantages and disadvantages of stress breakers will be considered in detail in Chapter 11.

Only the retentive arm of the clasp, however, should be made of wrought metal. Reciprocation and stabilization against lateral movement must be obtained through the use of rigid cast elements which make up the remainder of the clasp. This is called a combination clasp, being a combination of both cast and wrought materials incorporated into one direct retainer. It is more frequently used for the free-end partial denture. However, in addition to its greater flexibility, the combination clasp has further advantages of adjustability, minimal tooth contact, and better esthetics, which justifies its occasional use in tooth-borne designs also.

ESSENTIALS OF PARTIAL DENTURE DESIGN

The design of the partial denture framework should be carefully planned and outlined on an accurate study cast. Following the making of necessary mouth changes to provide for occlusal rests and guiding planes, the master cast is made and carefully surveyed to determine the location of undercut areas which are either to be blocked out or utilized for retention. The design should provide for occlusal rests and rigid reciprocal arms on all abutment teeth to assure vertical and horizontal stability of the partial denture.

Fig. 43. Removable bridge-type partial denture in a maxillary Class III arch. The design consists of anterior and posterior palatal bar major connectors, resin-supported denture teeth, and bar clasp arms throughout. (From McCracken, W. L.: Contemporary Partial Denture Designs, J. Pros. Den. 8:71-84, 1958.)

Fig. 44. Removable bridge-type partial denture in a maxillary Class III arch. The design consists of an anatomic replica palatal plate major connector, bar and circumferential clasp arm, and resin-supported denture teeth. (From McCracken, W. L.: Contemporary Partial Denture Designs, J. Pros. Den. 8:71-84, 1958.)

Fig. 45. Removable bridge-type partial denture in a mandibular Class III arch. The design consists of a lingual bar major connector, metal bases and tube teeth, and bar clasp arms. Note the mesially inclined left third molar with onlay-type reciprocal clasp arm. (From Mc-Cracken, W. L.: Contemporary Partial Denture Designs, J. Pros. Den. **8:**71-84, 1958.)

Fig. 46. A, A carefully designed tooth-borne denture framework outlined on the master cast, in this particular instance to support anterior teeth in the mouth of a musician being traumatized by constant trumpet playing. **B,** The cast framework as returned from the laboratory, following precisely the design prescribed by the dentist.

The design must include provision for adequate indirect retention which will function to counteract any lifting of the free end of the base away from the tissues. The indirect retainers should be placed in relation to a line drawn through the occlusal rests of the two principal abutments, which is the axis of rotation, or the *fulcrum line.* The indirect retainer may be in the form of an auxiliary occlusal rest, a secondary lingual bar in combination with terminal rests, a lingual plate with terminal rests, or an incisal or embrasure hook on an anterior tooth. The indirect retainer should be placed as far as possible from this fulcrum line and should not terminate on a tooth incline, such as the lingual surface of an anterior tooth.

Some retentive lugs for the attachment of the impression waxes and later the resin saddles must be provided for to complete the partial denture framework.

The Class III Removable Bridge Type of Partial Denture (Figs. 43 to 48). The Kennedy Class III removable bridge type of partial denture, being entirely tooth supported, may be made entirely to fit the anatomic form of the teeth and surrounding structures. It does not require an impression of the functional form of the ridge tissues nor does it require indirect retention. Cast clasps of either the circumferential or bar type may be used, or the combination clasp may be used if preferred. Unless a need for later rebasing is anticipated, as in

Fig. 47. An upper Class III partial denture framework designed for maximum periodontal support. The posterior occlusal rest and clasp arm on the nonedentulous side are added for stabilization and to prevent settling of the major connector at that point. A partial metal base is used to avoid any display of base metal anteriorly.

Fig. 48. Maxillary Class III, modification 1, denture designed as a periodontal splint. Full crowns on the patient's right premolar and molar are splinted together with continuous lingual ledges. The patient's left premolar is a full crown with lingual ledge. The left molar abutment is unrestored but altered somewhat by regrinding. All gold guiding plane surfaces, lingual and proximal, were machined parallel to the path of insertion. Unilateral fixed partial dentures would not provide the bilateral stabilization needed in this case.

the case of recently extracted teeth, the denture base may be made of metal, as it has several advantages.

The Class III partial denture can frequently be utilized as a valuable aid to periodontal treatment, because of its stabilizing influence on the remaining teeth (Fig. 47).

The Class I, Bilateral, Free-End Partial Denture. The Class I, bilateral, free-end partial denture is just about as unlike the removable bridge type as any two dental restorations could be. Since it derives its principal support from the tissues underlying its base, a Class I partial denture made to anatomic ridge form cannot have uniform and adequate support. Yet, unfortunately, many Class I partial dentures are being made from a single hydrocolloid impression. In such cases, both the abutment teeth and the residual ridges suffer because the occlusal load placed upon the remaining teeth is inevitably made greater by the lack of adequate posterior support.

Many dentists, recognizing the need for some type of impression registration which will record the supporting form of the residual ridge, attempt to record this form with a metallic oxide, rubber base, or silicone impression material. Such materials actually only record the anatomic form of the ridge, except for that displacement of tissues caused by the viscosity or confinement of the material. Others prefer to place a base that was made to fit the anatomic form of the ridge under some pressure at the time it is related to the remaining teeth, thus obtaining functional support. Any impression record will be influenced by the consistency of the impression material and the amount of hydraulic pressure exerted by its confinement within the impression tray. Still others, believing that a properly compounded mouth-temperature wax will displace only those tissues that are incapable of providing support to the denture base, use a wax secondary impression to record the supporting, or functional, form of the edentulous ridge.

The Class II Partial Denture (Figs. 49, 50, and 51). The Kennedy Class II partial denture may actually be a combination of both tissue-borne and tooth-

Fig. 49. Lower Class II, modification 1, partial denture utilizing a resin free-end base and a tubed denture tooth in the tooth-borne modification space. The indirect retainers serve also to provide stabilization against horizontal movement of the restoration and to prevent tissueward movement of the lingual bar major connector.

Fig. 50. A lower Class II partial denture with metal free-end base. Resin attachment of the denture teeth to the metal base is with suitable mechanical retention (nailheads, loops, or spurs plus an undercut finishing line). Embrasure clasps are used on the nonedentulous side, with an indirect retainer located favorably in relation to the fulcrum line.

Fig. 51. An upper Class II partial denture utilizing broad palatal coverage. Embrasure clasps are used on the nonedentulous side. Indirect retention is not used because of the retention provided by broad palatal coverage.

borne restorations. The free-end base must have adequate tissue support, whereas tooth-borne bases elsewhere in the arch may be made to fit the anatomic form of the underlying ridge. Indirect retention must be provided for, but occasionally the anterior abutment on the tooth-borne side will serve to satisfy this requirement. If additional indirect retention is needed, provisions must be made for it.

Cast clasps are usually used on the tooth-borne side, whereas some clasp design must be used on the abutment tooth adjacent to the free end which will prevent the application of torque to that tooth. A thorough understanding of the advantages and disadvantages of various clasp designs is necessary in determining which type of direct retainer is to be used for each abutment tooth.

The steps in the completion of the Class II partial denture follow closely those of the Class I partial denture, except that the free-end base is usually made of a resin material, whereas the base for any tooth-borne areas is frequently made of metal. This is permissible because the residual ridge beneath tooth-borne bases is not called upon to provide support for the denture and later rebasing is not likely to be necessary.

COMPONENT PARTS OF THE PARTIAL DENTURE

All partial dentures have two things in common: (1) they must be supported by oral tissues and (2) they must be retained against reasonable dislodging forces.

In the removable bridge-type of partial denture, three components are necessary: the connectors, the retainers, and the bracing or stabilizing components.

The partial denture that does not have the advantage of tooth support at each end of each edentulous space still must have support, but in this instance, the support comes from both the teeth and the underlying ridge tissues rather than from the teeth alone. This is a composite support, and the prosthesis must be so fabricated as to coordinate the resilient support provided by the edentulous ridge and the more stable support offered by the abutment teeth. The three essentials— connectors, retainers, and stabilizing components—must be even more carefully designed and executed because of the movement of tissue-supported denture base areas. In addition, provision must be made for three other essentials, as follows:

1. The best possible support must be obtained from the resilient ridge tissues. This is accomplished by the impression technique more than by the partial denture design, although the amount of area covered by the partial denture is a contributing factor in such support.

2. The method of direct retention must take into account the inevitable tissueward movement of the free-end base(s) under the stresses of mastication and occlusion. Either some kind of stress breaker must be used or direct retainers must be designed so that some flexing or stress-breaking under occlusal loading will occur to prevent the direct transmission instead of leverage to the abutment teeth.

3. The partial denture having one or more free-end denture bases must be so designed that movement of the unsupported and unretained end away from the tissues will be prevented or minimized. This is often referred to as indirect retention and is best described in relation to an axis of rotation through the occlusal rest areas of the principal abutments. However, retention from the partial denture base itself can frequently be made to prevent this movement of the denture base away from the tissues and, in such instances, may be spoken of as direct-indirect retention.

The support of the partial denture by the abutment teeth is dependent upon the alveolar support of those teeth, the rigidity of the partial denture framework in that area, and the design of the occlusal rests. Through clinical and roentgenographic interpretation, the dentist may evaluate the abutment teeth and decide whether or not they will provide adequate support. In some instances, the splinting of two or more teeth is advisable, either by fixed bridges or by soldering two or more restorations together. In other instances, a tooth may be deemed too weak to be used as an abutment, and extraction is indicated in favor of obtaining better support from an adjacent tooth.

Having decided upon the abutments, the dentist is responsible for the preparation of the abutment teeth, for the design of cast restorations, and for the form of the occlusal rest seats. These may be prepared either in sound tooth enamel or in the cast restorations. The technician cannot be blamed for inadequate occlusal rest support. On the other hand, the technician is solely to blame if he extends the casting beyond or fails to include the total prepared area. If a definite occlusal rest form with the floor of the rest inclined toward the center of the tooth is faithfully recorded in the master cast and delineated in the penciled design, no excuse can be made for poor occlusal rest form on the partial denture.

Major Connectors. A major connector should be properly located in relation to gingival and moving tissues and should be of such design as to be rigid. Rigidity in a major connector is necessary to provide proper distribution of forces to and from the supporting components.

A lingual bar connector should be tapered superiorly with a half-pear shape in cross section and should be relieved sufficiently but not excessively over the underlying tissues. The addition of a secondary (or Kennedy) bar or a lingual plate does not alter the basic design of the lingual bar. These are added solely for reasons of support and protection to the anterior teeth and specifically are neither connectors nor indirect retainers.

Rigidity of a palatal major connector is just as important and its location and design just as critical as a lingual bar. A horseshoe-shaped palatal connector is rarely justified except to avoid a palatal torus. Neither can the routine use of a single palatal bar be justified. The anterior and posterior palatal bar is mechanically and biologically sound if it is so located that it does not impinge upon tissues. The anatomic palatal strap or palatal plate is frequently preferred because of its rigidity, better acceptance by the patient, and greater stability without tissue damage. In addition, the palatal plate provides direct-indirect retention which frequently eliminates altogether the need for separate indirect retainers.

Direct Retainers for Tooth-Borne Partial Dentures. Retainers for tooth-borne partial dentures have only one function, and that is to retain the prosthesis against reasonable dislodging forces without damage to the abutment teeth. There can be no movement of the prosthesis tissueward because each terminus is supported by an occlusal rest. There can be no movement away from the tissues, and therefore no rotation about a fulcrum, because each terminus is secured by a direct retainer.

Any type of direct retainer is acceptable as long as the abutment tooth is not jeopardized by its presence. Intracoronal (frictional) retainers are ideal for tooth-borne appliances and offer esthetic advantages not to be had with extracoronal (clasp) retainers. Nevertheless, the circumferential and bar-type clasp retainers are mechanically effective and are more economically constructed than are intracoronal retainers. Therefore, they are more universally used.

Vulnerable areas on the abutment teeth must be protected by restorations with either type of retainer. The clasp retainer must not impinge upon gingival tissues. The clasp must not exert excessive torque upon the abutment tooth during insertion and removal. It must be placed the least distance into the tooth undercut for adequate retention, and it must be designed with a minimum of bulk and tooth contact.

The bar clasp arm should be used only where the area for retention lies close to the gingival margin of the tooth and little tissue blockout is necessary. If the clasp must be placed high occlusally, or if an objectional space would exist beneath the bar due to blockout of tissue undercuts, the bar clasp should not be used.

Direct Retainers for Free-End Base Partial Dentures. Retainers for free-end partial dentures, while retaining the prosthesis, must also be able to flex when the denture base moves tissueward under function. Thus, the retainer may act as a stress breaker. Mechanical stress breakers accomplish the same thing, but they do so at the expense of horizontal stabilization. When some kind of mechanical stress breaker is used, the denture flange must be able to act to prevent horizontal movement. Clasp designs that allow for flexing of the retentive clasp arm may be designed to accomplish the same purpose as that of mechanical stress breakers, without sacrificing horizontal stabilization and generally with less complicated techniques.

In evaluating the ability of a clasp arm to act as a stress breaker, one must realize that flexing in one plane is not enough. Rather, the clasp must be freely flexible in any direction, as dictated by the stresses applied. Bulky, half-round clasp arms cannot do this, and neither can a bar clasp engaging an undercut on the side of the tooth away from the denture base. Round clasp forms offer advantages of greater and more universal flexibility, less tooth contact, and better esthetics. Either the round (preferably wrought wire) circumferential clasp or the carefully located and properly designed bar clasp should be used on all abutment teeth adjacent to free-end denture bases.

Stabilizing Components. Stabilizing or bracing components of the partial denture framework are those rigid components that assist in stabilizing the denture against horizontal movement. The purpose of all stabilizing components should be to distribute stresses equally to all supporting teeth without overworking any one tooth.

All minor connectors that contact vertical tooth surfaces (and all reciprocal clasp arms) act as stabilizing components. It is necessary that minor connectors have sufficient bulk to be rigid and yet that they present as little bulk to the tongue as possible. This means that they should be confined to interdental embrasures wherever possible. When minor connectors are located on vertical tooth surfaces, it is best that these surfaces be parallel to the path of insertion. When cast restorations are used, these surfaces of the wax patterns should be made parallel on the surveyor prior to casting.

Reciprocal clasp arms must also be rigid, and they must be placed above the height of contour of the abutment teeth where they will be nonretentive. By their rigidity these clasp arms reciprocate the opposing retentive clasp and they also prevent horizontal movement of the prosthesis under functional stresses. For a reciprocal clasp arm to be placed favorably, some reduction of the tooth surfaces involved is frequently necessary to increase the suprabulge area.

Where crown restorations are used, a lingual reciprocal clasp arm may be inset into the tooth contour by providing a ledge on the crown upon which the clasp arm may rest. This permits the use of a wider clasp arm and restores a more nearly normal tooth contour, at the same time maintaining its strength and rigidity.

Ridge Support. Support for the tooth-borne partial denture or the tooth-borne modification space comes entirely from the abutment teeth by means of occlusal rests. Support for the free-end denture base comes primarily from the resilient soft tissues overlying the residual alveolar bone. In the latter, occlusal rest support is effective only at the abutment end of the denture base.

The effectiveness of tissue support is dependent upon four things: (1) the quality of the residual ridge, (2) the total occlusal load applied, (3) the accuracy of the denture bases, and (4) the accuracy of the impression registration.

The quality of the ridge cannot be influenced, except to modify it or improve it by surgical intervention. Such modification is infrequently advisable and even less frequently done.

The total occlusal load applied to the residual ridge may be influenced by reducing the occlusal area. This is done by the use of fewer, narrower, and more effectively shaped denture teeth.

The accuracy of the denture base is influenced by our choice of materials and by the exactness of the processing techniques. Inaccurate and warped denture bases influence adversely the support of the partial denture. Materials and techniques should be selected which will minimize the possibility of processing errors and assure the greatest dimensional stability.

The accuracy of the impression technique is entirely in the hands of the dentist. Maximum tissue coverage for support should be the primary objective in any partial denture impression technique. The manner in which this is accomplished should be based upon a biologic comprehension of what happens beneath a free-end denture base when an occlusal load is applied.

The true partial denture is unique in that its support is derived from both abutment teeth which are comparatively unyielding and from resilient soft tissues which are comparatively yielding under occlusal forces. Resilient tissues, being unable to provide support for the denture base comparable to that offered by the abutment teeth, are displaced by the occlusal load. Only the projections of the underlying residual bone remain to be traumatized by occlusal forces. This problem of support is further complicated by the fact that the patient has natural teeth remaining upon which he may exert far greater force than he would were he completely edentulous. This fact is clearly evident from the damage commonly occurring to an edentulous ridge when it is opposed by a few remaining anterior teeth in the other arch.

Ridge tissues recorded in their resting or nonfunctioning form are incapable of providing the composite support needed for a denture that derives its support from both hard and soft tissue. It is necessary that two factors be taken into consideration in the acceptance of an impression technique for free-end partial dentures: (1) the material should record the resilient tissues in their supporting form and (2) the total area covered by the impression should be as great as possible, in order to distribute the load over as large an area as can be tolerated by the patient. This is an application of the principle of the snowshoe. Waxes that are moldable at mouth temperature are the materials of choice for the impression, because they are the only impression materials available that have the combined advantages of controlled displacement of fluid tissues and correctability under functional loading.

Anyone who has had the opportunity of comparing two master casts for the same partially edentulous arch, one cast having the distal extension area recorded in its anatomic or resting form and the other cast having the distal extension area recorded in its functional form, has been impressed by the differences in the two. A denture base processed to the functional form is generally less irregular, and it has greater areal coverage than a denture base processed to the anatomic or resting form. Moreover, and of far greater significance, a denture base made to anatomic form exhibits less stability under rotating forces than a denture base processed to functional form and thus fails to maintain its occlusal relation with the opposing teeth. By having the patient close onto strips of soft wax it is evident that occlusion is maintained at a point of equilibrium over a long period of time when the denture base has been made to the functional form. In contrast, there is evidence that there has been a rapid settling of the denture base when it has been made to the anatomic form, with an early return of the occlusion to natural tooth contact only. Such a denture not only fails to distribute the occlusal load equitably but it also allows rotational movement which is damaging to the abutment teeth and their investing structures.

Indirect Retainers. An indirect retainer must be placed as far anteriorly from the fulcrum line as adequate tooth support permits if it is to function to restrict movement of a free-end base away from the tissues. It must be placed on a rest seat prepared in an abutment tooth that is capable of withstanding the stresses placed upon it. An indirect retainer cannot function effectively on an inclined tooth surface, nor can a single weak incisor tooth be used for this purpose. Either a canine or a premolar tooth should be used for the support of an indirect retainer, and the rest seat must be prepared with as much care as any other occlusal rest. An incisal rest or a cingulum rest may be used on an anterior tooth, provided a definite seat can be obtained either in sound enamel or on a cast restoration.

Indirect retainers serve a second purpose in partial denture design, that of occlusal rest support for major connectors. A long lingual bar or an anterior palatal bar is thereby prevented from settling into the tissues. Even in the absence of a need for indirect retention, provision for such auxiliary support is sometimes indicated.

Contrary to common usage, a secondary lingual bar (Kennedy bar) or a lingual plate does not in itself act as an indirect retainer. Since these are located on inclined tooth surfaces, they serve more as an orthodontic appliance than as support for the partial denture. Where they are used, terminal occlusal rests should always be provided at either end to stabilize the denture and to prevent orthodontic movement of the teeth contacted. Such terminal rests may function also as the indirect retainers, but these would function equally well in that capacity without the added bar or plate.

The use of a lingual plate is indicated where the lower anterior teeth are subject to calculus formation or are weakened by periodontal disease. Calculus may then form on the plate instead of forming on the teeth. Experience with the lingual plate has shown that with adequate oral hygiene the underlying tissues remain healthy and there are no harmful effects to the tissues from the metallic coverage per se. However, adequate relief must be provided wherever a bar or plate crosses the gingival margins and the adjacent gingivae. This should be accomplished by using at least a .002-inch tin foil in these areas, and in addition there should be a wax or clay blockout of the gingival crevices. Excessive relief should be avoided because tissues tend to fill a void, resulting in the overgrowth of abnormal tissue. The amount of relief used, therefore, should be only the minimum necessary to avoid gingival impingement.

It does not seem that there are any advantages to be found in the use of the secondary lingual, or Kennedy, bar that are not enhanced by the use of a lingual plate. In rare instances, where a lingual plate would show through multiple interproximal embrasures, the Kennedy bar may be preferred for esthetic reasons only. In others, where a single diastema exists, a lingual plate may be cut out in this area to avoid display of metal, without sacrificing its use where otherwise indicated.

Chapter 7

Component parts of the partial denture: major and minor connectors

FACTORS INFLUENCING THE DESIGN OF THE PARTIAL DENTURE

As a direct result of examination and diagnosis, the design of the partial denture must originate on the study cast so that all mouth preparations may be planned and performed with a specific design in mind. This will be influenced by many factors, some of which are listed below:

1. Which arch is to be restored and if both, their relationship to one another.

2. Whether or not the denture will be entirely tooth borne. If one or more free-end bases are involved, the following must be considered:

(a) The need for indirect retention

(b) The clasp designs that will best minimize the forces applied to the abutment teeth during function

(c) The need for later rebasing, which will influence the type of base material used

(d) The secondary impression method to be used.

3. The materials to be used, both for the framework and for the bases.

4. The type of replacement teeth to be used. This may be influenced by the opposing dentition.

5. The need for abutment restorations, which may influence the type of clasp arms to be used and their specific design.

6. The patient's past experience with a partial denture and the reasons for making a new denture. If, for example, a lingual bar has been objectionable, was it due to its design, fit, or the patient's inability to accept it? Frequently, this alone justifies the use of a contoured lingual plate rather than al ingual bar. Or, if an anterior palatal bar has proved objectionable, was it due to its bulk, it loca-

tion, or its flexibility, or to tissue irritation? A design using a thin palatal plate located more posteriorly may be preferable to an anterior bar or palatal horseshoe located anteriorly.

7. The periodontal condition of the remaining teeth, the amount of abutment support remaining, and the need for splinting. This may be accomplished either by means of fixed restorations or by the design of the denture framework.

8. The method to be used for replacing single teeth or missing anterior teeth. The decision to use fixed restorations for these spaces instead of replacing them with the removable denture must be made at the time of treatment planning. Such a decision will necessarily influence the design of the denture framework.

COMPONENT PARTS OF THE PARTIAL DENTURE

A typical partial denture will have the following components:
1. One or more major connectors
2. Several minor connectors
3. Two or more occlusal rests
4. Two or more direct retainers
5. Two or more reciprocal or bracing arms
6. One or more indirect retainers (if the prosthesis has one or more free ends)
7. One or more bases, each supporting one to several replacement teeth

These will now be considered separately as to their function, their location, and the acceptable designs, keeping in mind both biologic and mechanical considerations.

Major Connectors

A major connector is that unit of the partial denture that connects the parts of the prosthesis located on one side of the arch with those on the opposite side. It is that unit of the partial denture to which all other parts are directly or indirectly attached.

The major connector may be compared to the frame of an automobile, and in the construction of a partial denture it is just as essential. It might also be compared to the foundation of a building for the same reasons. It must be rigid so that stresses applied to any one portion of the denture may be effectively distributed over the entire supporting area, including abutment teeth and the supporting subjacent tissue areas. Being rigid, the major connector resists torque that would otherwise be transmitted to the abutment teeth as leverage.

It is only through the rigidity of the major connector that all other component parts of the partial denture may be effective. If they are attached to or originate from a flexible major connector, the effectiveness of these components is jeopardized to the detriment of the oral structures and the discomfort of the patient. Many partial dentures have failed to serve comfortably and effectively only because the major connector failed to provide rigid support to the rest of the prosthesis. Any partial denture design utilizing a nonrigid major connector is doomed to failure, either by causing discomfort to the patient or by subjecting the remaining structures to trauma. Trauma may be manifested by damage to the periodontal support of the abutment teeth, injury to the supporting ridge areas, or impingement of underlying tissues due to flexure of the major connector.

The major connector should be located in a favorable relation to moving tissues and at the same time should avoid impingement of gingival tissues. It should also be so located that areas of bony and tissue prominence are not encountered during insertion and removal. Sufficient relief must be provided beneath a major connector to avoid settling into hard areas such as a mandibular torus, a palatal torus, or the median suture line. Location and relief must also take into consideration possible impingement of gingival tissues.

Adequate relief beneath the major connector avoids the need for later adjustments to provide relief of the prosthesis after tissue damage has occurred. Not only is this time-consuming but also frequently the connector is so weakened by grinding that flexibility and sometimes fracture result. It seems that tissues once impinged by the connector require more relief to avoid recurrence than would have been required originally. To accomplish this, the connector is seriously weakened by adjustment because the original bulk did not provide for the possibility of future reduction.

Where adjustments in the future to compensate for denture settling into hard areas may be anticipated, the connector should be given added bulk in this area to allow for future relief. This is particulary true where a palatal connector lies over a maxillary torus or prominent median suture line or where settling into a mandibular torus may be anticipated.

Margins of major connectors adjacent to gingival tissues should be located far enough from those tissues to avoid any possible impingement. The upper border of a lingual bar connector should be located at least 3 mm. below the gingival margin and more if possible (Fig. 52). The limiting factor is the height of the moving tissues in the floor of the mouth. Since the connector must have

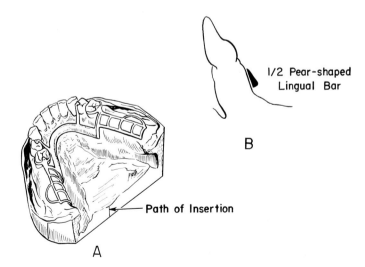

1/2 Pear-shaped
Lingual Bar

B

Path of Insertion

A

Fig. 52. A lingual bar major connector should be located at least 3 mm. below the gingival margins and more if possible.

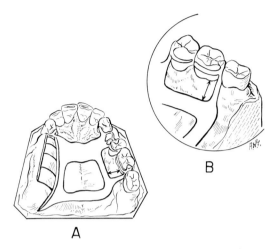

Fig. 53. A palatal major connector should be located at least 6 mm. away from gingival margins and parallel to their mean curvature. All adjoining minor connectors should cross gingival tissues abruptly and should join major connectors at nearly a right angle.

sufficient width and bulk to provide rigidity, the superior border must sometimes be placed closer to gingival tissues than is desirable.

The closer to gingival attachments the connector is placed, the greater the relief necessary to provide an escape for food which would otherwise be irritating to gingival tissues. A common cause of gingival irritation is a small circular or rectangular space occurring between the major connector and the bounding minor connectors. Such spaces should be avoided whenever possible, but if unavoidable they should be compensated for by providing adequate clearance beneath the major connector for food escape.

In the maxillary arch, since there are no moving tissues in the palate as in the floor of the mouth, the borders of the major connector may be placed well away from gingival tissues. There is no justification for impinging gingival tissues if adequate support for the connector is available elsewhere. Structurally, the tissues covering the palate are well suited for support of the connector and have adequate deep blood supply. The gingival tissues, on the other hand, must have an unrestricted superficial blood supply to remain healthy. The borders of the palatal connector should be placed a minimum of 6 mm. away from gingival margins and should be located parallel to their mean curve. Minor connectors that must cross gingival tissues should do so abruptly, joining the major connector at nearly a right angle (Fig. 53). In this way, the maximum freedom of gingival tissues is assured.

Except for a palatal torus or median suture line, palatal connectors ordinarily require no relief, nor is relief desirable. Intimate contact between the connector and the supporting tissues adds much to the retention and stability of the denture. Except for gingival areas, intimacy of contact elsewhere in the palate is not of itself detrimental to the health of the tissues, if supported against settling by occlusal rests on abutment teeth.

Where it is necessary for the palatal connector to make contact with the teeth for reasons of support, definite tooth support should be provided. Anterior tooth support is sometimes necessary, particularly where the denture includes anterior replacements. This is best accomplished by establishing shoulders or ledges on gold restorations using veneer crowns, three-quarter crowns, or pin-ledge restorations. However, where the abutment teeth are sound, caries activity is low, and oral hygiene habits are favorable, enamel ledges may be used effectively. Multiple enamel ledges extending over several teeth may be considered to be just as effective as lesser areas of greater depth. These should be located far enough above the gingival attachment to provide for bridging the gingival crevice with blockout. At the same time they should be low enough on the tooth to avoid unfavorable leverage, and low enough on maxillary incisors and canine teeth to avoid occlusal interference at the cingulum of the tooth. Experience with ledges placed in sound enamel has been entirely satisfactory, all other factors being favorable.

Connector borders resting on unprepared tooth surfaces can lead only to slippage of the denture along tooth inclines, or orthodontic movement of the tooth, or both. In any case, settling into gingival tissues is inevitable. When the needed occlusal support ceases to exist, the health of the surrounding tissues is usually impaired. Similarly, interproximal projections resting upon the gingival third of the tooth and upon gingival tissues that are structurally unable to render support can only cause impingement to the detriment of the health of those tissues.

A cardinal rule, then, for the location of the major connector in relation to the remaining teeth and their surrounding gingivae is this: *Either support the connector by definite rests on the teeth contacted, bridging the gingivae with adequate relief, or locate the connector far enough away from the gingivae to avoid any possible restriction of blood supply and entrapment of food debris.* All gingival crossings should be abrupt and at right angles to the major connector, and these should bridge the gingivae with adequate relief.

The major connector must be so contoured that it does not present sharp margins to the tongue and cause irritation or annoyance by its angular form. The superior border of a lingular bar connector should be tapered to the tissues above, with its greatest bulk at the lower border. This results in a contour that is known as a half-pear shape, being flat on the tissue side, tapered superiorly, and the greatest bulk in the inferior third. Lingual bar patterns, both wax and plastic, are made in this conventional shape. Frequently, additional bulk is necessary to provide rigidity, particularly when the bar is long or an alloy of lesser rigidity is used. This is accomplished by underlying the ready-made form with one or two sheets of 28-gauge casting wax rather than altering the original half-pear shape.

Sharp, angular form of any portion of a palatal connector should be avoided, and all borders should be tapered slightly toward the tissues. A posterior palatal bar should be half-round in shape and located as far posteriorly as possible to avoid interference with the tongue. A posterior bar or the posterior border of any palatal connector should never be placed on moving tissues and should be located on the hard palate anterior to the line of flexure formed by the junction of the hard and soft palates.

Fig. 54. An anterior palatal bar or the anterior margin of a palatal plate should be located as far posteriorly on the rugae as possible, with its anterior border following the natural valley between rugae crests.

An anterior palatal bar or the anterior border of a palatal plate should also be located as far posteriorly as possible to avoid interference with the tongue in the rugae area. It should be flat or straplike rather than half-round and should be so located that its anterior border follows existing valleys between or behind the crests of the rugae (Fig. 54). The anterior border of either an anterior bar or a palatal plate will therefore be irregular in outline as it follows the valleys between the rugae. The tongue may then pass from one rugae prominence to another without encountering the border of the denture lying between. Where a rugae crest must be crossed by the connector border, it should be done abruptly, avoiding the crest as much as possible.

A rule to be followed throughout partial denture design is as follows: *Try to avoid adding any part of the denture framework to an already convex surface. Rather, try to utilize existing valleys and embrasures for the location of component parts of the framework. All components should be tapered where they join convex surfaces.*

Mandibular Major Connectors. The basic form of a mandibular major connector is the *half-pear-shaped lingual bar*, located above moving tissues but as far below the gingival tissues as possible. It is usually made of a 6-gauge, half-pear-shaped wax or a similar plastic pattern. Fortunately, there are few cases where extreme lingual inclination of the remaining lower premolar and incisor teeth prevents the use of a lingual bar connector. Usually by conservative mouth preparations in the form of disking and by blockout a lingual bar connector can almost always be used. Lingually inclined teeth may sometimes have to be reshaped by means of crowns. Although the use of a labial major connector may be necessary

Fig. 55. A secondary lingual bar located above the cingulum of the anterior teeth may be added for one reason or another, but only when it provides needed stabilization for the teeth or the denture.

Fig. 56. A lingual plate or lingual apron is used where the space between bounding connectors is better filled in than left open. Such an apron does not serve to replace those connectors but, instead, is sometimes added to the fundamental denture design.

in rare instances, this should be avoided by resorting to necessary mouth preparations rather than accepting a condition that is otherwise correctable. The same applies to the use of a labial bar where a mandibular torus interferes with the placement of a lingual bar. Unless surgery is definitely contraindicated, interfering mandibular tori should be removed rather than a labial bar connector used.

A secondary lingual bar located above the cingulum of the anterior teeth may be added to the lingual bar for one reason or another, but this should never be done without good reason (Fig. 55).

If the rectangular space bounded by the two lingual bars and the bounding minor connectors is filled in, a *lingual plate* or *lingual apron* results (Figs. 56 and 57). Again, this should only be done for good reason. The following rule applies:

No component of a partial denture should be added arbitrarily or conventionally. Each component should be added for good reason and to serve a definite purpose. The reason for adding a component may be for stabilization, retention, patient comfort, the preservation of the health of the tissues, esthetics, or any one of several other reasons, but the dentist alone should be responsible for the choice of design used and he should have good reasons, both biologic and mechanical, for doing so.

A lingual plate should be made as thin as is technically feasible and should be contoured to follow the contours of the teeth and the embrasures. The patient should be made as little aware of added bulk and altered contours in this area as possible. The upper border should follow the natural curvature of the supracingular surface of the teeth and should not be located above the middle third of the lingual surface. All gingival crevices and deep embrasures should be blocked out to avoid gingival irritation and any wedging effect between the teeth.

The lingual plate should be something that is added to, not something replacing the conventional lingual bar. The half-pear shape of a lingual bar should still be present, with the greatest bulk and rigidity at the inferior border. The lingual plate does not in itself serve as an indirect retainer. Where indirect retention is required, definite tooth rests must be provided for this purpose. Both the lingual plate and the secondary lingual bar must always have a terminal tooth rest at each end regardless of the need for indirect retention. But where indirect retainers are necessary, it is incidental that these rests may serve also as terminal rests for the lingual plate or secondary lingual bar. In such case, it is the rests and not the lingual plate or bar that function as indirect retainers.

A   B

Fig. 57. Two views of a lower Class I design with contoured lingual plate added to the lingual bar. The lingual plate is made as thin as possible and follows the contours of the teeth contacted. It is bounded inferiorly by the half-pear-shaped lingual bar, superiorly by a secondary lingual bar, and distally by the minor connectors supporting auxiliary occlusal rests, in this case serving also as indirect retainers. Whether or not these are used for indirect retention, any lingual plate or secondary lingual bar must have a terminal rest in a prepared seat at each end. A, The design as submitted to the laboratory. B, The cast framework as returned from the laboratory. Note how faithfully the original design is reproduced in the casting.

The lingual plate may be described as being bounded as follows: inferiorly by the lingual bar; superiorly by contact with the supracingular surface of the anterior teeth, terminating within the middle third of their lingual surface; and distally on each side by a vertical minor connector originating from the lingual bar, passing vertically in the embrasure between two teeth, and terminating in a definite prepared rest seat.

Indications for the Use of a Lingual Plate. The indications for the use of a lingual plate may be listed as follows:

1. *For the purpose of stabilizing periodontally weakened lower anterior teeth.* While not as effective as fixed splinting and not as effective as when a labial bar is added, lingual splinting can be of definite value when used in conjunction with definite rests on sound adjacent teeth. A secondary lingual bar may be used to accomplish the same purpose, since it is actually the upper border of a lingual plate without the gingival apron. The secondary lingual bar accomplishes stabilization alone without the other advantages of a lingual plate. It is frequently more objectionable to the patient's tongue than the contoured apron.

2. *To prevent calculus formation on the lingual surfaces of the lower anterior teeth.* Heavy calculus formation with its periodontal implications can be avoided by causing it to be precipitated upon the lingual plate, where it can be removed daily, rather than on the teeth themselves. Tissues that were formerly kept irritated by rapid calculus formation will remain healthy beneath a clean lingual plate if they are given daily stimulation by toothbrushing.

3. *Where the lingual frenum is high or the space available for a lingual bar is slight.* In either case, the superior border of a lingual bar would have to be placed objectionably close to gingival tissues. Irritation could only be avoided by generous relief, which would be annoying to the tongue. By using a lingual plate, the gingivae may be bridged and the superior border tapered to tooth contact, permitting the use of a high lingual bar without tongue and gingival irritation.

4. *Where the patient has found a lingual bar objectionable in the past.* It is usually either the superior border of the lingual bar or the space caused by excessive relief that has been found objectionable. Experience with the use of a thin, contoured lingual apron has shown patient acceptance in preference to the lingual bar alone.

5. *Where the future replacement of one or more incisor teeth will be facilitated by the addition of retention loops to an existing lingual plate.* Mandibular incisors which are periodontally weak may thus be retained, with the knowledge that future additions to the partial denture are possible.

The same reasons for using a lingual apron anteriorly apply also to its use elsewhere in the lower arch. If a lingual bar alone is to be used anteriorly, there is no reason for adding an apron elsewhere. But where auxiliary splinting is used for stabilization of the remaining teeth and/or for horizontal bracing of the prosthesis, small rectangular spaces sometimes remain. Such small spaces are better bridged with an apron than left open. Generally, this is done for the purposes of avoiding gingival irritation, the entrapment of food debris, or to cover generously relieved areas which would be irritating to the tongue (Fig. 58).

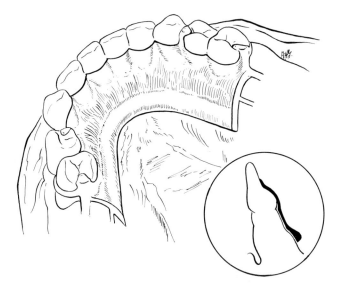

Fig. 58. A lingual apron may be extended to include all open spaces lying between the major connector and other component parts of the denture. This should never be done arbitrarily but only where open spaces would be less desirable.

Fig. 59. Saddle-Lock's "Splint Bar" mandibular major connector. (Courtesy Saddle-Lock, Inc., Brooklyn, N. Y.)

Saddle-Lock's "Splint Bar." The term *splint bar* is used elsewhere in this chapter to designate a fixed bar continuous with abutment crowns for the purpose of providing support to the anterior portion of a removable partial denture. Therefore, the use of the same term by the Saddle-Lock Company to designate a type of major connector is confusing terminology.

About the time of the first edition of this book, Dr. Victor Jaffe of Washington, D. C., called my attention to the use of a "cingulum bar" as a major connector for mandibular partial dentures. More recently, this design is offered as an exclusive Saddle-Lock design under the name "Splint Bar." Basically, the conventional lingual bar major connector is replaced with a type of lingual plate alone, contoured to cover the cingulum and gingival two-thirds of the mandibular anterior teeth. One must assume that positive occlusal rest support is provided to prevent gingival impingement due to settling. (Fig. 59.)

The "cingulum bar" or "splint bar," although it eliminates the patient's obvious objections to the presence of a conventional lingual bar, cannot be made rigid enough to function as a proper major connector without objectionable bulk in the region of normal tongue activity. Therefore, employment of this type of major connector must be at the expense of rigidity and bilateral transfer of forces. It should be used only with full awareness of this lack of rigidity.

Maxillary Major Connectors. Four basic types of maxillary major connectors will be considered: (1) single palatal bar, (2) U-shaped palatal horseshoe, (3) anterior and posterior palatal bar, and (4) palatal strap or palatal plate.

Single Palatal Bar. This is perhaps the most widely used and yet the least logical of all the palatal major connectors. It is difficult to say whether this or the palatal horseshoe is the more objectionable of palatal connectors.

For a single palatal bar to have the necessary rigidity, it must have concentrated bulk. The latter may be avoided only by ignoring the need for rigidity, which is unfortunately too frequently done. For a single palatal bar to be rigid enough to be effective, it must be centrally located between the two halves of the denture. This means that a single palatal bar must always be centrally located with concentrated bulk. Mechanically, this practice may be sound enough, but from the standpoint of patient comfort, it is highly objectionable.

A partial denture made with a single palatal bar is frequently either too flexible or too objectionable to the patient's tongue, or both. The decision to use a single palatal bar should be based on the size of the denture areas being con-

Fig. 60. A major connector for a surgically mutilated mouth. This is actually a "T" beam, designed to provide strength and rigidity without excessive bulk, bridging the edentulous span without contacting the underlying tissues.

nected and whether or not a single connector located between them would be rigid without objectionable bulk. Bilateral tooth-borne restorations of short span may be effectively connected with a single bar, particularly where the edentulous areas are located posteriorly.

For reasons of torque and leverage, a single palatal bar should not be used to connect anterior replacements with free-end bases. To be rigid enough to resist torque and to provide adequate horizontal and vertical support as well, a single bar would have to be objectionably bulky. When placed anteriorly, this bulk becomes even more objectionable to the patient as it interferes with speech formation.

U-Shaped Palatal Horseshoe. From both the patient's standpoint and a mechanical standpoint, the palatal horseshoe is a poor palatal connector. It should

Fig. 61. A U-shaped palatal horseshoe is a poor major connector that should be used only where a large palatal torus prevents the use of a palatal plate or anterior and posterior palatal bars.

Fig. 62. A common partial denture design utilizing an objectionable palatal horseshoe major connector. Such a connector lacks necessary rigidity, places bulk where it is most objectionable to the patient, and impinges gingival tissues lingual to the remaining teeth, resulting in chronic inflammation. This denture failed primarily because of lack of the rigidity in the major connector that is so necessary if all other components are to function effectively.

never be used arbitrarily. Where a large palatal torus exists and occasionally where several anterior teeth are to be replaced, the palatal horseshoe may have to be used (Fig. 61). In most instances, however, other designs will serve more effectively.

To be rigid, the palatal horseshoe must have bulk where the tongue needs the most freedom, which is in the rugae area. Without sufficient bulk, the U-shaped design leads to increased flexibility and movement at the open ends. In free-end dentures, where posterior tooth support is nonexistent, movement is particularly noticeable and is traumatic to the residual ridge. Many maxillary partial dentures have failed for no other reason except the flexibility of a U-shaped major connector (Fig. 62). No matter how well the free-end base is supported or how harmonious the occlusion, when horizontal movement under function is not resisted by a rigid major connector, the residual ridge suffers.

The wider the coverage of a U-shaped major connector, the more it resembles a palatal plate with its several advantages. But when used as a narrow horseshoe, the necessary rigidity is usually lacking. A U-shaped connector may be made rigid by providing multiple tooth support on definite tooth rests. A common error in the design of a U-shaped connector, however, is its proximity to, or actual contact with, gingival tissues. This principle has been given previously, that the borders of major connectors should either be placed on prepared tooth rests or be located well away from gingival tissues. The majority of U-shaped connectors fail to do either, with resulting gingival irritation and periodontal damage to the tissues adjacent to the remaining teeth.

Anterior and Posterior Palatal Bar (A-P Bar). Structurally, the most rigid of palatal major connectors, the anterior and posterior palatal bar combination, may be used in almost any maxillary partial denture design (Figs. 63, 64, and 65).

Fig. 63. The anterior and posterior palatal bar is the most rigid of palatal major connectors and, when properly designed, is neither objectionable to the patient nor harmful to the adjacent tissues.

The only condition preventing its use is when there is a maxillary torus extending posteriorly to the soft palate which prevents the use of a posterior bar. In this situation, a U-shaped major connector must be used.

The strength of the A-P bar connector lies in the fact that the half-round posterior bar and the flat anterior bar are joined together by longitudinal con-

Fig. 64. Anterior and posterior palatal bar major connectors. The anterior bar is a flat strap located as far posteriorly as possible to avoid rugae coverage and tongue interference. The anterior border of this bar should be located just posterior to a rugae crest or in the valley between two crests. The posterior bar is half-round (approximately 6-gauge) and is located as far posteriorly as possible yet entirely on the hard palate. It should be located at right angles to the midline rather than on a diagonal, even though its two wings must curve inward as it connects with other components of the denture framework.

Fig. 65. An upper Class II, modification 2, partial denture with anterior and posterior palatal bar major connectors, before and after denture teeth have been added. Except for a short free end, this is essentially a tooth-borne restoration. Since a lateral incisor was necessarily used as an abutment on one side, double cingulum rests were used on enamel ledges prepared on both the central and lateral incisors. Denture teeth that would be visible anteriorly are abutted to the ridge to avoid any visible display of the denture base material. Note the posterior location of the half-round posterior bar crossing the midline at a right angle rather than on a diagonal.

nectors on either side, forming a square or rectangular frame. Each component braces the other against possible torque and flexure. Flexure is practically non-existent in a well-designed connector of this design.

Ordinarily, both the anterior and posterior bars should be placed as far posterior as possible to avoid interference with the tongue. The anterior bar may be extended anteriorly to support anterior tooth replacements, or it may be widened to form a thin palatal plate with a posterior brace. In this form, a U-shaped connector is made rigid because of the added horizontal brace posteriorly. Frequently, a maxillary torus may thus be encircled by the major connector without sacrificing rigidity.

The A-P connector may be used with any Kennedy Class of partially edentulous arch. It is used most frequently in Classes II and IV, whereas the single wide palatal bar or strap is more frequently used in Class III cases and the palatal plate or full coverage most frequently in Class I cases for reasons to be explained subsequently.

Both anterior and posterior bars, and also the anterior and posterior borders of a palatal plate, should cross the midline at a right angle rather than on a diagonal. This is for reasons of symmetry. The tongue, being a bilateral organ, will accept symmetrically placed components far more readily than those placed without regard for bilateral symmetry. Therefore, any curves in the connector should be placed to one side of the midline, so that the connector may pass from one side to the other at right angles to the saggital plane.

Palatal Strap or Plate. For lack of better terminology, the terms strap and plate are used to designate any thin, contoured palatal coverage used as a maxillary major connector. The older types of thin castings, usually made of 26-gauge wax, were of indefinite thickness. This was due to the wax being thinned during adaptation to the cast and to polishing with abrasive wheels (Fig. 66). Newer techniques have resulted in the production of anatomic replica palatal castings which have uniform thickness and strength by reason of their corrugated contours. Thinner castings possessing greater rigidity are possible by this method. Through the

Fig. 66. Full palatal coverage with a full lingual apron provides maximum retention and stability in a surgically mutilated mouth. Each remaining tooth is used for support, and all but two incisors for retention to resist the leverage from the edentulous space. This must be considered an entirely tooth-borne restoration despite the length of the edentulous span.

use of electrolytic polishing, uniformity of thickness can be maintained and the anatomic contours of the plate faithfully reproduced in the finished denture.

The anatomic replica strap or plate has several advantages over other types of palatal major connectors. Some of these are as follows:

1. It permits the making of a uniformly thin metal plate that reproduces faithfully the anatomic contours of the patient's own palate. Because of its uniform thinness, the fact that it feels familiar to the patient's tongue, and the thermal conductivity of the metal, the palatal plate is accepted more readily by the tongue and underlying tissues than any other type of connector.

2. The corrugation in the anatomic replica adds strength to the casting; a thinner casting with adequate rigidity is thus possible than was formerly possible with adapted sheet wax.

Fig. 67. An upper Class III partial denture with anatomic replica palatal plate major connector. Such a denture is used where bilateral stabilization of abutment teeth is needed. Note the posterior extension of the palatal plate to provide broader coverage and to extend the margin posteriorly where it will be less noticeable to the tongue. Partial metal bases are used with loops and undercut finishing lines for retention, but without visible display of metal anteriorly.

Fig. 68. Upper Class I partial denture with anatomic replica palatal strap. Indirect retainers are not necessary because of the added retention obtained by broad palatal coverage. Combination clasps are used with wrought-wire wide retentive arms on the buccal side of the abutment teeth. Note the modification of stock resin teeth, carved to restore occlusal anatomy after being ground to fit an occluding template.

3. Surface irregularities are intentional rather than accidental; therefore, electrolytic polishing is all that is needed. The original uniform thickness of the plastic pattern is thus maintained.

4. Interfacial surface tension between metal and tissues provides the prosthesis with greater retention. Thus, less direct retention is needed, and in many instances the need for indirect retention is eliminated entirely. Retention must be adequate to resist the pull of sticky foods, the action of moving border tissues against the denture, the forces of gravity, and the more violent forces of coughing and sneezing. These are all resisted by the retention of the base itself in proportion to the total area of denture contact. The amount of both direct and indirect retention required will depend upon the amount of retention provided by the denture base.

The palatal plate may be used in one of two ways. It may be used as a plate of varying width covering the area between two or more edentulous areas (Figs. 67 and 68), or it may be used as a full or partial cast palate extending posteriorly to a palatal seal area (Figs. 69 and 70).

In most Class II and Class III cases, the palatal plate will be located anterior to the posterior palatal seal area. Only in extensive Class I cases will it be extended posteriorly to the vibrating line of the soft palate. Little posterior seal is ever necessary with a metal palate because of the accuracy and stability of the cast metal. This is in contrast to the broad posterior palatal seal needed with resin denture bases. The location of the posterior seal, at the junction of the movable and immovable soft palate, is the same for both.

Where the last remaining abutment tooth on either side of a Class I arch is the canine or first premolar tooth, full palatal coverage is not only advisable but

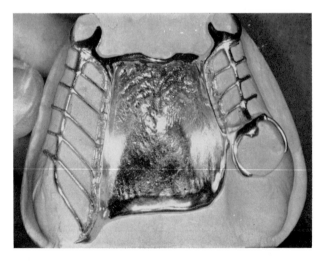

Fig. 69. Tru-Rugae palatal major connector for a Class II, modification 1, partial denture. The anterior border avoids coverage of the anterior rugae; the posterior border lies well back on the immovable hard palate, crossing the midline at a right angle. Total contact provides excellent auxiliary retention without objectionable bulk. The finishing lines are parallel to the crest of the ridge. All retention in this case is buccal wrought wire.

Fig. 70. Three views of an upper Class I, modification 1, partial denture with full palatal plate extending posteriorly to the vibrating line. Note the apron anteriorly terminating an enamel ledge prepared on all the anterior teeth. Note the clearance lingual to the premolar and molar abutments. **A,** The design as submitted to the laboratory. **B,** The casting as returned from the laboratory. Note the partial metal base with diagonal spurs and undercut finishing line parallel to the crest of the residual ridge. **C,** The completed restoration. The replaced lateral incisor, canine, and first premolar are abutted to the ridge; but from the second premolar distally a buccal flange of resin is used.

is also practically mandatory. This may be accomplished in one of two ways. One method is to use a casting anteriorly with retention posteriorly for the attachment of a resin palate which then extends posteriorly to a palatal seal (Fig. 71). The other is to utilize a full cast palate extending to the posterior palatal seal area (Figs. 70 and 72). The several advantages of a cast palate over a full resin palate make the full cast palate sufficiently preferable to offset the slight additional cost. However, where the cost and fee must be held to a minimum, the former method may be used satisfactorily. The partial metal palate may also be used when later rebasing is anticipated. In such case, the posterior seal can be redone as part of the rebasing procedure.

While it is not a connector that may be used universally, the palatal plate

Fig. 71. An upper Class I major connector to which a full resin palate will be added, extending posteriorly to the palatal seal area. A thin anatomic replica palatal plate is designed to avoid, as much as possible, coverage of the rugae area and to provide thinness in the functioning area of the tongue. Retention for the resin base is provided over the ridge crests, with an undercut finishing line across the midline.

has become accepted as the most satisfactory palatal connector for the majority of maxillary partial dentures. Both the dentist and the technician should be familiar with its use and, at the same time, with its limitations, so that it may be used intelligently and to fullest advantage.

The Use of a Splint Bar for Denture Support. In Chapter 13 under the heading Missing Anterior Teeth, mention is made of the fact that missing anterior teeth are best replaced with a fixed bridge rather than with a removable partial denture that replaces posterior teeth elsewhere in the arch. The following is quoted from that chapter: "From a biomechanical standpoint, . . . a partial denture should replace only the missing posterior teeth, *after* the remainder of the arch has been made intact by means of fixed restorations."

Occasionally, a situation is found where, economics aside, it is necessary that a number of missing anterior teeth be replaced with the partial denture rather than by fixed bridgework. This may be due to the length of the edentulous span, or to the loss of sufficient residual ridge by resorption, accident, or surgery, or in a case where the amount of vertical space prevents the use of fixed bridgework, or where esthetic requirements can better be met through the use of teeth added to the denture framework. In such instances, it is necessary that the best possible support for the replaced anterior teeth be provided. Ordinarily, this is done through the placement of occlusal and/or cingular rests on the adjacent natural teeth, but where the edentulous span is too large to assure adequate support from the adjacent teeth, another method must be used. This is included in this chapter only because it influences the design of the major connector which must then be used.

An anterior splint bar may be attached to the adjacent abutment teeth in such a manner that a fixed bridge results, but with a smooth, contoured bar resting lightly on the gingival tissues for the purpose of supporting the partial denture. As with any fixed bridge, the type of abutment retainers and the deci-

Fig. 72. Four views of an upper Class I partial denture with palatal plate major connector extending posteriorly to the palatal seal area. **A,** The design as drawn on the master cast submitted to the laboratory. **B,** The cast framework returned following the original design. **C,** The completed denture with resin bases overlaying partial metal bases, retained by diagonal spurs and undercut lingual finishing lines. **D,** The partial denture in the mouth. The anatomic replica palatal strap major connector is extended posteriorly to the palatal seal area. Direct-indirect retention is sufficient to eliminate the necessity for separate indirect retainers placed anteriorly, thus leaving the anterior palate free of encumbrance. (**D,** From McCracken, W. L.: Contemporary Partial Denture Designs, J. Pros. Den. 8:71-84, 1958.)

sion to use multiple abutments will depend upon the length of the span and the stability of the teeth being used as abutments. Irregardless of the type of abutment retainers used, the connecting bar must be cast separately of a very rigid alloy and attached to the abutments by soldering. Rather than rely upon soldered junctions alone, it is best that recesses be formed in the abutment pieces and the connecting bar, which rest lightly on the tissues, be cast to fit into these recesses; they are then attached by soldering.

Because of the greater rigidity of the chromium-cobalt alloys, the splint bar is preferably cast in one of these materials and then attached to the gold abutment pieces by electric soldering. The complete assembly (abutment pieces and connecting bar) is then cemented permanently to the abutment teeth the same as a fixed bridge (Fig. 73, *A*). The impression for the partial denture is then made and a master cast obtained which accurately reproduces the contours of the tissue bar. The denture framework is then made to fit this bar by extending the major connector to cover and rest upon the tissue bar. Either retention for the attachment of a resin base or any other acceptable means of attaching the replaced anterior teeth is incorporated into the denture design. (Fig. 73, *B* and *C*.)

The resulting partial denture will have the esthetic and other advantages of

A

B   C

Fig. 73. A, A splint bar attached to double abutments on either side of the arch. Although this may be made of a hard gold alloy, its rigidity is better assured by making the bar of a chromium-cobalt alloy which fits into recesses prepared in the abutment pieces, attaching it by electric soldering. **B** and **C,** Denture framework designed to fit and be supported by the splint bar.

removable anterior replacements but will have positive support from the under-lying splint bar.

Internal Clip Attachment. The internal clip (or grip) attachment differs from the splint bar in that the internal clip attachment provides both support and retention at the connecting bar.

The connecting bar is made of 11-gauge platinum alloy wire, and the female grip is made of 27-gauge plate metal. Instead of resting on the tissues of the residual ridge as does the splint bar, the wire bar is located approximately above the tissues. Retention is provided by the plate metal grip which is con-toured to fit the bar and is partially embedded by means of retention spurs or loops into the overlying resin denture base.

The internal clip attachment thus provides both support and retention for the anterior modification area and may serve to eliminate both occlusal rests and retentive clasps on the adjacent abutment teeth.

Minor Connectors

Arising from the major connector, the minor connector joins the major con-nector with other parts of the denture. For example, each direct retainer and each occlusal rest are joined to the major connector by a minor connector. In many instances, a minor connector may be identified even though continuous with some other part of the denture. For example, an occlusal rest at one end of a lingual plate is actually the terminus of a minor connector, even though that minor connector is continuous with the lingual plate. Similarly, the portion of a denture base frame that supports the clasp and the occlusal rest is the minor connector joining the major connector with the clasp proper.

Functions of the Minor Connectors. In addition to joining denture parts, the minor connector serves two other purposes. These are diametric in function.

One function is to *transfer functional stress to the abutment teeth.* Occlusal forces applied to the artificial teeth are transmitted through the base to the underlying ridge tissues, if that base is primarily tissue supported. Occlusal forces applied to the artificial teeth nearer to an abutment are transferred to that tooth through the occlusal rest. Similarly, occlusal forces are transferred to other abut-ment teeth supporting auxiliary occlusal rests and to the abutment teeth support-ing a partial denture that is entirely tooth borne. The minor connectors arising from a rigid major connector makes possible this transfer of functional stress throughout the dental arch. This, then, is a *prosthesis-to-abutment* function of the minor connector.

Another function of the minor connector is to *transfer the effect of the re-tainers, occlusal rests, and stabilizing components to the rest of the denture.* This is an *abutment-to-prosthesis* function of the minor connector. The effect of oc-clusal rests on supporting tooth surfaces, the action of retainers, and the effect of reciprocal clasp arms, guiding planes, and other stabilizing components are transferred to the rest of the denture by the minor connectors and then through-out the dental arch. Thus, forces applied on one portion of the denture may be resisted by other components placed elsewhere in the arch for that purpose. A bracing or stabilizing component on one side of the arch may be placed for the specific purpose of resisting horizontal forces originating on the opposite side. This is possible only because of the transferring effect of the minor connector, which supports that stabilizing component, and by the rigidity of the major connector.

Form and Location of the Minor Connector. Like the major connector, the minor connector must have sufficient bulk to be rigid; otherwise, the transfer of the stresses and of the effect of other components cannot be effective. At the same time, the bulk of the minor connector must be as unobjectionable as possible.

A minor connector should not be located on a convex surface but, instead, should be located in an embrasure where it will be the least noticeable to the tongue. It should conform to the interdental embrasure, passing vertically from the major connector to the other components. It should be thickest toward the lingual surface, tapering toward the contact area. The deepest part of the interdental embrasure should have been blocked out to avoid interference during insertion and removal and to avoid any wedging effect on the teeth contacted.

Generally, the minor connector should form a right angle with the major connector so that the gingival crossing may be abrupt and cover as little of the gingival tissues as possible. All gingival crossings should be relieved, first with a blockout of the gingival crevice, followed by a relief of at least .002-inch tin foil over the adjacent tissues.

Where the minor connector contacts tooth surfaces on either side of the embrasure in which it lies, it should be tapered to the teeth so that the tongue may encounter a smooth surface. Sharp angles should be avoided, and spaces should not exist for the trapping of food debris.

It is the minor connector that contacts the guiding plane surfaces of the abutment teeth. Here the minor connector must be wide enough to utilize the guiding plane to fullest advantage. Where it gives rise to a clasp arm, it should be tapered to the tooth below the origin of the clasp. If no clasp arm originates, such as where a bar clasp arm is originating elsewhere, it should be tapered to a knife edge the full length of its buccal aspect.

Where a denture tooth will be placed against it, the greatest bulk of the minor connector should be located toward the lingual aspect of the abutment tooth. In this manner, sufficient bulk is assured with the least interference to the placement of the denture tooth. Ideally, the artificial tooth should contact the abutment tooth with only a thin layer of metal intervening buccally. Lingually, the bulk of the minor connector should lie in the interdental embrasure the same as between two natural teeth.

The minor connector, then, should be located so as to pass vertically in an interdental embrasure whenever possible. Its form should conform to the interdental embrasure, with sufficient bulk to be rigid but tapered to the tooth surface where exposed to the tongue, and it should be so designed that it will not interfere with the placement of an artificial tooth.

Chapter 8

Occlusal rests

Occlusal support for the partial denture must be provided by some kind of occlusal rests placed on the abutment teeth. These should always be located upon tooth surfaces properly prepared to receive the occlusal rest.

It is a reflection upon the ability and the integrity of the dentist if, for the purpose of fabricating a partial denture, he sends to the laboratory a cast or an impression of a dental arch without having first prepared occlusal rest areas, for this is the very least that should be done in the way of mouth preparations. The laboratory that fabricates partial dentures for dentists who make no attempt at mouth preparations shares in this dereliction of professional responsibility, because it encourages a continuation of such practices.

Any unit of a partial denture that rests upon a tooth surface for the purpose of providing vertical tooth support to the denture may be called an *occlusal rest*. An occlusal rest may be placed upon the occlusal surface of a premolar or molar tooth, upon the prepared lingual surface of an anterior tooth that is capable of withstanding the forces applied, or upon an incisal surface of an anterior tooth. Occlusal support is sometimes obtained upon a tooth surface inclined occlusally from its greatest convexity, but any rest so placed upon an unprepared surface is subject to slippage along tooth inclines. This violates one of the basic rules for occlusal rest design: *an occlusal rest should be so designed that transmitted forces are directed toward the long axis of the supporting tooth.* A second rule is that *an occlusal rest must be so placed that it will prevent movement of the appliance in cervical direction.*

In an all-tooth-borne denture, the occlusal rest should be capable of transferring *all* of the occlusal stresses to the abutment teeth. In addition to preventing movement of the partial denture in a cervical direction, this is one of the principal functions of an occlusal rest. A tooth-supported denture may therefore function just as effectively as a fixed bridge, the occlusal rest serving the same purpose as the soldered union of the bridge pontic with the abutment piece. For this degree of stability to exist, it is obvious that the occlusal rest must be rigid and must receive positive support from the abutment tooth.

In a true partial denture having one or more free-end bases, the denture becomes increasingly tissue supported as the distance from the abutment increases. Closer to the abutment, however, the occlusal load is transmitted to the abutment tooth by means of the occlusal rest. The load is thereby distributed proportionately between the abutment and the supporting ridge tissues.

In addition to distributing the occlusal load, the occlusal rest serves other purposes. It acts to maintain the occlusal relationship with the opposing teeth by preventing settling of the partial denture. At the same time, settling of the denture against gingival tissues is prevented, thereby avoiding any impingement of the gingival tissues adjacent to the abutment teeth.

By preventing movement of the denture in a cervical direction, the position of the retentive portion of the clasp arm is maintained in its intended relation to the tooth undercut. Although passive when in its terminal position, the retentive portion of the clasp arm should remain in contact with the tooth ready to resist a vertical dislodging force. Then, when a dislodging force is applied, the clasp arm should immediately become active to resist vertical displacement. If, due to settling of the denture, the clasp arm is standing away from the tooth, some vertical displacement is possible before the retainer can become functional. The occlusal rest serves to prevent such settling and thereby helps to maintain the vertical stability of the partial denture.

Location and Form of the Occlusal Rest. Whenever possible, an occlusal rest should be located upon the occlusal surface of a molar or premolar tooth that has been prepared to receive it (Fig. 74). The marginal ridge should be lowered to permit enough bulk of metal for strength and rigidity without interfering with the occlusion.

The floor of the occlusal rest seat should be inclined slightly toward the center of the tooth and should be concave or *spoon-shaped*. The angle formed by the occlusal rest and the vertical minor connector from which it originates should be less than a right angle, or less than 90 degrees (Figs. 75 and 76). Only in this way can the occlusal forces be directed toward the long axis of the abutment tooth. An angle greater than 90 degrees fails to transmit occlusal forces along the supporting axis of the abutment tooth. It also permits slippage

deepest part of
rest preparation

Fig. 74. The deepest part of an occlusal rest preparation should be inside the lowered marginal ridge at **X.** The marginal ridge is lowered to accommodate the origin of the occlusal rest with the least occlusal interference without sacrificing bulk. (From McCracken, W. L.: Mouth Preparations for Partial Dentures, J. Pros. Den. **6:**39-52, 1956.)

Fig. 75. An occlusal rest should be spoon-shaped and inclined slightly toward the center of the tooth on an occlusal surface properly prepared to receive it.

Fig. 76. The floor of the occlusal rest should be inclined slightly from the lowered marginal ridge toward the center of the tooth. Any angle less than 90 degrees is acceptable so long as the disking of the proximal surface and the lowering and rounding of the marginal ridge precede the completion of the rest seat itself.

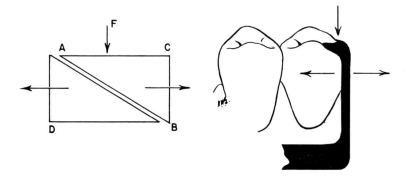

Fig. 77. The resultant of a force applied to an inclined plane where the floor of an occlusal rest preparation inclines away from instead of toward the center of the abutment tooth. **F,** Occlusal force applied to abutment tooth. **AB,** Relationship of occlusal rest with abutment tooth when angle is greater than 90 degrees. **ABC,** Partial denture framework. **ABD,** Abutment tooth.

of the prosthesis away from the abutment and causes orthodontic forces to be applied, which are the resultant of forces applied to an inclined plane (Fig. 77).

Where an existing occlusal rest preparation on enamel or on an existing cast restoration cannot be modified or deepened for fear of perforation of the enamel or gold, yet the existing floor is inclined away from the center of the tooth, a secondary occlusal rest must be employed to prevent slippage of the primary rest and orthodontic movement of the abutment tooth. Such a rest should pass over the lowered marginal ridge on the side of the tooth opposite the primary rest and should, if possible, be inclined slightly toward the center of the tooth. However, two opposing occlusal rests on diverging tooth inclines will function to prevent unfavorable forces if all related connectors are sufficiently rigid.

In any tissue-supported partial denture, the relation of the occlusal rest to the abutment should be that of a shallow ball-and-socket joint, so shaped to prevent a possible transfer of horizontal stresses to the abutment tooth. The occlusal rest should provide only occlusal support. Stabilization against horizontal movement of the prosthesis must be provided by other components of the partial denture rather than by any locking effect of the occlusal rest which might cause the application of leverages to the abutment tooth.

Internal Occlusal Rests. A partial denture which is totally tooth-supported by means of cast retainers on all of the abutment teeth may utilize internal occlusal rests for both occlusal support and horizontal stabilization (Figs. 78, 79, and 80).

An internal occlusal rest is not in any way a retainer and therefore should not be confused with an internal attachment. The term "precision" is applied to both, but any element of a partial denture should possess the accuracy and exactness synonymous with precision.

Occlusal support is derived from the floor of the rest and an additional occlusal bevel if such is provided. Horizontal stabilization is derived from the

Fig. 78. Mandibular internal occlusal rest partial denture. **A,** Abutment crowns with precision rests. Both the dovetail design and a gingival well prevent horizontal movement. **B,** Completed partial denture framework with cast lingual retention on all four abutments. A short buccal stabilizing and removal arm is used on the molar abutments.

Fig. 79. Mandibular internal occlusal rest partial denture. **A,** Precision rests in four abutment crowns. **B,** Occlusal view showing proximal guiding planes. **C,** Buccal view showing the machined parallelism of the proximal surface. **D,** Completed gold alloy casting with wrought-wire lingual retention on all four abutments. Use of a buccal stabilizing arm is optional.

near-vertical walls. The form of the rest should be parallel to the path of insertion, tapered slightly occlusally, and slightly dovetailed to prevent dislodgement proximally. The original Neurohr rest is thus modified to provide support and stabilization for the partial denture (Fig. 115, A).

The principal advantage of the internal occlusal rest is that it facilitates the elimination of a visible clasp arm buccally. Retention is provided by a lingual clasp arm, either cast or of wrought wire, lying in a natural or prepared infrabulge area on the abutment tooth. Wrought wire is preferable because it can be satisfactorily adjusted to increase or decrease retention by raising or lowering its terminus in relation to the height of contour and the magnitude of the cervical convergence.

Technical obstacles to the use of internal occlusal rests are gradually being overcome. Such a rest cannot satisfactorily be carved in wax or machined in gold. Ready-made plastic rest patterns are generally too bulky. Assembly of a ready-made rest similar to an internal attachment necessitates soldering operations and added cost. The best solution seems to be the use of a machined mandrel made of chrome-cobalt alloy* which can be waxed into the crown or inlay pattern, invested, and cast to. The mandrel is easily tapped out leaving the internal occlusal rest formed in the abutment casting. Further developments of this technique promise more widespread use of the internal occlusal rest

---

*Ticon PRP mandrel and surveyor fixture, Ticonium Division, CMP Industries, Inc., Albany, N. Y.

Fig. 80. Maxillary internal occlusal rest partial denture. **A,** Precision rests in four abutment crowns. **B,** Completed partial denture, pressed-on resin teeth. Lingual retention on premolar abutments. **C** and **D,** Buccal views of the completed restoration showing abutted resin teeth and absence of visible clasp arms on the premolar abutments.

but only for tooth-supported partial dentures unless some form of stress breaker is used between the abutment tooth and the free-end denture base.

Possible Movements of the Partial Denture. There are at least three possible movements of a free-end partial denture. One is rotation about an axis formed by the two prinicpal occlusal rests (Fig. 81, A). This axis, known as the *fulcrum line,* is the center of rotation as the free end moves *toward* the supporting tissues when an occlusal load is applied. It is also the center of rotation as the free-end base moves *away* from the supporting tissues as an occlusal load is released and vertical dislodging forces become effective. These dislodging forces are the vertical pull of food between opposing tooth surfaces, the effect of moving border tissues, and the forces of gravity against a maxillary denture. Presuming that the direct retainers are functional and that the occlusal rests remain seated, rotation instead of total displacement occurs. This movement is resisted in one direction by the tissues of the residual ridge, in proportion to the supporting quality of those tissues, the accuracy of the fit of the denture base, and the total amount of occlusal load applied. It is resisted in the opposite direction by the action of occlusal rests serving as *indirect retainers.*

A second movement is rotation about a longitudinal axis as the free-end base moves in a rotary direction about the residual ridge (Fig 81, B). This movement is resisted primarily by the rigidity of the major connector and its ability to resist torque. If the major connector is not rigid or if a "stress breaker" exists between the free-end base and the major connector, this rotation about a longitudinal axis either applies undue stress to the sides of the supporting ridge or causes horizontal shifting of the denture base.

A third movement is rotation about an imaginary perpendicular axis located near the center of the dental arch (Fig. 81, *C*). This movement occurs under function as diagonal and horizontal occlusal stresses are brought to bear upon the partial denture. It is resisted by stablizing or bracing components, such as reciprocal clasp arms and minor connectors which are in contact with vertical tooth surfaces. Such stabilizing components are essential to any partial denture design regardless of the manner of support and the type of direct retention employed. Bracing components on one side of the arch act to stabilize the partial denture against horizontal forces being applied from the opposite side. It is obvious that rigid connectors must be employed to make this effect possible.

Horizontal forces will always exist to some degree, due to lateral stresses occurring during mastication and bruxism. The magnitude of lateral stress may be minimized by fabricating an occlusion that is in harmony with the oppos-

Fig. 81. Three possible movements of a free-end partial denture. **A,** Rotation around the fulcrum line passing through the two principal occlusal rests. **B,** Rotation around a longitudinal axis formed by the crest of the residual ridge. **C,** Rotation around a perpendicular axis located near the center of the arch.

ing dentition and free of lateral interference during excursive jaw movements. The amount of horizontal shift occurring in the partial denture will therefore depend upon the magnitude of lateral stresses applied and the effectiveness of the stabilizing components.

In a tooth-borne partial denture, movement of the base *toward* the edentulous ridge is prevented by the occlusal rests on the abutment teeth. Movement *away* from the edentulous ridge is prevented by the action of direct retainers on the abutments situated at each end of each edentulous space. Therefore, the first of the three possible movements is nonexistent in the tooth-borne denture. The second possible movement, which is about a longitudinal axis, is prevented by the rigid components of the direct retainers on the abutment teeth as well as by the ability of the major connector to resist torque. This movement is much less in the tooth-borne denture, due to the presence of posterior abutments. The third possible movement occurs in any partial denture; therefore, bracing components against horizontal movement must be incorporated into any partial denture design.

The functions of the occlusal rest are not directly involved in either of the latter two movements. Instead, the occlusal rest should provide occlusal support only. All movements of the partial denture other than in a gingival direction should be resisted by other components. For the occlusal rest to enter into a bracing function would result in a direct transfer of torque to the abutment tooth. Since three movements are possible in a free-end partial denture, an occlusal rest for a free-end partial denture should not have steep vertical walls or locking dovetails which could possibly cause horizontal and torque stresses to be applied intracoronally to the abutment tooth.

In the tooth-borne denture, the only movements of any significance are horizontal, and these may be resisted by the stabilizing effect of bracing components placed on the several abutments. Therefore, in the tooth-borne denture, the use of intracoronal precision rests is permissible. In such usage the precision rests provide not only occlusal support but also horizontal stabilization.

Stress distribution in a tooth-supported partial denture is, or should be, such that each abutment tooth is assisted by others in the dental arch, and possible movements of the partial denture under function are held within acceptable physiologic limitations. It is therefore possible and acceptable to utilize an intracoronal type of occlusal rest if desired in any tooth-supported situation. In such case, vertical walls of an internal occlusal rest may be utilized to transfer horizontal forces to the abutment teeth and, by so doing, stabilize the partial denture against horizontal movement. An internal occlusal rest can thus be substituted for an external stabilizing clasp arm and, by utilizing a retentive clasp arm on the lingual surface of an abutment tooth, eliminate altogether the necessity for a visible clasp arm buccally or labially. This will be discussed further in the chapter on direct retainers.

The use of intracoronal precision rests and intracoronal direct retainers is optional with the tooth-borne denture. But with the free-end denture, the ball-and-socket type of rest is preferable and should be used wherever possible. In the absence of molar and premolar abutments, any occlusal rest preparations or occlusal rest designs on canine and incisor teeth that might apply torque and tipping forces to the abutment due to the length of the lever arm should be avoided.

Location of Occlusal Rests. Occlusal rests may be placed upon sound enamel, cast restorations, or amalgam alloy restorations. The use of an amalgam alloy restoration as support for an occlusal rest is the least desirable because of its tendency to flow under pressure and also because of the weakness of a marginal ridge made of amalgam alloy.

Occlusal rests placed on sound enamel are not conducive to caries in a mouth with a low caries index, provided good oral hygiene is maintained. Proximal tooth surfaces are much more vulnerable to caries attack than are the occlusal surfaces supporting an occlusal rest. The decision to use abutment coverage is usually based upon proximal and cervical vulnerability of the tooth rather than upon the vulnerability of an occlusal rest area. Where pre-carious fissures are found in occlusal rest areas in teeth that are otherwise sound, they may be removed and filled with amalgam alloy or gold foil without resorting to more extensive abutment protection.

While it cannot be denied that the best protection for an abutment tooth is full coverage, it must be presumed that such crowns will be properly contoured to provide support and retention for the partial denture and that full coverage restorations will provide subgingival protection to the tooth. Little is accomplished by the placement of full crowns if the more vulnerable cervical areas of an abutment tooth are not fully protected.

In making the decision whether or not to use unprotected enamel surfaces for occlusal rests, future vulnerability must be considered, for it is not easy to fabricate full crowns later to accommodate occlusal rests and clasp arms. In many instances, sound enamel may be safely used for the support of occlusal rests. In such cases, the patient should be advised that future caries susceptibility is not predictable and that much will depend upon his oral hygiene and possible future changes in his caries susceptibility. Although the decision to use unprotected abutments should logically be left up to the dentist, economic factors may influence the final decision. The patient should be made aware of the risks involved and of his responsibility for maintaining good oral hygiene and for returning periodically for observation and repair should caries ensue.

Rest Preparations in Sound Enamel. In most instances, disking of proximal tooth surfaces is necessary to provide proximal guiding planes and to eliminate undesirable undercuts where rigid parts of the denture casting must pass during insertion and removal. The preparation of occlusal rests *must always follow proximal disking,* never precede it. Only after the disking is completed may the location of the occlusal rest in relation to the marginal ridge be determined. When disking follows the preparation of the occlusal rest, the inevitable consequence is that the marginal ridge is too low and too sharp, with the center of the floor of the rest too close to the marginal ridge. Therefore, it is often not possible to correct the rest preparation without making it too deep, and irreparable damage has then been done to the tooth.

Occlusal rests in sound enamel should be prepared with round diamond points of approximately the size of Nos. 6 and 8 round burs. The larger of the two diamonds is used first to lower the marginal ridge and to establish the outline form of the occlusal rest. The resulting occlusal rest seat is then complete except that the floor is not deepened sufficiently to be inclined slightly toward the center of the tooth. The smaller diamond point is then used to deepen the floor of the occlusal rest to a gradual incline toward the center of the tooth, at the same time forming the desired spoon shape inside the lowered marginal ridge. Smoothing the enamel rods by the planing action of a round bur of suitable size revolving at moderate speed is usually the only polishing needed.

When a small enamel defect is encountered in the preparation of an occlusal rest, it is usually best to ignore it until the rest preparation has been completed, and then prepare the remaining defect with small burs to receive a small gold foil or amalgam alloy restoration. This may then be finished flush with the floor of the rest preparation previously established.

Occlusal rest preparations in existing restorations are treated the same as those in sound enamel. Any proximal disking must be done first, for if the oc-clusal rest is placed first and then the proximal surface is disked, the outline form of the occlusal rest is sometimes irreparably altered.

There is always a possibility that an existing restoration may be perforated in the process of preparing an ideal occlusal rest seat. While some compromise is permissible, the effectiveness of the occlual rest should not be jeopardized for fear of perforating an existing inlay or crown. The rest may be widened to com-pensate for its shallowness, but the floor of the rest should still be inclined slightly toward the center of the tooth. Where this is not possible, a secondary occlusal rest should be used on the opposite side of the tooth to prevent slipping of the primary rest.

When perforation does occur, it may be filled with gold foil, but occasionally the making of a new restoration is unavoidable. In such case, the original crown or inlay preparation should be modified to accommodate the occlusal rest, which is then placed in the wax pattern to avoid risking again the perforation of the completed restoration.

Occlusal rests in new restorations should always be placed in the wax pat-tern. The location of the occlusal rest should be known at the time the tooth is prepared for a crown or an inlay, so that sufficient clearance may be provided in the preparation for the rest. The final step in the preparation of the tooth should be to make sure that such clearance exists, and, if not, to make a depres-sion to accommodate the depth of the rest.

Occlusal rests in wax patterns are best made with round steel burs of suitable sizes. A perfectly round rest seat is thus possible, whereas carving with an instru-ment frequently results in an angular or irregular rest preparation. Although a round steel bur in a straight handpiece becomes partially clogged with wax dur-ing the first few revolutions, it may be used with light pressure to form the rest seat. The larger of two sizes is used first to create the outline form and to lower the marginal ridge. A slightly smaller bur is then used to deepen the floor of the rest, moving it around sufficiently to make one smooth concavity. After casting, an occlusal rest thus formed in a wax pattern needs only to be cleaned and burnished with a small finishing bur. Further polishing is usually un-necessary.

Occlusal rests in crowns and inlays are generally made somewhat larger and deeper than those in enamel. Those made in abutment crowns supporting tooth-borne dentures may be made slightly deeper than those in free-end abutments, thus approaching the effectiveness of boxlike precision rests.

Precision rests also should be created first in wax, either with suitable burs in a handpiece holder or by waxing around a lubricated mandrel held in the surveyor. In either case, the rest preparation must be finished on the casting with burs in a handpiece holder or with a precision drill press. Plastic shoes which fit over a mandrel are also available for this purpose, thus assuring a smooth casting and eliminating the need for finishing the inside of the precision rest with burs. Sufficient clearance must have been provided in the preparation of the abutment to accommodate the depth of the precision rest.

Occlusal Rests on Canine and Incisor Teeth. While the preferred site for an occlusal rest is the occlusal surface of a molar or premolar tooth, an anterior tooth may be the only abutment available for occlusal support of the denture. Also, an anterior tooth must occasionally be used to support an indirect retainer or an auxiliary occlusal rest.

A canine tooth is much preferred over an incisor for this purpose. When a canine tooth is not present, multiple rests spread over several incisor teeth are preferable to the use of a single incisor. Root form, root length, the inclination of the tooth, and the ratio of the length of the clinical crown to the alveolar support must all be considered in determining the site and form of the incisor rests.

Types of Canine Rests. The preparation of a canine tooth to receive an occlusal rest may be accomplished in one of several ways. Generally, the same applies to rest preparations on incisor teeth. These are as follows:

1. If a canine tooth is sound and the lingual slope is gradual rather than perpendicular, an occlusal rest may be placed at or just above the cingulum in much the same manner as a rest is placed upon an occlusal surface (Fig. 82, A). This type of occlusal rest may be used successfully on a maxillary canine with a gradual lingual incline and a prominent cingulum. The lingual slope of the mandibular canine is usually too steep for this type of rest, and some other provision for occlusal rest support must be made.

The proximal marginal ridge is lowered and the deepest part of the rest is made toward the center of the tooth. The path of insertion of the partial denture must be kept in mind in preparing the rest. The occlusal rest must not be prepared as though it were going to be approached from a direction perpendicular to the lingual slope. Instead, the floor of the rest should be toward the cingulum rather than on the axial wall. Care must be taken not to create an enamel undercut which would interfere with insertion of the denture.

2. If a canine tooth is sound, a circumferential lingual shoulder may be prepared in the enamel at or below the cingulum (Fig. 82, B). Since such a shoulder is formed at right angles to the path of insertion, it does not satisfy all of the requirements of an occlusal rest. Nevertheless, by including the entire mesiodistal width of the tooth, a narrow ledge will provide adequate occlusal support if the denture casting is accurate.

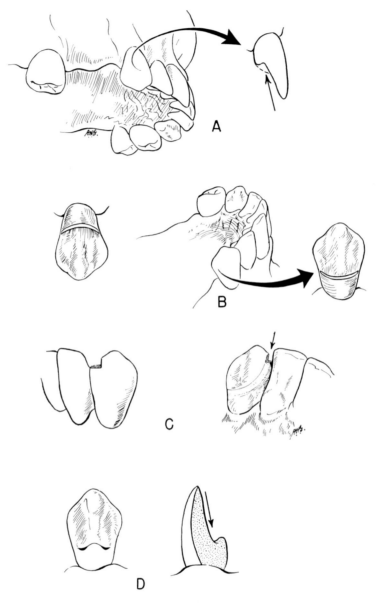

Fig. 82. Various types of canine rests. **A,** An occlusal rest placed in the enamel just above the cingulum. **B,** A circumferential lingual shoulder prepared in the enamel at the cingulum. **C,** An incisal rest. **D,** A cingulum rest on a cast restoration.

The lingual ledge may be used on both mandibular and maxillary canine teeth and also on incisor teeth. If in the maxillary arch incisor rests only must be used, several adjacent teeth rather than a single tooth should be prepared so as to distribute the load and avoid orthodontic stresses on any single tooth. The lingual shoulder or circumferential ledge may also be used where multiple cast restorations are being used on the anterior teeth. In gold, a slight incline of the ledge toward the center of the tooth is possible and desirable, whereas on enamel the ledge should be made at a right angle only to prevent accumulation of debris upon the enamel surface.

3. If a canine tooth is sound and a more positive rest than the circumferential shoulder is desired, some sort of incisal rest may be used (Fig. 82, C). There are two disadvantages to this type of rest. One is the display of metal incisally. The other is that occlusal and lateral forces applied to the tooth are magnified by the length of the lever arm. To avoid possible orthodontic movement, such a rest should form a hook over the incisal edge, yet by doing so a locking effect may result which may cause tipping forces to be applied to the tooth.

While the incisal rest may be used on a canine abutment in either arch, it is more applicable to the mandibular canine. This type of rest provides definite support with relatively little loss of tooth structure and little display of metal. Esthetically, it is preferable to the three-quarter crown. The same criteria apply in deciding whether to use this type of rest in preference to the three-quarter crown as in deciding whether or not to use unprotected enamel for an occlusal rest on a molar or premolar tooth. On incisor teeth, however, an incisal rest inevitably leads to some orthodontic movement of the tooth, due to the root form and the unfavorable leverage applied. Where an occlusal rest on an incisor tooth must be used, multiple lingual shoulders on several teeth is generally pre ferred over a single incisal rest.

The incisal rest (sometimes called an incisal notch or an embrasure hook) should be located at the mesio-incisal angle of the abutment farthest from the point of origin of the rest arm. The incisal notch should be beveled both labially and lingually, and the lingual enamel should be shaped to accommodate the rest arm. This arm is actually a minor connector terminating at the incisal rest and therefore must be rigid.

It is, of course, essential that both the master cast and the casting be accurate if the rest is to seat properly. The incisal rest should be overcontoured slightly to allow for labial and incisal finishing to the adjoining enamel in much the same manner as a three-quarter crown or inlay margin is finished to enamel. In this way, minimal display of metal is possible without jeopardizing the effectiveness of the rest.

Although all of the preceding three canine and incisor rest preparations have their disadvantages and do not satisfy all of the requirements of an occlusal rest, they may be used successfully in selected cases where the abutment is sound and where a cast restoration is not otherwise indicated. Care in selecting the type of rest to be used and care in its preparation and in the fabrication of the casting do much to assure the success of such an occlusal rest.

4. The most satisfactory canine or incisor rest is one placed on a prepared seat in a cast restoration (Fig. 82, D). This is done most effectively by planning and executing a rest seat in the wax pattern rather than by attempting to cut a rest in a cast restoration in the mouth. Two types of rests on canine and incisor teeth are possible with cast restorations. One is the circumferential lingual ledge located in the vicinity of the cingulum. The contour of the denture cast-

ing may then form the cingulum of the tooth. This type of rest is most applicable where multiple ledges are to be used in conjunction with an apron bridging the adjacent gingivae.

The most effective of all canine rests is a cingulum rest located at the lower third of the lingual surface of a cast restoration. By accentuating the cingulum in the wax pattern, the floor of the rest may be made to incline toward the center of the tooth. A saddle is thus formed which provides a positive rest seat located favorably in relation to the long axis of the tooth. In either of these rest forms, the denture casting may be made to fill out the continuity of the lingual surface so that the tongue contacts a smooth surface without being conscious of any bulk or irregularity.

The cingulum rest may be placed on the lingual surface of a cast veneer crown, a three-quarter crown, or some type of pin-ledge inlay. The latter displays less metal than the three-quarter crown, especially on the mandibular canine where the cingulum rest is most frequently used. The three-quarter crown may be used if the labial surface of the tooth is sound and retentive contours are satisfactory. But, if the labial surface presents inadequate or excessive contours for the placement of a retentive clasp arm, or if gingival decalcification or caries is present, a veneered full crown must be used.

Because of its steep lingual surface, the cingulum rest is more often necessary on a mandibular canine than on a maxillary canine and maxillary incisors. On the maxillary canine the lingual ledge is usually used, especially where the occlusal load may be distributed over two or more teeth.

Chapter **9**

Direct retainers

A partial denture must have *support*, derived from the abutment teeth through the use of occlusal rests and from the residual ridge through well-fitting bases. It must be *stabilized against horizontal movement* through the use of rigid bracing components such as reciprocal clasp arms and the contact of minor connectors with vertical tooth surfaces. It must be *stabilized against rotational movement and resulting torque* through the use of rigid connectors, indirect retainers, and other bracing components. In addition, the partial denture must have sufficient *retention* to resist reasonable dislodging forces.

Retention for the partial denture is accomplished mechanically by retaining elements on the abutment teeth and physiologically by the intimate relationship of denture bases and connectors with the underlying tissues. The latter is identical to the retention of complete dentures and is proportionate to the accuracy of the impression registration, the accuracy of the fit of the denture bases, and the total area of contact involved.

Retention of denture bases has been described as the result of the following forces: (1) adhesion, which is the attraction of the saliva to the denture and to the tissues; (2) cohesion, which is the attraction of the molecules of the saliva for each other; (3) atmospheric pressure, which is dependent upon a peripheral seal and results in a partial vacuum beneath the denture base when a dislodging force is applied; (4) the plastic molding of the tissues around the polished surfaces of the denture; and (5) the effect of gravity upon the mandibular denture. Boucher, writing on the subject of complete denture impressions, describes these forces as follows:

> Adhesion and cohesion are effective when there is perfect apposition of the impression surface of the denture to the mucous membrane surface. These forces lose their effectiveness if there is any horizontal displacement of the dentures that breaks the continuity of this contact. Atmospheric pressure is effective primarily as a rescue force when extreme dislodging forces are applied to the denture. It depends on a perfect peripheral seal to keep the pressure applied on only one side of the denture. The presence of air on the impression surface would neutralize the pressure of the air

against the polished surface. Since each of these forces is directly proportional to the area covered by the dentures, the dentures should be extended to the limits of the oral cavity.

The plastic molding of the soft tissues around the polished surfaces of dentures helps to perfect the peripheral seal. Also, it forms a mechanical lock at certain locations on the dentures, provided these surfaces are prepared for it. This lock is developed automatically and without effort by the patient if the impression is built with an understanding of the anatomic possibilities.*

Although few partial dentures are made without some mechanical retention, retention from the denture bases may contribute significantly to the over-all retention of the partial denture and therefore must not be discounted as a major retentive force. Denture bases should be so designed and so fabricated that they will contribute as much retention to the partial denture as possible.

Mechanical retention of removable partial dentures is accomplished by means of direct retainers of one type or another. A direct retainer is any unit of a removable dental prosthesis that engages an abutment tooth in such a manner as to resist *vertical displacement* of the prosthesis. This may be accomplished by frictional means, by engaging a depression in the abutment tooth, or by engaging a tooth undercut lying below the height of contour.

TYPES OF DIRECT RETAINERS

There are two basic types of direct retainers. One is the *intracoronal* retainer which engages vertical walls built into the crown of the abutment tooth so as to create frictional resistance to removal. The other is the *extracoronal* retainer which engages an external surface of the abutment tooth in an area cervical to the greatest convexity or in a depression created for that purpose. Rather than creating frictional resistance to removal, a flexible arm is forced to deform, or a spring device is compressed, thereby generating resistance to removal. The most common extracoronal attachment is the *retentive clasp arm.*

The intracoronal retainer is usually spoken of as an *internal attachment,* or a *precision attachment.* The principle of the internal attachment was first formulated by Dr. Herman E. S. Chayes in 1906 and the attachment manufactured commercially carries his name. While it may be fabricated by the dental technician as a cast dovetail fitting into a counterpart receptacle in the abutment crown, the alloys used in manufactured attachments and the precision with which they are constructed make the ready-made attachment much preferable to any that can be fabricated in the dental laboratory. Much credit is due the manufacturers of precious metals used in dentistry for their continued improvements in the design of internal attachments and to the development of precise techniques for their use.

Some of the better-known internal attachments are the *Ney-Chayes attachment,* the *Stern-Goldsmith attachment,* the *Brown attachment,* the *Baker attachment,* and the *Williams attachment.* Descriptive literature and technique manuals are available from the manufacturers.

---

*From Boucher, C. O.: Complete Denture Impressions Based Upon the Anatomy of the Mouth, J.A.D.A. 31:1174-1181, 1944.

Internal Attachments

The internal attachment has one major advantage over the extracoronal attachment, which is the elimination of a visible retentive component. For this reason the internal attachment may be preferable in selected cases. It provides some horizontal stabilization similar to that of a precision rest, but some additional bracing extracoronally is usually desirable. It has been claimed that stimulation to the underlying tissues is greater where internal attachments are used, due to intermittent vertical massage. This is probably no more than is possible with extracoronal retainers of similar construction.

Some of the disadvantages of internal attachments are that (1) they require prepared abutments and castings, (2) they require somewhat complicated clinical and laboratory procedures, (3) they eventually wear, with resulting loss of frictional resistance to denture removal, (4) they are difficult to repair and replace, (5) they are effective in proportion to their length and are therefore least effective on short teeth, and (6) it is difficult to place an internal attachment completely within the circumference of an abutment tooth.

Since the internal attachment must be built within the coronal limits of the tooth, a large pulp may be jeopardized by the depth of the receptacle. Since it depends upon frictional resistance for retention, crown length must be sufficient to provide adequate frictional surfaces. The cost of an internal attachment prosthesis is necessarily higher than an appliance of similar construction utilizing extracoronal retainers, even where the latter utilizes abutment castings. Limitations to the use of internal attachments are (1) size of the pulp, which is usually related to age of the patient, (2) length of the clinical crown, which may prevent use on short or abraded teeth, and (3) greater cost to the patient.

Since the very principle of the internal attachment does not permit horizontal movement, all horizontal, tipping, and rotational movements of the prosthesis are transmitted directly to the abutment tooth. The internal attachment may therefore not be used in conjunction with tissue-supported free-end denture bases unless some form of stress breaker is used between the movable base and the rigid attachment. While stress breakers may be used, they do have some disadvantages, which will be discussed later, and their use adds further to the cost of the partial denture. It is doubtful that the several advantages of the stress-broken, internal-attachment denture are available to but a small percentage of the population needing partial denture service.

Clasp Retainers

While the extracoronal or clasp direct retainer is used many times more frequently than the internal attachment, it is also all too frequently misused. It is hoped that a better understanding of the principles of clasp design will lead to more intelligent use of this retainer in the future.

Clasp retention is based upon the resistance of metal to deformation. For a clasp to be retentive, it must be placed in an undercut area of the tooth where it is forced to deform when a vertical dislodging force is applied. It is this resistance to deformation that generates retention. Such resistance is proportionate to the flexibility of the clasp arm.

It should be clearly understood that a retentive undercut exists only in relation to a given path of insertion and removal, for if the path of escapement of the retentive clasp is parallel to the path of removal of the prosthesis, no retentive undercut exists.

A positive path of insertion and removal is made possible by the contact of rigid parts of the denture framework with parallel tooth surfaces that act as guiding planes. It is also made possible, to some extent, by simultaneous tooth contact on either side of the dental arch as the prosthesis is inserted and removed. But if some degree of parallelism does not exist during insertion and removal, trauma to the teeth and supporting structures, as well as strain on the denture parts, is inevitable. This ultimately results either in damage to the teeth and their periodontal support, or to the denture itself, or both. Therefore, without guiding planes clasp retention will either be detrimental or nonexistent. If clasp retention is only frictional, due to an active relationship of the clasp to the teeth, orthodontic movement and/or damage to periodontal tissues will result. Instead, a clasp should bear a passive relationship to the teeth except when a dislodging force is applied.

To be retentive, a tooth must have a height of contour cervical to which the surface converges. Although any single tooth, when surveyed, will have a height of contour or an area of greatest convexity, areas of cervical convergence may not exist when that tooth is viewed in relation to a given path of insertion. Also, certain areas of cervical convergence may not be available for the placement of retentive clasps, due to their proximity to gingival tissues.

This is best illustrated by mounting a spherical object such as an egg on the adjustable table of a dental surveyor (Fig. 83, *A*). The egg now represents the cast of a dental arch or, more correctly, one tooth of a dental arch. The egg is first placed perpendicular to the base of the surveyor and surveyed to determine the height of convexity. The vertical arm of the surveyor represents the path of insertion that a denture would take and, conversely, its path of removal.

With a carbon marker, a circumferential line is drawn on the egg at its greatest circumference. This line is its greatest convexity, which Kennedy called the *height of contour*. Cummer spoke of it as the *guide line,* since it is used as a guide in the placement of retentive and nonretentive clasps. To this, DeVan added the terms *suprabulge,* denoting the surfaces sloping superiorly, and *infrabulge,* denoting the surfaces sloping inferiorly. Prothero proposed that the height of convexity of a tooth be considered as the common base of two cones, the apex of one cone being somewhere above the occlusal surface and the apex of the other being somewhere below the cervical circumference of the tooth.

Any areas inferior to the height of contour may be utilized for the placement of retentive clasp arms, whereas any areas superior to the height of contour may be utilized for the placement of nonretentive reciprocating or stabilizing components. Obviously, only flexible components may be placed inferior to the height of contour, for if rigid elements were to be so placed, the undercut areas would be areas of interference to insertion and removal rather than areas of retention.

With the original guide lines on the egg, the egg is now tilted from the perpendicular to an angular relation with the base of the surveyor (Fig. 83, *B*).

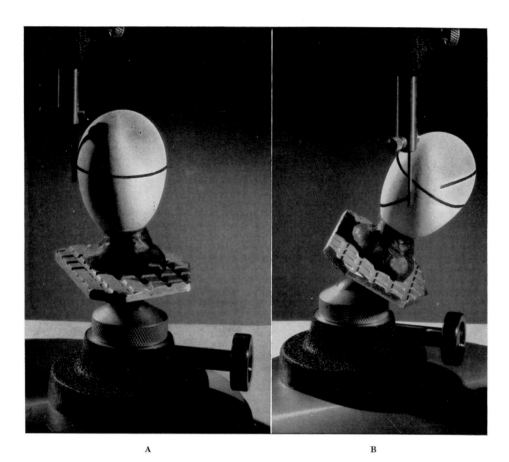

A   B

Fig. 83. A, When an egg is placed with its long axis parallel to the surveying tool, the height of contour is found at its greatest circumference. Similarly, the height of contour may be identified on a single tooth when its long axis is placed parallel to the surveying tool. Rigid parts of the partial denture framework may be located in the suprabulge areas above the height of contour, whereas only the flexible portions of clasp retainers may be placed in the infrabulge areas below. Those infrabulge surfaces that will be crossed by rigid parts of a partial denture framework must be eliminated either during mouth preparations or by blockout. **B,** If the same egg is tilted in relation to the vertical arm of the surveyor, areas formerly infrabulge are now found to be suprabulge and will accommodate nonretentive denture components. At the same time, however, areas formerly suprabulge or only slightly infrabulge are found to be so severely undercut that the design and location of clasp retainers must be changed. Unfortunately, no single tooth in a partially edentulous arch may govern the relation of the cast to the surveyor and thus the path of insertion of the partial denture. A compromise position must be found which, following reasonable mouth preparations, will satisfy all four factors: (1) no interference to insertion, (2) effective location of retentive components, (3) the most esthetic placement of all component parts, and (4) the existence of guiding planes that will assure a definite path of insertion and removal. (Courtesy the J. M. Ney Co., Hartford, Conn.)

Its relation to the vertical arm of the surveyor has now been changed, just as a change in the position of a dental cast would bring about a different relationship with the surveyor. The vertical arm of the surveyor still represents the path of insertion, but its relation to the egg is totally different.

Again, the carbon marker is used to delineate the greatest convexity or the height of contour. It will be seen that areas which were formerly infrabulge are now suprabulge, and vice versa. A retentive clasp arm placed below the height of contour in the original position may now be either excessively retentive or totally nonretentive, whereas a nonretentive reciprocal arm located above the height of contour in the first position may now be located in an area of undercut.

The location and degree of a tooth undercut available for retention is therefore relative to the path of insertion and removal of the partial denture; at the same time, nonretentive areas upon which rigid components of the clasp may be placed exist for a given path of insertion only.

When the theory of clasp retention is applied to the abutment teeth in a dental arch, each tooth may be considered as an entity so far as the design of retentive and reciprocating components is concerned. This is possible because its relationship to the rest of the arch and to the design of the rest of the prosthesis has previously been considered in selecting the most suitable path of insertion. Once the relation of the cast to the surveyor has been established, the height of contour on each abutment tooth becomes fixed, and the clasp design for each may be considered separately.

When the surveyor blade contacts a tooth on the cast at its greatest convexity, a triangle is formed. The apex of the triangle is at the point of contact of the surveyor blade with the tooth, and the base is the area of the cast representing the gingival tissues (Fig. 37). The apical angle is called the angle of cervical convergence (Fig. 84). This angle may be measured as described in Chapter 5, Surveying, or it may be estimated by observing the triangle of light visible between the tooth and the surveyor blade. For this reason, a wide surveyor blade

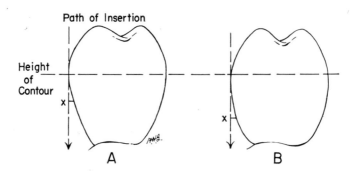

Fig. 84. The angle of cervical convergence on two teeth presenting dissimilar contours. The greater angle of cervical convergence on tooth **A** necessitates the placement of a clasp terminus nearer the height of contour than where a lesser angle exists, as in **B.** It is apparent that uniform clasp retention depends upon the degree of tooth undercut rather than on the distance below the height of contour at which the clasp terminus is placed.

rather than a small cylindrical tool is used, so that the triangle of light may be more easily seen.

The following factors determine the amount of retention that a clasp is capable of generating:

1. The size of the angle of cervical convergence.
2. How far into the angle of cervical convergence the clasp terminal is placed.
3. The flexibility of the clasp arm. Flexibility of a clasp arm is the product of:

(a) Its length, measured from its point of origin to its terminal end.

(b) Its relative diameter, regardless of its cross-sectional form.

(c) Its cross-sectional form or shape, i.e., whether it is round, half-round, or some other form.

(d) The material of which the clasp is made, i.e., whether it is made of a cast gold alloy, cast chrome alloy, wrought gold alloy, or wrought chrome alloy. Each alloy has its own characteristics in both cast or wrought form.

Uniformity of Retention. The size of the angle of convergence will determine how far into that angle a given clasp arm will be placed. Disregarding, for the time being, variations in clasp flexibility, uniformity of retention will depend upon the location of the clasp terminal—not in relation to the height of contour but in relation to the angle of cervical convergence.

The retention on all principal abutments (of which there will be two in Class I and Class II cases and three or more in Class III cases) should be as nearly equal as possible. While esthetic placement of clasp arms is desirable, it may not be possible to place all clasp arms in the same occlusocervical relationship, due to variations in tooth contours. The only exceptions are where retentive surfaces may be made similar by altering tooth contours or where two cast restorations are made with similar contours.

Instead, the clasp arms must be so located that they lie in the same degree of undercut on each abutment tooth. In Fig. 84, this is at point *X* on both teeth, *A* and *B*, despite the variation in the distance below the height of contour. Should both clasp arms be placed equidistantly below the height of contour, the higher location on tooth *B* would have too little retention, whereas the lower location on tooth *A* would be too retentive.

The measurement of the degree of undercut, either by visual or mechanical means, is therefore most important. I believe that visual evaluation of a tooth undercut, when based on experience, is at least as reliable as blind reliance upon a mechanical device, due to the many variable factors involved. While experience with undercut gauges is desirable, the student should graduate with a thorough comprehension of all the factors influencing clasp retention and be able to apply them intelligently.

Flexibility of the Clasp Arm. The following factors influence the flexibility of a clasp arm.

LENGTH. The longer the clasp arm the more flexible it will be, all other factors being equal. The length of a circumferential clasp arm is *measured from the point at which a uniform taper begins,* either at its origin from the minor connector or just before it crosses the height of contour to engage a tooth undercut. For example, in a unilateral removable bridge prosthesis, each clasp arm must provide both bracing and retention. This is because there is no cross-arch stabilization from the opposite side. In such case, the origin of the clasp arm must be rigid, and the flexible component begins just above the height of contour. In a bilateral prosthesis where bracing is accomplished from the opposite side of the arch through a rigid major connector, the circumferential clasp arm should be tapered uniformly from its point of origin. The length of this uniform taper is the full length of the clasp arm.

The length of a bar clasp arm also is measured from the point at which a uniform taper begins. The origin of the bar clasp arm ahead of the tapered portion must be considered a connector rather than a part of the clasp arm itself. Generally, the taper of a bar clasp arm should begin at its point of origin from a metal base or at the point at which it emerges from a resin base. While a bar clasp arm will usually be longer than a circumferential clasp arm, its flexibility will be less because of the fact that its half-round form lies in several planes, which prevents its flexibility from being proportionate to its total length.

DIAMETER OF THE CLASP ARM. The greater the average diameter of a clasp arm, the less flexible it will be, all other factors being equal. If its taper is absolutely uniform, the average diameter will be at a point midway between its origin and its terminal end. If its taper is not uniform, a point of flexure and therefore a point of weakness will exist which will then be the determining factor in its flexibility regardless of the average diameter of its entire length.

CROSS-SECTIONAL FORM OF THE CLASP ARM. Flexibility may exist in any form, but it is limited to only one direction in the case of the flat, oval, or half-round form. The only universally flexible form is the round form, which is practically impossible to obtain by casting and polishing.

Since all cast clasps are essentially half-round in form, they may flex away from the tooth, but edgewise flexing (and edgewise adjustment) is very limited. For this reason, cast retentive clasp arms are more acceptable in tooth-borne partial dentures in which they are called upon to flex only during insertion and removal of the prosthesis. A retentive clasp arm on an abutment adjacent to a free end must not only flex during insertion and removal but must also be capable of flexing during functional movement of the free-end base. It must have universal flexibility to avoid transmission of tipping stresses to the abutment tooth. A round clasp form is the only clasp form that may be safely used to engage a tooth undercut on the side of an abutment tooth away from the free-end base. The location of the undercut is perhaps the most important single factor in selecting a clasp for use with free-end partial dentures.

MATERIAL USED FOR CLASP ARM. While all cast alloys used in partial denture construction possess flexibility, their flexibility is proportionate to their bulk. If this were not true, other components of the partial denture could not have the necessary rigidity. The only disadvantage, other than cost, of cast gold partial dentures is that their bulk must be increased to obtain rigidity where needed at the expense of added weight. It cannot be denied that greater rigidity with less bulk is possible through the use of chrome alloys.

Although cast gold alloys may have greater resiliency than cast chrome alloys, the fact remains that the structural nature of the cast clasp does not approach the flexibility and adjustability of the wrought-wire clasp. Having been formed by being drawn into a wire, the wrought-wire clasp arm has toughness exceeding that of a cast clasp arm. It may therefore be used in smaller diameters to provide greater flexibility without fatigue and ultimate fracture.

Advantages and Disadvantages of Any Given Clasp Design. In selecting a particular clasp arm for a given situation, its advantages must be weighed against its disadvantages. The dentist should not expect the technician to make the decision as to which clasp design is to be used. The choice of clasp design must be both biologically and mechanically sound, based upon the diagnosis and treatment plan previously established.

The advantages of any particular clasp design should lie in an affirmative answer to most or all of the following questions:

1. Is it flexible enough for the purpose it is being used? (On an abutment adjacent to a free end, will tipping and torque be avoided?)

2. Does the clasp arm cover a minimum of tooth surface?

3. Will the clasp arm be as inconspicuous as possible?

4. Will tooth dimension not be increased which would increase the width of the occlusal table?

5. Is the clasp design applicable to malposed or rotated abutment teeth?

6. Can it be used despite the presence of tissue undercuts?

7. Can the clasp terminal be adjusted to increase or decrease retention?

8. Will adequate stabilization be provided to prevent horizontal and rotational movements?

9. Will rigidity be provided where it is needed?

10. Is the clasp arm likely to become distorted or broken? If so, can it be replaced?

The disadvantages of any given clasp design are generally the opposite of the advantages listed above. These are as follows:

1. The retentive arm is too rigid for a free-end abutment.

2. Too much tooth surface is covered, resulting in the trapping of food debris and possible caries attack and/or abrasion of enamel surfaces.

3. There will be an objectionable display of metal, resulting in poor esthetics.

4. Tooth dimension will be increased, resulting in an increased functional load on the abutment.

5. Tooth undercuts on malposed teeth cannot be approached without encountering other disadvantages.

6. Tissue undercuts would have to be blocked out excessively, resulting in poor esthetics, annoyance to cheek and tongue, and the trapping of debris.

7. Edgewise adjustment to increase or decrease retention is impossible.

8. Orthodontic movement of the abutment tooth is possible due to inadequate stabilization.

9. Horizontal stabilization of the partial denture is inadequate due to insufficient rigidity of stabilizing components.

10. The clasp arm may be easily distorted by careless handling.

11. If broken, the clasp arm may be difficult to replace.

With this background, the various types of clasps will be considered. The choice of clasp is like the choice of a tool to be used in a given situation. Knowing what types are available and being familiar with their various advantages and disadvantages, a clasp design may be selected which best meets the needs of the individual situation.

Although there are some rather complex designs for clasp arms, they may all be classified as falling into one of two categories. One is the *circumferential clasp arm,* which approaches the retentive undercut from an occlusal direction. The other is the *bar clasp arm,* which approaches the retentive undercut from a cervical direction.

Circumferential clasp designs include the Akers clasp arm, the embrasure clasp, the ring clasp, the back-action clasp, and the combination clasp.

Bar clasp designs include the DeVan infrabulge clasp, all of the Roach clasp

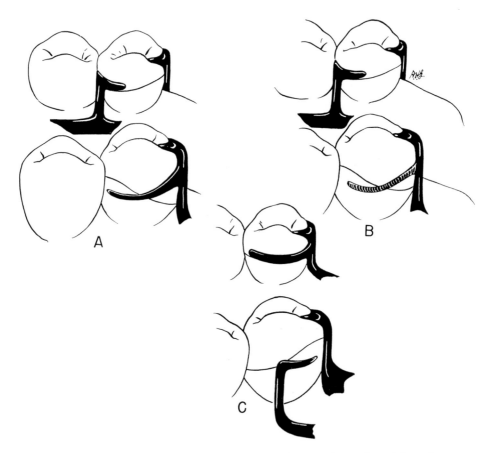

Fig. 85. A clasp assembly may be a combination of circumferential and bar clasp arms in one of several possible combinations. **A,** A cast circumferential retentive clasp arm with a nonretentive bar clasp arm on the opposite side for reciprocation. **B,** A wrought-wire circumferential retentive clasp arm with a nonretentive bar clasp arm on the opposite side for reciprocation. **C,** A retentive bar clasp arm with a nonretentive cast circumferential clasp arm on the opposite side for reciprocation.

designs, such as the T, Y, L, C, I, U, E, and S clasp arms, and the mesiodistal clasps.

A clasp assembly may be a combination of circumferential and bar clasp arms in one of several possible combinations, some of which are (1) a cast circumferential retentive clasp arm with a nonretentive bar clasp on the opposite side for reciprocation (Fig. 85, *A*); (2) a wrought-wire circumferential retentive clasp arm with a nonretentive bar clasp arm on the opposite side for reciprocation (Fig. 85, *B*); and (3) a retentive bar clasp arm with a nonretentive cast circumferential clasp arm on the opposite side for reciprocation (Fig. 85, *C*).

There should be no confusion between the choice of clasp arm and the purpose for which it is used. Either type of cast clasp arm may be made tapered and retentive or rigid and nonretentive, depending upon whether it is used for retention or reciprocation. A clasp assembly should consist of (1) one or more minor connectors from which the clasp arms originate; (2) a principal occlusal rest; (3) a retentive clasp arm engaging a tooth undercut with a retentive terminal; (4) a nonretentive clasp arm on the opposite side of the tooth for purposes of reciprocation and stabilization against horizontal movement of the prosthesis. Rigidity of this clasp arm is essential to its purpose. An auxiliary occlusal rest may be used instead of a reciprocal clasp arm if it is so located to accomplish the same purpose (Fig. 86). The addition of a lingual apron to a cast reciprocal clasp arm does not alter its primary purpose nor the need for proper location to accomplish that purpose.

Basic Principles of Clasp Design. Any clasp assembly must satisfy the basic principle of clasp design, which is that *more than 180 degrees of the circumference of the tooth must be included.* This may be in the form of continuous

Fig. 86. An auxiliary occlusal rest may be used instead of a reciprocal clasp arm without violating any principle of clasp design. Its greatest disadvantages are that a second rest seat must be prepared and an enclosed tissue space results. An auxiliary occlusal rest is also sometimes used to prevent slippage where the principal occlusal rest cannot be inclined toward the center of the tooth.

contact where circumferential clasp arms are used or broken contact where bar clasp arms are used. There must be at least three areas of tooth contact embracing more than one half the tooth circumference. These are the occlusal rest area, the retentive terminal area, and the reciprocal terminal area.

Other principles to be considered in the design of a clasp are as follows:

1. The occlusal rest must be so designed that movement of the clasp arms cervically is prevented.

2. Each retentive terminal should be opposed by a reciprocal arm capable of resisting any orthodontic pressures exerted by the retentive arm.

3. Unless guiding planes will positively control the path of removal, retentive clasps should be bilaterally opposed, i.e., buccal retention on one side of the arch should be opposed by buccal retention on the other, or lingual on one side opposed by lingual on the other. In Class II cases, the third abutment may have either buccal or lingual retention. In Class III cases, retention may be either bilaterally or diametrically opposed.

4. The path of escapement of each retentive clasp terminal must be other than parallel to the path of removal of the prosthesis.

5. Retention should always be the minimum necessary to resist reasonable dislodging forces.

6. Clasp retainers on abutment teeth adjacent to free-end bases should be so designed that they will avoid direct transmission of tipping and rotational forces to the abutment. In effect, they must act as "stress breakers," either by their design or by their construction. This is accomplished by proper placement of the retentive terminal or by the use of a more flexible clasp arm.

Except for unilateral removable bridges, in which case each clasp arm must provide both bracing and retention, only one clasp arm on an abutment tooth should be retentive. The other clasp arm should be nonretentive and should be made rigid enough to provide adequate reciprocation and bracing.

The reciprocal clasp arm has two, sometimes three, functions. First, the reciprocal clasp arm should provide reciprocation against the action of the retentive arm. This is particularly important should the retentive arm be accidentally distorted toward the tooth where it would become an active orthodontic force. Normally, the retentive clasp arm should be passive until a dislodging force is applied.

During insertion and removal, reciprocation is most needed as the retentive arm flexes over the height of contour. Unfortunately, the reciprocal clasp arm does not usually come into contact with the tooth until the denture is fully seated and the retentive clasp arm has again become passive. A momentary tipping force is thus applied to the abutment during each insertion and removal. This may not be a damaging force, since it is very transient, so long as the force does not exceed the normal elasticity of the periodontal attachments. True reciprocation during insertion and removal is possible only through the use of crown surfaces made parallel to the path of insertion. The use of a ledge on a cast restoration permits the paralleling of the surfaces to be contacted by the reciprocal arm in such a manner that true reciprocation is made possible. This will be discussed in Chapter 12, Mouth Preparations.

Second, the reciprocal clasp arm should be so located that the denture is stabilized against horizontal movement. This is possible only through the use of rigid clasp arms, rigid minor connectors, and a rigid major connector. Horizontal forces applied on one side of the dental arch are resisted by the stabilizing components on the opposite side. These are not only the reciprocal clasp arms but also all rigid components contacting vertical tooth surfaces. Obviously, the greater the number of such components, within reason, the greater will be the distribution of horizontal stresses.

Third, the reciprocal clasp arm may act to a minor degree as an indirect retainer. This is only true when it rests on a suprabulge surface of an abutment tooth lying anterior to the fulcrum line. Lifting of a free end away from the tissues is thus resisted by a rigid arm which is not easily displaced cervically. The effectiveness of such an indirect retainer is limited by its proximity to the fulcrum line, which gives it a relatively poor leverage advantage, and by the fact that slippage along tooth inclines is always possible. The latter may be prevented by the use of a ledge on a cast restoration, but enamel surfaces are not ordinarily so prepared.

Circumferential Clasp Arms. While a thorough knowledge of the principles of clasp design should lead to a logical application of those principles, it is better that some of the more common clasp designs be considered individually. The circumferential clasp will be considered first as an all-cast clasp.

The cast circumferential clasp is the most logical clasp to use with all tooth-supported partial dentures because of its ease of construction and its effectiveness. Only when the retentive undercut may be approached better with a bar

Fig. 87. An example of the two types of cast clasps in use. The molar abutment is engaged by a circumferential clasp originating above (or occlusal to) the height of contour, whereas the premolar abutment is engaged by a bar clasp originating from the metal base below (or gingival to) the height of contour.

clasp arm or esthetics will be enhanced should the latter be used (Fig. 87). The circumferential clasp arm does have some disadvantages, as follows:

1. More tooth surface is covered than with a bar clasp arm, due to its occlusal direction of approach.

2. On some tooth surfaces, particularly the buccal surface of mandibular teeth and the lingual surfaces of maxillary teeth, its occlusal approach may increase the width of the occlusal surface of the tooth.

3. In the mandibular arch, more metal may be displayed than with a bar clasp arm.

4. As with all cast clasps, its half-round form prevents edgewise adjustment to increase or decrease retention. Adjustments in the retention afforded by a clasp arm should be made by moving a clasp terminal cervically into the angle of cervical convergence or occlusally into a lesser area of undercut. Tightening a clasp against the tooth or loosening it away from the tooth increases or decreases frictional resistance rather than adjusting the retentive potential of the clasp. True adjustment is, therefore, impossible with most cast clasps.

Despite its disadvantages, the cast circumferential clasp arm may be used effectively, and many of these disadvantages may be minimized by proper design. Adequate mouth preparations will permit its point of origin to be placed far enough below the occlusal surface to avoid poor esthetics and increased tooth dimension (Fig. 88). Although some of the other disadvantages listed imply that the bar-type clasp may be preferable, the circumferential-type clasp is actually superior to a bar clasp arm that is improperly used or poorly designed. Experience has shown that the possible advantages of the bar clasp arm are too often negated by faulty application and design, whereas the circumferential clasp arm is less easily misused.

Fig. 88. A cast circumferential retentive clasp arm properly designed. It originates on and above the height of contour, which it then crosses approximately midway, and engages a retentive undercut progressively as its taper decreases and its flexibility increases.

The basic form of the circumferential-type clasp is a buccal and lingual arm originating from a common body, sometimes called an *Akers clasp* (Fig. 89). This clasp is used improperly when two retentive clasp arms originate from the body and occlusal rest areas and approach bilateral retentive areas on the side of the tooth away from the point of origin. The correct form of this clasp has only one retentive clasp arm, opposed by a nonretentive reciprocal arm on the opposite side. A common error of laboratory technicians is to use this clasp improperly by making both clasp terminals retentive. This is not only unnecessary but also disregards the need for reciprocation and bilateral stabilization.

Fig. 89. A cast circumferential retentive clasp arm.

Fig. 90. A ring clasp encircling nearly all of the tooth from its point of origin. **A,** The clasp originates on the mesiobuccal surface and encircles the tooth to engage a mesiolingual undercut. **B,** The clasp originates on the mesiolingual surface and encircles the tooth to engage a mesiobuccal undercut. In either case a supporting strut is used on the nonretentive side. (Drawn both as a direct view of the near side of the tooth and as a mirror view of the opposite side.)

In addition to the Akers clasp, the circumferential-type clasp may be used in several other forms. One is the *ring clasp*, which encircles nearly all of a tooth from its point of origin (Fig. 90). It is used where a proximal undercut cannot be approached by other means. For example, where a mesiolingual undercut on a lower molar abutment cannot be approached directly, due to its proximity to the occlusal rest area, yet cannot be approached with a bar clasp arm, due to lingual inclination of the tooth, the ring clasp encircling the tooth allows the undercut to be approached from the distal aspect of the tooth.

The ring clasp should never be used as an unsupported ring (Fig. 91), for if it is free to open and close as a ring, it cannot provide either reciprocation or bracing. Instead, the ring clasp should always be used with a supporting strut on the nonretentive side, with or without an auxiliary occlusal rest on the opposite marginal ridge. The advantage of an auxiliary rest is that further movement of a mesially inclined tooth is prevented by the presence of a distal rest. In any case, the supporting strut should be thought of as being a minor connector from which the flexible retentive arm originates. Reciprocation then comes from the rigid portion of the clasp lying between the supporting strut and the principal occlusal rest. (Figs. 92 and 93.)

The ring clasp should be used on protected abutments whenever possible because it covers such a large area of tooth surface. Esthetics usually need not be considered on such a posteriorly located tooth.

A ring clasp may be used in reverse on an abutment located anterior to an edentulous space (Fig. 94). While potentially an effective clasp, this clasp covers an excessive amount of tooth surface and is esthetically objectionable. The only justification for its use is when a distobuccal or distolingual undercut cannot be approached directly from the occlusal rest area, yet tissue undercuts prevent its approach from a gingival direction with a bar clasp arm.

Fig. 91. An improperly designed ring clasp lacking necessary support. Such a clasp lacks any reciprocating or stabilizing action, since the entire circumference of the clasp is free to open and close. Instead, a supporting strut should always be added on the nonretentive side of the abutment tooth, which then becomes, in effect, a minor connector from which a tapered and flexible retentive clasp arm originates.

Fig. 92. A buccal strut supporting a mesially originating ring clasp. The flexible retentive arms begins at the distal occlusal rest and engages a mesiolingual undercut. Despite its resemblance to a bar-type clasp, this is a circumferential clasp by reason of its point of origin, the strut being actually an auxiliary minor connector.

Fig. 93. A ring clasp engaging a mesiobuccal undercut on a mesially inclined lower right molar requires a supporting bar on the lingual surface to limit flexure to only the retentive portion of the clasp.

Fig. 94. A ring clasp may be used in reverse on an abutment located anterior to an edentulous space.

Fig. 95. A back-action circumferential clasp used on a premolar abutment anterior to an edentulous space.

The *back-action* and *reverse back-action* clasps are modifications of the ring clasp, with all of its disadvantages and no apparent advantages (Fig. 95). It is difficult to ever justify their use. The undercut can usually be approached just as well with an Akers clasp, with less tooth coverage and less display of metal. With the Akers clasp, the proximal tooth surface can be used properly as a guiding plane, as it should be, and the occlusal rest can have the rigid support it requires. An occlusal rest should always be attached to some rigid minor connector and should never be supported by a clasp arm alone. If the occlusal rest is part of a flexible assembly, it cannot function adequately as an occlusal rest. Unfortunately, the back-action clasp is still being used, despite the fact that it is biologically and mechanically unsound.

In the construction of an unmodified Class II or Class III partial denture, there are no edentulous spaces on the opposite side of the arch to aid in clasping. Mechanically, this is a disadvantage—so much so, in fact, that a second premolar or first molar tooth may be extracted with the slightest provocation to provide a modification space for more advantageous clasping. However, when the teeth are sound and retentive areas are available or when multiple restorations are justified, clasping is accomplished by means of a double Akers clasp, called an *embrasure clasp* (Figs. 96 and 97).

Sufficient space must be provided between the abutment teeth in their occlusal third to make room for the common body of the two Akers clasps (Fig. 98), yet the contact area should not be eliminated entirely. Since vulnerable areas of the teeth are involved, abutment protection with inlays or crowns is indicated in almost every case. The decision to use unprotected abutments must be made at the time of oral examination and should be based on the age of the patient, caries index, and oral hygiene, as well as on whether or not existing tooth contours are favorable.

The embrasure clasp should always be used with double occlusal rests, even where definite proximal shoulders can be established. This is to avoid inter-proximal wedging due to setting of the prosthesis, which could cause separation of the abutment teeth and result in food impaction and clasp displacement. In addition to providing support, occlusal rests also serve to shunt food away from

Fig. 96. An embrasure clasp is used where no edentulous space exists. Although in this drawing both retentive clasp arms are located on the buccal surface, and the nonretentive arms on the lingual surface, retention and reciprocation can be reversed on both teeth or on either tooth.

Fig. 97. Multiple clasping in a surgically mutilated mouth. On the right are an embrasure clasp, a bar clasp arm, and an Akers clasp engaging lingual undercuts on three abutment teeth. On the left is a well-designed ring clasp engaging a lingual undercut, with supporting strut on the buccal surface and auxiliary occlusal rest to prevent mesial tipping. Note the rigid design of the major connector.

Fig. 98. Embrasure and hairpin circumferential retentive clasp arms. The terminus of each engages a suitable retentive undercut. Use of the hairpin-type clasp on the second molar is made necessary by the fact that the only available undercut lies directly below the point of origin of the clasp arm.

Fig. 99. Two examples of the use of embrasure clasps for Class II partially edentulous arches. **A,** Mandibular Class II. Embrasure clasps on two left molar abutments, buccal wrought-wire retention on the right second premolar, and indirect retainer on the left first premolar and canine. **B,** Maxillary Class II. Embrasure clasps on left premolar and first molar with additional occlusal rest and lingual stabilizing arm on the second molar. Buccal wrought-wire retention on the right premolar. No indirect retention is needed, because of the "direct-indirect" retention obtained from broad palatal coverage. The palatal connector avoids the palatal rugae and unnecessary contact with gingival tissues. Posteriorly the connector crosses the midline symmetrically just anterior to the posterior limit of immobile palatal tissues.

contact areas. For this reason, occlusal rests should always be used wherever food impaction is possible.

Embrasure clasps should have two retentive clasp arms and two reciprocal clasp arms, either bilaterally or diagonally opposed. An auxiliary occlusal rest or a bar clasp arm can be substituted for a circumferential reciprocal arm so long as definite reciprocation and bracing result. A lingually placed retentive bar clasp arm may be substituted, if a rigid circumferential clasp arm is placed on the buccal surface for reciprocation.

Other modifications of the cast circumferential clasp are the multiple clasp, the half-and-half clasp, and the reverse action clasp. The *multiple clasp* is simply two opposing Akers clasps joined at the terminal end of the two reciprocal arms (Fig. 100). It is used where additional retention is needed, usually on tooth-borne partial dentures. It may be used for multiple clasping in cases where the partial denture replaces an entire half of a dental arch. It may be used instead of an embrasure clasp where the only available retentive areas are adjacent to each other. Its disadvantage lies in the fact that two embrasure approaches are necessary rather than a single common embrasure for both clasps.

The *half-and-half clasp* consists of a circumferential retentive arm arising

Fig. 100. A multiple clasp is actually two opposing Akers clasps joined at the terminal end of the two reciprocal arms.

Fig. 101. A half-and-half clasp consists of one circumferential retentive arm arising from the distal and a second circumferential arm arising from the mesial on the opposite side, with or without a secondary occlusal rest. The dotted line illustrates a nonretentive reciprocal clasp arm used without a secondary occlusal rest.

from one direction and a reciprocal arm arising from another (Fig. 101). Since the second arm must arise from a second minor connector, this arm is actually a bar clasp used with or without an auxiliary occlusal rest. Reciprocation arising from a second minor connector can usually be accomplished with a short bar or with an auxiliary occlusal rest, thereby avoiding so much tooth coverage. Thus, it is apparent there is little justification for the use of the half-and-half clasp in bilateral dentures. Its design was originally intended to provide dual retention, a principle which should be applied only to unilateral denture design.

The *reverse action* or *hairpin clasp arm* is designed to permit engaging a proximal undercut from an occlusal approach (Fig. 102). Other methods of accomplishing the same thing are with a ring clasp originating on the opposite side of the tooth or with a bar clasp arm originating from a gingival direction. However, when a proximal undercut must be used on a posterior abutment and tissue undercuts or high tissue attachments prevent the use of a bar clasp arm, the reverse action clasp may be used successfully. Although the ring clasp would be preferable, lingual undercuts may prevent the placement of a supporting strut without tongue interference. In this limited situation, the hairpin clasp arm serves adequately, despite its several disadvantages. The clasp covers considerable tooth surface and may trap debris; its occlusal origin may increase the functional load on the tooth, and its flexibility is limited. Esthetics usually need not be considered where the clasp is used on a posterior abutment, but the hairpin clasp arm does have the additional disadvantage of displaying too much metal for use on an anterior abutment.

Properly designed, the reverse action clasp should make a hairpin turn to engage an undercut below the point of origin (Fig. 102). The upper arm of this clasp should be considered a minor connector giving rise to the tapered lower arm. Therefore, only the lower arm should be flexible, with the retentive portion beginning beyond the turn. Only the lower arm should flex over the height of

Fig. 102. A reverse-action or hairpin clasp arm may be used where a proximal undercut lies below the point of origin of the clasp. It can be used on any posterior abutment, but it may be esthetically objectionable and covers considerable tooth surface.

contour to engage a retentive undercut. The clasp should be designed and fabricated with this in mind.

These are the various types of cast circumferential clasps. As mentioned previously, they may be used in combination with bar clasp arms so long as differentiation is made by their location and bulk between retention and reciprocation. Circumferential and bar clasp arms may be made either flexible (retentive) or rigid (reciprocal) in any combination as long as each retentive clasp arm is opposed by a rigid reciprocal arm. The only exception is in the case of the unilateral removable bridge prosthesis, where each clasp arm must provide both bracing and retention.

The use of many of the less desirable clasp forms can be avoided by changing the crown forms of the abutments with full restorations. In fabricating abutment coverage, tooth contours should be established which will permit the use of the most desirable clasp forms rather than reproduce a form that makes necessary the use of less desirable clasp designs.

Bar Clasp Arms. The term *bar clasp arm* is generally preferred over the less descriptive term *Roach clasp arm*. Reduced to its simplest terms, the bar clasp arm arises from the denture framework or a metal base and approaches the retentive undercut from a gingival direction (Fig. 87).

The bar clasp arm has been classified by the shape of the retentive terminal. Thus, it has been identified as a T, modified T, Y, C, I, U, E, R, or S clasp arm. All have the same things in common: they originate from the framework or base and approach the undercut from a gingival direction. The form the terminal takes is of little significance so long as it is mechanically and functionally effective, covers as little tooth surface as possible, and displays as little metal as possible.

The T and Y clasp arms are the most frequently misused. It is unlikely that the full area of a T or Y terminal is ever necessary for adequate clasp retention. While the larger area of contact would provide greater frictional resistance, this is not true clasp retention and only that portion engaging an undercut area should be considered retentive. Usually, only one terminal of such a clasp arm is placed in an undercut area. The remainder of the clasp arm is therefore superfluous, because it adds neither retention nor bracing to the denture. If the bar clasp arm is made to be flexible for retentive purposes, it is impossible for any suprabulge portion of that clasp to provide stabilization and bracing, since it is also part of the flexible arm. Therefore, the suprabulge portion of a T or Y clasp arm should be dispensed with and the clasp terminal placed in a retentive undercut. It matters little whether the arm takes the form of a modified T, the curve of a C, of the more direct approach of an I.

The L clasp is simply an I clasp with a longer arm and the U merely a double I. In the S clasp, the arm is given an S turn, supposedly for the purpose of making it more flexible; actually, its only purpose should be to avoid a tissue undercut. The terminal of the bar clasp should be designed to be biologically and mechanically sound rather than to conform to any alphabetical connotation.

With only one exception, the bar clasp arm should be used only with tooth-borne partial dentures or tooth-borne modification areas. This exception is where

Fig. 103. A bar clasp arm properly used on a free-end abutment. A mesial extension or "T" is neither advantageous nor desirable.

Fig. 104. A bar clasp arm on a free-end abutment must be made light enough to be flexible and may be used only when it can engage a proximal undercut adjacent to the free-end base. (From McCracken, W. L.: Contemporary Partial Denture Designs, J. Pros. Den. **8:**71-84, 1958.)

Fig. 105. A bar clasp arm on a maxillary free-end abutment. Note the uniform taper from the point where it will emerge from a resin base, and the fact that it engages the tooth undercut on the *side adjacent* to the free-end base.

an undercut which can logically be approached with a bar clasp arm lies on the side of an abutment tooth adjacent to a free-end base (Figs. 103, 104, and 105). Should a tissue undercut prevent such use of a bar clasp arm, a mesially originating ring clasp or a cast or wrought-wire reverse action clasp may be used.

A bar clasp arm should never be used on a free-end abutment if the undercut lies on the side of the tooth away from the free end. The bar clasp arm is not a particularly flexible clasp arm because of the effect of its half-round form and its several planes of origin. Although the cast circumferential clasp arm can be made more flexible than the bar clasp arm, the combination clasp is much preferred for use on all free-end abutments where torque and tipping are possible due to engaging an undercut away from the free end. Occasionally, however, a situation exists where a bar clasp arm may be used to advantage without jeopardizing a free-end abutment. In this instance alone, a bar clasp arm swinging distally into the undercut is a logical choice, since movement of the abutment, as the free-end base moves tissueward, is avoided by the distal location of the clasp terminal.

The specific indications for the use of a bar clasp arm may be stated as follows: *Where a small degree of undercut exists in the cervical third of the abutment tooth, which may be approached from a gingival direction, and with a single exception, only on abutment teeth supporting tooth-borne partial dentures or tooth-borne modification areas* (Fig. 106). Thus, use of the bar clasp arm is contraindicated where a deep cervical undercut exists or where a severe tissue undercut exists, either of which must be bridged by excessive blockout. The bar clasp arm must always be located below gingival attachments. Where severe tooth and tissue undercuts exist which must be blocked out, the presence of a bar clasp arm usually results in annoyance to tongue and cheek, the trapping of food debris, and poor esthetics.

Fig. 106. A bar clasp arm on a lower molar abutment engaging a mesiobuccal undercut. Note the proper utilization of parallel proximal guiding planes.

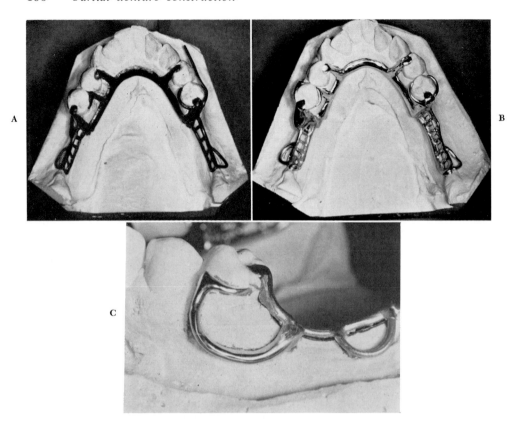

Fig. 107. Bar clasps used for both retention and reciprocation on a rotated premolar abutment. Contours of the opposite abutment on the right side permitted the use of a combination clasp. **A,** Wax pattern. The extension of the wrought wire on the right side will be held by the outer investment. **B,** Completed cast framework. The lingual reciprocal clasp arm on the left abutment is a mesially originating bar located at and above the height of contour. **C,** The bar retentive clasp arm on the buccal aspect engages a distobuccal undercut. Note the guiding plane contact of the minor connector with adequate relief over the free gingival margins.

The Combination Clasp. The combination clasp consists of a wrought-wire retentive clasp arm and a cast reciprocal clasp arm (Fig. 108). While the latter may be in the form of a bar clasp arm, it is usually a circumferential arm. The retentive arm is almost always circumferential, but it also may be used in the manner of a bar, originating gingivally from the denture base.

The advantages of the combination clasp lie in the *flexibility,* the *adjustability,* and the *appearance* of the wrought-wire retentive arm. It is used where maximum flexibility is desirable, such as on an abutment tooth adjacent to a free-end base or on a particularly weak abutment. It may be used for its adjustability where precise retentive requirements are unpredictable and later adjustment to increase or decrease retention may be necessary. A third justification for its use is its esthetic advantage over cast clasps. Being wrought in structure, it

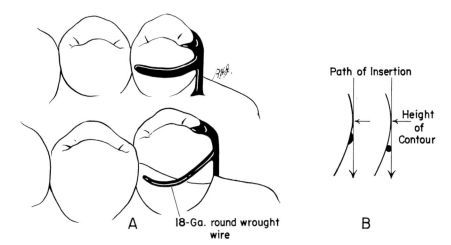

A

18-Ga. round wrought
wire

Path of Insertion

Height
of
Contour

B

Fig. 108. **A,** The combination clasp consists of a cast reciprocal clasp arm and a wrought-wire retentive clasp arm. The latter is either cast to or soldered to the cast framework. **B,** In addition to the advantages of flexibility, adjustability, and appearance, the wrought-wire retentive arm makes only a line contact with the abutment tooth, rather than the broader contact of the cast clasp.

may be used in smaller diameters than a cast clasp with less danger of fracture. Being round in form, light is refracted in such a manner that the display of metal is less noticeable than with the broader surfaces of a cast clasp.

The most common use of the combination clasp is on an abutment tooth adjacent to a free-end base. Where a distal undercut exists which may be approached with a properly designed bar clasp arm or with a ring clasp (despite its several disadvantages), a cast clasp can be so located that it will not cause abutment tipping as the free end moves tissueward. But where the undercut is on the side of the abutment away from the free end, the wrought-wire retentive arm offers greater flexibility than the cast clasp arm and therefore better dissipates functional stresses. For this reason, the combination clasp is preferred (Fig. 109).

The combination clasp has two disadvantages: (1) the extra steps in fabrication, particularly when high-fusing chrome alloys are used, and (2) the fact that it is easily distorted by careless handling on the part of the patient. The disadvantages of the wrought-wire clasp are offset by its advantages, which are (1) its flexibility, (2) its adjustability, (3) its esthetic advantage over other circumferential clasp arms and most bar clasp arms, and (4) the fact that a minimum of tooth surface is covered because of its line contact with the tooth rather than the surface contact of a cast clasp arm.

Experience with the combination clasp has shown its superiority over other clasp designs for use with free-end abutments. The disadvantages listed above should not prevent its use regardless of the type of alloy being used for the cast framework. Technical problems are minimized by selecting the best wrought wire for this purpose and then either casting to it or soldering it to the cast framework. Eighteen-gauge round Ticonium wrought wire has proved to be the best

Fig. 109. Four types of clasp arms which may be used on an abutment adjacent to a free-end base. A bar clasp arm, **A**, a ring clasp arm, **B**, or a hairpin clasp arm, **C**, may be used only where the undercut lies on the side of the abutment tooth adjacent to the edentulous space. None of these is flexible enough to be used where the undercut lies on the side of the abutment tooth away from the edentulous space. In this situation the combination clasp with its wrought-wire retentive arm, **D**, should be used because of its greater flexibility.

material up to the present time. It is tough, yet flexible enough, and not expensive. Gold alloys and Ticonium may be cast to it, and it may be soldered to the higher fusing chrome alloys. The technique for adapting wrought-wire clasp arms will be given in Chapter 17, Laboratory Procedures.

The patient may be taught to avoid distortion of the wrought wire by explaining that the fingernail should always be applied to its point of origin where it is held rigid by the casting rather than at the flexible terminal end. Frequently, lingual retention may be used instead of buccal retention, especially on a mandibular abutment, so that the wrought-wire arm is never touched by the patient during removal of the denture. Instead, removal may be accomplished by lifting against the cast reciprocal arm located on the buccal side of the tooth. However, this negates the esthetic advantage of the wrought-wire clasp arm, and esthetics may be given preference where the choice must be made between buccal and lingual retention. Frequently, however, retention must be used where it is found and the clasp designed accordingly.

It is unfortunate that most dental laboratories have not looked upon the combination clasp as an essential clasp form in partial denture design. This is probably due to a lack of understanding of its biologic significance and to the fact that it is not easily incorporated into mass production procedures. It is also probably due to the fact that there are relatively few requests for this type of clasp. The responsibility for clasp design has been relegated to the dental laboratory far too much in the past. This responsibility should be reassumed by the dentist and should be based upon his diagnosis and upon an established treatment plan.

Lingual Retention in Conjunction With Internal Occlusal Rests. The internal occlusal rest has been covered in Chapter 8, Occlusal Rests. It has been pointed out that the internal occlusal rest is not utilized as a retainer, but that its near-vertical walls provide for reciprocation against a lingually placed retentive clasp arm. For this reason, visible clasp arms may be eliminated, thus meeting one of the principal objections to the extracoronal retainer.

Such a retentive clasp arm, terminating in an existing or prepared infra-bulge area on the abutment tooth, may be of any acceptable design. It is usually a circumferential arm arising from the body of the denture framework at the occlusal rest area. It may be either cast or wrought, but the advantage of adjustability makes the wrought clasp arm preferable. It may be made of either platinum-gold-paladium or of chrome-cobalt alloy and may be cast to with gold or Ticonium or be assembled by soldering to one of the higher-fusing chrome-cobalt alloys. In any case, future adjustment or repair is facilitated.

The use of lingual extracoronal retention avoids much of the cost of the internal attachment yet disposes of a visible clasp arm where esthetics must be considered. Frequently its use with a tooth-supported partial denture is employed only on the anterior abutments, and the posterior abutments, where esthetics is not a consideration, are clasped in the conventional manner. (Figs. 78, 79, and 80.)

Other Types of Clasps. Several other types of clasps will be considered briefly. One is the *mesiodistal clasp*. It is sometimes used on isolated abutments where some retention is desired. It should never be used where a free end is involved, because tipping of the abutment would be inevitable.

In most instances, the tooth must be prepared to receive this type of clasp. Its flexibility lies in its ability to open and close as it engages bilateral proximal undercuts. It must be kept thin and flexible. To be effective, the tips of the clasp must engage part of the labial or buccal surface, but they should be made wide and flat interproximally so as to display as little metal as possible. Since adjoining tooth replacements would prevent the intended action of the clasp, the

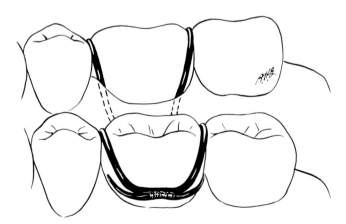

Fig. 110. The Crozat-type clasp used in removable orthodontic appliances and temporary partial dentures.

mesiodistal clasp may only be used where interproximal spaces exist which are not to be filled by other parts of the denture.

The *crib*, or *modified Crozat-type*, *clasp* is a wrought-wire clasp frequently used in removable orthodontic appliances (Fig. 110). Retention from the Crozat clasp is not obtained from the crib alone but rather from the retentive terminals attached to it by soldering.

The *DeVan*, or *infrabulge, clasp* is a bar clasp arm arising from the periphery of the base, either as an extension of a cast base or attached to the periphery of a resin base (Fig. 111). It is made more flexible than the usual bar clasp arm by separating that portion of the cast base which gives rise to the clasp arm from the clasp arm itself, either by making a saw cut or by casting against a separating shim of matrix metal which is later removed with acid. It may be made more flexible through the use of wrought wire, which is either attached to a metal base by soldering or embedded in the periphery of a resin base.

Some of the advantages attributed to the DeVan clasp are (1) its interproximal location, which may be used to esthetic advantage, (2) increased retention without tipping action on the abutment, and (3) less chance of accidental distortion due to its proximity to the denture periphery. The DeVan clasp is not a very hygienic clasp design, due to the narrow separation that tends to trap debris, and is therefore not readily cleaned by tongue and saliva. The wearer should be

Fig. 111. The DeVan infrabulge clasp. In **A** the clasp arm arises from the periphery of a metal base and is separated from it with a saw cut or by having been cast against a separating shim which is later removed. A wrought-wire retentive arm may be soldered to the metal base to serve the same purpose. In **B** the clasp arm is attached to the periphery of a resin base. This is usually a wrought-wire clasp arm partially embedded in the resin base at the periphery.

Fig. 112. The Saddle-Lock principle of hidden clasp retention. This effectively conceals retentive clasps but may do so at the expense of proximal guiding planes and unprotected tooth surfaces. These objections can be overcome by providing parallel guiding surfaces on protective crown or inlay restorations occlusal to the area used for retentive purposes. The vertical minor connector supporting the occlusal rest is separated from the retentive clasp arm by applying a protective coating over the clasp pattern and then waxing the vertical minor connector over it. (Courtesy Saddle-Lock, Inc., Brooklyn, N. Y.)

Fig. 113. Utilization of a proximal undercut provides excellent and esthetically acceptable retention but prevents effective use of a proximal guiding plane and may jeopardize a surface vulnerable to caries attack unless the crown is protected with a cast restoration. (Courtesy Saddle-Lock, Inc., Brooklyn, N. Y.)

meticulous in his care of a denture so made, not only for reasons of oral hygiene but also to prevent cariogenic debris being held against tooth surfaces.

Mesiodistal Clasping of Posterior Abutment Teeth. Several dental laboratory companies have stressed the esthetic advantages of mesiodistal clasping (Figs. 112 and 113). While esthetics is desirable, it should not be given precedence over biologic considerations. Such mesiodistal clasping utilizes the very areas on abutment teeth that are the most vulnerable to caries attack and also those surfaces that ordinarily should be utilized for guiding planes.

Where enamel surfaces are sound and other factors are favorable, where the use of guiding planes is not jeopardized, and where adequate reciprocation is provided, proximal undercuts may be used to obtain better esthetic placement of clasp retainers. Such clasps should be designed to include more than half of the tooth circumference, which is difficult to accomplish without some display of metal.

Mesiodistal clasping is most effective when used in conjunction with cast restorations and precision rests. Precision rests eliminate the need for the clasp to include 180 degrees of the tooth, since the boxlike rest provides adequate stabilization of the abutment tooth. On cast restorations, proximal undercuts may be created without fear of jeopardizing areas that would be vulnerable on the natural tooth. On cast restorations also, guiding planes need not be ignored altogether, even when a proximal undercut is utilized for retention.

In some modern clasp designs, the occlusal rest is separated from the clasp retainer to allow flexing into interproximal areas. While accomplishing its intended purpose of better esthetics, this design ignores the need for guiding planes and results in an unhygienic clasp, due to the trapping of debris. Such clasps are mechanically sound but biologically objectionable. Moreover, the technician frequently leaves the clasp terminal embedded in resin, rendering it totally inactive as a retentive clasp arm.

The choice of clasp designs should be based upon biologic as well as mechanical principles. The dentist responsible for the service being rendered to the patient must be able to justify the clap design used for each abutment tooth in keeping with these principles.

*The Hart-Dunn Attachment for Unilateral Free-End Partial Dentures.** Objections to the use of embrasure clasp retainers on the nonedentulous side of a Kennedy Class II partially edentulous arch can be met with the use of the Hart-Dunn attachment partial denture. Retention is by an embrasure hook consisting of 18- or 19-gauge round wrought wires placed just beneath the contact areas in the mesial and distal areas of the selected abutment tooth, slightly curved to allow easy insertion from the lingual direction and protection of the interdental papillae. Stabilization is provided by occlusal rests mesially and distally, which also serve to prevent the wires from settling into the interdental papillae (Fig. 114).

Mann has pointed out that, because the Hart-Dunn attachment is inserted in a horizontal direction just prior to seating the clasp on the opposite or denture

---

*Dunn, A. L.: A Safe Temporary Partial Denture, J.A.D.A. **23**:96-99, 1936.

Fig. 114. Hart-Dunn attachment for free-end partial dentures. **A,** Mandibular Class II free-end partial denture retained by circumferential clasping on the free-end abutment and embrasure wires on either side of the left second premolar. **B,** The partial denture off of the cast, showing the occlusal rests and embrasure wires. **C,** Maxillary Class II free-end partial denture of similar design with split palatal bar stress breaker leading from the clasp retainer on the free-end abutment.

base side, conventional surveying of the abutment teeth cannot be used. This is to say that guiding planes to insertion and removal are not used. Instead, a divider is used for surveying the cast. Mann is quoted directly, as follows:

> One point of the divider is placed on the center of rotation for the attachment (at a point midway between the embrasure hook and the occlusal rests), and the other end of the divider is swept over the buccal and lingual surfaces of the abutment tooth on the opposite side and over the lingual denture base area on the study cast. Either a precision attachment or a circumferential clasp can be used on the denture base side to lock the partial denture in position. However, *these retainers must be on the arc scribed by the divider* in order that the attachment can first be seated horizontally, then the clasp or attachment on the denture base side is seated occlusogingivally. If the abutment on the denture base side is inclined toward the

buccal, it presents an undercut problem. This can be solved best by constructing a cast crown to eliminate the undercut. . . .*

Either a precision attachment or conventional clasp on the denture base side may be used. On the opposite side, the hook may be fitted into the pontic casting of a fixed bridge instead of embrasure hooks. A prefabricated hook suggested and designed by Dr. George Hollenback for this purpose is commercially available.†

Other Types of Retainers

Numerous other types of retainers for partial dentures have been devised that cannot be classified as being primarily of the intracoronal or extracoronal type. Neither can they be classified as relying primarily on frictional resistance or placement of an element in an undercut to prevent displacement of the denture. However, all of these utilize some sort of locking device, located either inter-coronally or extracoronally, for the purpose of providing retention without visible clasp retention. While the motivation behind the development of other types of retainers has usually been a desire to eliminate visible clasp retainers, the desire to minimize torque and tipping stresses on the abutment teeth has also been given consideration.

The few of these retainers that will be discussed herein all have merit, and much credit is due those who have developed specific devices and techniques for the retaining of partial dentures. Unfortunately, not all can be included without devoting considerable space to the history and development of parital denture re-

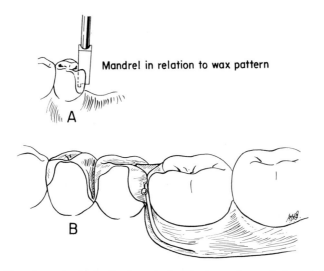

Fig. 115. The Neurohr spring-lock attachment. **A,** The tapered mandrel used in the surveyor to form the vertical rest. **B,** The spring wire lock soldered to the denture base, engaging a depression in the abutment tooth casting.

---

*From Mann, A. W.: The Lower Distal Extension Partial Denture Using the Hart-Dunn Attachment, J. Pros. Den. **8:**282-288, 1958.
†Williams hook attachment, Williams Gold Refining Co., Buffalo, N. Y.

taining devices. Also, the use of patented retaining devices and precision techniques falls in the same limited category as the internal attachment prosthesis and is, for economic and technical reasons, available to only a small percentage of those patients needing partial denture service.

Neurohr Spring-Lock Attachment. One of the earlier attempts at eliminating partial denture clasp and at the same time providing adequate extracoronal retention was the spring wire lock system of attachment devised by Dr. F. G. Neurohr and patented in 1930 (Fig. 115). The Neurohr method employs tapered

Fig. 116. The Sherer spring-lock attachment. The tapered male, **A**, attached to the partial denture, slides into the counterpart female at **A1**, which is part of the abutment casting. When these are firmly in place, they are held by the spring lock, **B**, attached to the male, which engages a seat, **B1**, ground into the gold faceplate of the abutment casting. (Courtesy J. F. Jelenko & Co., Inc., New York, N. Y.)

vertical rests retained within the contours of the abutment tooth. A single buccal clasp arm engages an undercut in the abutment casting and locks the partial denture in place. Occlusal stress is transmitted to the abutment tooth in a vertical direction. However, without an external embracing arm on the lingual surface of the abutment tooth or teeth, some distal tipping force may be applied to the abutment when this attachment is used with a free-end denture, because of the locking effect of the tapered rest seat. For this reason, the Neurohr attachment is usually used in conjunction with multiple abutments splinted together or in conjunction with a stress breaker.

Sherer Spring-Lock Attachment. The Sherer spring-lock attachment also uses a tapered vertical rest but utilizes a dovetail rather than a locking seat to prevent displacement (Fig. 116). This attachment was developed by Dr. J. W. Sherer in 1938. An L-shaped flat spring arm is soldered close to the keyed rest where it engages an undercut in the abutment casting.

Clark Attachment. The Clark method of attachment, developed by Dr. E. B. Clark in 1938, makes use of the Neurohr-Williams rest shoe, which provides a thin-gauge platnium box for the tapered Neurohr-type rest. The rest shoes are placed in the several abutment castings with the aid of a mandrel held in the surveyor related to the master cast according to a predetermined path of insertion. This differs little from the original Neurohr technique and the technique for plac-

Fig. 117. The Neurohr-Williams shoe No. 2 with step and corresponding mandrel and a unilateral view of the skeleton of a lower bilateral distal extension partial denture using the Neurohr shoe as a precision rest. A, Lingual bar. B, Lingual clasp arm. C, Male portion of the attachment which is cast as part of the skeleton. (Courtesy Williams Gold Refining Co., Inc., Buffalo, N. Y.)

Fig. 118. Bilateral dowel rest attachments used on a Kennedy Class I (bilateral distal extension) cast gold partial denture skeleton. **A,** Stabilizing bar. **B,** Lug rest which fits into notch **F** of the abutment. **C,** Slit made with a gold saw to provide spring for the stabilizing bar. **D,** Boss which fits into round recess **H** of the abutment. **E,** Dowel which fits into well **G** of the abutment. **F,** Notch into which the lug rest fits. **G,** Well into which dowel fits. **H,** Round recess into which the boss fits. (From Thompson, M. J.: Solution for Specific Problems in Replacing Missing Teeth With Partial Dentures, Illinois State Dental Society's Seminar Manual, 1957.)

ing other types of internal attachments. Rather than use a spring lock for retention, however, a lingual clasp arm on the denture casting is used to engage an undercut that has been created in the abutment casting on the side of the tooth away from the tapered rest (Fig. 117). Thus, occlusal support, stability, and retention are provided without the use of a visible clasp arm. Some tipping of the abutment tooth is possible when this attachment is used in conjunction with a free-end base denture, thus imposing the same limitations to the use of this attachment as other combinations utilizing internal attachments. All of these are most applicable to tooth-borne restorations and should be used with free-end dentures only when some type of stress breaker is used in the design of the denture itself or when multiple splinted abutment crowns are used.

Rybeck* has presented the technique for the use of the Clark attachment in detail. In personal correspondence he has further emphasized the stress-breaking

*Rybeck, S. A.: Simplicity in a Distal Extension Partial Denture, J. Pros. Den. 4:87-92, 1954.

Fig. 119. **A,** Preparations for canine and molar abutment teeth upon which precision dowel rest attachments will be constructed. **B,** Precision dowel rest attachments constructed on canine and molar abutment teeth. Note the tapered nonlocking precision rest seat and dimple recessed in the lingual surface which will be engaged by a corresponding boss on the retentive arm of the denture framework. (From Harris, F. N.: The Precision Dowel Rest Attachment, J. Pros. Den. **5:**43-48, 1955.)

action of this design by pointing out that the sidewalls of the attachment are perpendicular to the fulcrum line and thus permit the partial denture to rotate without placing a distal stress on the abutment tooth. He has also emphasized that the design of the clasp arm should be such that only minimal pressure is applied to the abutment tooth at any time.

Precision Dowel Rest Attachment. Dr. Morris J. Thompson and others have

Fig. 120. A maxillary partial denture framework with nonlocking precision rest and lingual retentive arm originating from the palatal major connector but separated from it with a fine saw cut. Note the boss on the spring arm which engages a corresponding dimple in the abutment restoration. (From Harris, F. N.: The Precision Dowel Rest Attachment, J. Pros. Den. **5:**43-48, 1955.)

developed a modification of the Clark attachment which is called the *precision dowel rest attachment* (Figs. 118, 119, 120, and 121). A boxlike occlusal rest seat is provided in the abutment casting for support of the partial denture, and a dimple is provided on the lingual surface of the abutment casting for the purpose of retention. This dimple is engaged by a boss on a lingual arm on the denture framework, thereby affording retention without the use of a visible clasp arm. The lingual arm is an extension of the major connector, separated from it by a saw cut in the completed casting.

This attachment is most applicable to maxillary partial dentures, where the saw cut may be made in the palatal plate or strap. A stainless steel shim may be used instead of a saw cut to provide the necessary separation, which is then removed from the casting with acid. Flexibility of the retentive arm will be in proportion to its length as determined by the distance the separation is carried into the major connector.

The advantages which are given for this attachment are (1) no contact of the prosthesis with tooth structure, (2) stress-breaking effect, due to the flexibility of the lingual arm engaging the dimple on the abutment casting, (3) hygienic contours, and (4) no visible clasp arms. One of the most obvious disadvantages of this type of attachment is the apparent lack of stabilization against horizontal movement of the partial denture. Abutment torque is avoided by making the rest seat free of any locking effect; but by so doing, since the only external arm is a flexible one, stabilization against horizontal movement may be almost totally absent. Thus, as with most stress-breaker designs, the edentulous ridge is called upon to resist horizontal movement of the prosthesis unaided by any rigid components located on the abutment teeth.

Coil Spring Attachment. Lenchner, Handlers, and Weissman have recently developed a spring retaining device for partial dentures, available as the *TACH E-Z coil spring attachment.* This is a prefabricated device consisting of a metal cylinder which contains a coil spring, a T-shaped cylindrical bar, and an adjustable screw collar. There is an opening in one end of the cylinder through which a portion of the bar protrudes under the action of the spring. This action

Fig. 121. A, Schematic drawing of precision dowel rest preparation in a lower premolar full crown (buccal view). B, Schematic drawing of proximal view of precision dowel rest preparation and lingual dimple in a lower left premolar full crown. C, Schematic drawing of a lingual view of the precision dowel rest attachment. The spring arm terminating in a boss which engages a dimple in the abutment crown is separated from the major connector by a saw cut, or a split lingual bar is cast around a metal shim which is later eliminated with acid. (Courtesy Dr. R. C. Van Dam.)

is limited by the screw collar that is set in the opening of the cylinder through which the bar protrudes. (Figs. 122 and 123.)

The attachment is either soldered or welded to the metal partial denture framework. It is set in such a position so that the tip of the bar protrudes and fits into a receptable (dimple) prepared in the abutment casting. When used with unrestored abutments, the tip of the bar engages the natural undercut of the tooth and requires no receptacle. However, in either case it is necessary to have an opposing occlusal rest in the opposite proximo-occlusal position from the attachment. The receptacle in the abutment casting is located and formed after the

CYLINDER _____

SCREW COLLAR _____

COILED SPRING _____

T-SHAPED BAR _____

ATTACHMENT
ASSEMBLED _____

Fig. 122. A detailed diagram of the modified coil spring attachment. (From Lenchner, N. H., Handlers, M., and Weissman, B.: A Modification of a Special Retaining Device for Partial Dentures, J. Pros. Den. **8:**973-980, 1958.)

denture framework is completed rather than being established previously as with the precision dowel rest attachment of Thompson.

The advantages claimed for this device are as follows:

1. The device maintains its relation to the abutment during function.

2. No part of the device extends onto the labial or buccal surfaces of the abutment teeth.

3. No special preparation of the abutment is necessary (although crown restorations are preferable); the use of prepared abutments and castings is optional.

4. It is unnecessary to overbuild abutment castings.

5. It can be used with very short abutments.

6. Reduction of contact area reduces the susceptibility to caries (on unprotected abutments).

7. Adjustments are rarely, if ever, necessary.

8. All parts are readily adjustable, removable, and replaceable.

9. Cleanliness is easily maintained by the patient. The exposed portion is readily accessible to brushing.

10. Insertion and removal of the denture is easy.

11. It is impossible for the patient to distort the denture during insertion and removal.

12. Adequate stabilization against horizontal movement is provided by a lingual stabilizing arm.

The disadvantages of the coil spring attachment are as follows:

1. The total cost will exceed that of a clasp-retained partial denture.

2. Proximal occlusal rests and guiding planes are not used with this device. However, proximal guiding planes are much more essential to clasp retention,

Fig. 123. **A,** A veneer crown designed for use with the coil spring attachment. **B,** The bar of the retaining device, which is attached to the framework, protrudes and engages a receptacle prepared in an abutment tooth casting; or it may engage a natural tooth undercut. **C,** A diagram of the device in the denture base. Note the relationship with the lingual stabilizing arm and the occlusal rest. **D,** An abutment casting, showing the relation of the rest seat and the inset for the lingual stabilizing arm. (From Lenchner, N. H., Handlers, M., and Weissman, B.: A Modification of a Special Retaining Device for Partial Dentures, J. Pros. Den. **8:**973-980, 1958.)

and the presence of a precision rest on the opposite side of the tooth from the retainer, plus paralleled lingual surfaces above a lingual shoulder, should provide all the stabilization and reciprocation needed.

3. The movable bar may eventually accumulate debris and clog. However, the device may be adjusted or disassembled for cleaning if necessary.

The laboratory technique for the use of the coil spring attachment is provided by the manufacturer. This attachment merits further consideration, and with some modifications it may prove to be a very satisfactory type of retainer for partial dentures, since it avoids a display of metal yet provides retention against reasonable dislodging forces.

Indirect retainers

Movement of the base of an entirely tooth-borne partial denture *toward* the edentulous ridge is prevented by occlusal rests placed on the abutment teeth located at each end of each edentulous space. Presuming that the denture framework is rigid and the occlusal rests are properly placed, occlusal forces are transmitted directly to the abutment teeth through the occlusal rests placed on those teeth. Movement of the base *away* from the edentulous ridge is prevented by the action of the direct retainers on the same abutment teeth. Horizontal movement of the partial denture and longitudinal rotational movement of the denture base are prevented by stabilizing components on the same abutment teeth plus any auxiliary abutments contacted for purposes of stabilization. Rotation of the tooth-borne partial denture is therefore nonexistent.

In contrast, all Kennedy Class I and Class II partial dentures, having one or more free-end bases, are not totally tooth supported; neither are they completely retained by bounding abutments. Any Class III or Class IV partial denture that does not have adequate abutment support falls in the same category. These latter derive some support from the edentulous ridge and therefore have a composite support from both teeth and ridge tissues.

Movement of a free-end base *toward* the ridge tissues will be proportionate to the quality of those tissues, the accuracy of the denture base, and the total functional load applied. Movement of a free-end base *away* from the ridge tissues will occur either as a rotational movement about an axis or as displacement of the entire denture. The forces that tend to displace any denture are also the forces that cause rotation of a free-end partial denture.

Denture Rotation About an Axis. Presuming that direct retainers are functioning to prevent total displacement, thus holding the occlusal rests in their seats, rotational movement will occur about an axis as the free-end base or bases lift away from the underlying tissues. This axis is an imaginary line drawn through the occlusal rest areas of the two principal abutments. It is called the *fulcrum line,* being the axis of rotation upon which denture movement occurs as the free end moves toward or away from the underlying ridge tissues.

The fulcrum line is identified on a Class I (Kennedy) partial denture as passing through the occlusal rest areas of the most posterior abutment on either side of the arch (Fig. 124, *A* and *B*). On a Class II partial denture the fulcrum line is always diagonal, passing through the occlusal rest area of the abutment on the free-end side and the occlusal rest area of the most distal abutment on the other side (Fig. 124, *C*). If a modification area is present on that side, the additional abutment lying between the two principal abutments may be used for support of the indirect retainer, if it is far enough removed from the fulcrum line (Fig. 124, *D*). In a Class IV partial denture the fulcrum line passes through the two abutments adjacent to the single edentulous space (Fig. 124, *E* and *F*). In a tooth-and-tissue-supported Class III partial denture, the fulcrum line is determined by considering the weaker abutment as nonexistent and that end of the base as being a free end (Fig. 124, *G* and *H*).

Movement of the denture about the fulcrum line is prevented by units of the partial denture framework which are located on definite tooth rests on the opposite side of the fulcrum line from the free-end base. These should be placed as far as possible from the free-end base so as to have the best possible leverage advantage against lifting of the free-end base. Such units are called indirect retainers.

An indirect retainer consists of one or more tooth rests and their supporting minor connectors. While it is customary to identify the entire assembly as the indirect retainer, it should be remembered that it is the tooth rest that is actually the indirect retainer, united to the major connector by a minor connector. This is to avoid interpreting any contact with tooth inclines as being part of the indirect retainer. *An indirect retainer should be placed as far from the free-end base as possible, in a prepared rest seat on a tooth capable of supporting its function.*

While the most effective location of an indirect retainer is frequently in the vicinity of an incisor tooth, that tooth may not be strong enough to support an indirect retainer and may have steep inclines which cannot be favorably altered to support a rest. In such case, the nearest canine tooth or the mesial occlusal surface of the first premolar may be the best location, despite the fact that it is not as far removed from the fulcrum line. Wherever possible, two indirect retainers closer to the fulcrum line are then used to compensate for the compromise in distance.

Factors Influencing Effectiveness of an Indirect Retainer. The factors influencing the effectiveness of an indirect retainer are as follows:

1. The effectiveness of the direct retainers. Unless the principal occlusal rests are held in their seats by the action of the direct retainers, rotation about the fulcrum line will not occur and therefore an indirect retainer cannot act to prevent lifting of the free-end base away from the tissues.

2. The distance from the fulcrum line. Three areas must be considered:

(a) The length of the free-end base.

(b) The location of the fulcrum line.

(c) How far beyond the fulcrum line the indirect retainer is placed.

3. The rigidity of the connectors supporting the indirect retainer. All connectors must be rigid if the indirect retainer is to function as intended.

4. The effectiveness of the supporting tooth surface. The indirect retainer must be placed on a definite rest where slippage or tooth movement will not

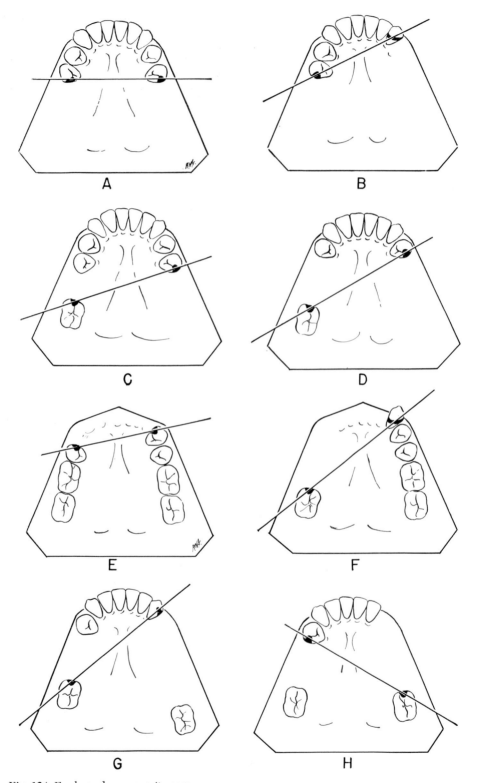

Fig. 124. For legend see opposite page.

occur. Tooth inclines and weak teeth should never be used for the support of indirect retainers.

Auxiliary Functions of an Indirect Retainer. In addition to preventing movement of a free end away from the tissues, an indirect retainer may serve the following purposes. These are auxiliary functions of an indirect retainer.

1. It tends to reduce anteroposterior tilting leverages on the principal abutments. This is particularly important where an isolated tooth is being used as abutment, a situation that should be avoided whenever possible. Ordinarily, proximal contact with the adjacent tooth prevents such tilting of an abutment as the base lifts away from the tissues.

2. Contact of its minor connector with vertical tooth surfaces aids in stabilization against horizontal movement of the denture. Such tooth surfaces, when made parallel to the path of insertion, may also act as auxiliary guiding planes

3. Anterior teeth supporting indirect retainers are splinted against lingual movement.

4. It may act as an auxiliary occlusal rest to support a portion of the major connector. For example, a lingual bar may be supported against settling into the tissues by the indirect retainer acting as an auxiliary occlusal rest. One must be able to differentiate between an auxiliary occlusal rest placed for reasons of support for a major connector, one placed for the purpose of indirect retention, and one serving a dual purpose. Some auxiliary occlusal rests are added solely for the purpose of providing occlusal rest support to a segment of the denture and should not be confused with indirect retention

Forms of Indirect Retainers. The indirect retainer may take any one of several forms. All are effective in proportion to their *support* and the *distance from the fulcrum line they are placed.*

Auxiliary Occlusal Rest. The most frequently used indirect retainer is an auxiliary occlusal rest located on an occlusal surface as far away from the free-end base as possible. In a mandibular Class I this is usually on the mesial marginal ridge of the first premolar on each side (Fig. 125). The longest perpendicular to the fulcrum line would be in the vicinity of the central incisors which are too weak and have lingual surfaces that are too perpendicular to support an occlusal rest. Bilateral rests on the first premolar are quite effective, even though located closer to the axis of rotation.

Fig. 124. The fulcrum line found in various types of partially edentulous arches. **A** and **B**, In a Class I arch the fulcrum line passes through the occlusal rest areas of the most posterior abutments. **C**, In a Class II arch the fulcrum line is diagonal, passing through the occlusal rest areas of the abutment on the free-end side and the most posterior abutment on the opposite side. **D**, If an abutment tooth anterior to a modification space lies far enough removed from the fulcrum line, it may be used effectively for the support of an indirect retainer. **E** and **F**, In a Class IV arch the fulcrum line passes through the two abutments adjacent to the single edentulous space. **G**, In a Class III arch with a posterior tooth on one side, which will eventually be lost, the fulcrum line is considered the same as though the posterior tooth were not present. Thus, its loss at some future date will not necessitate altering the design of the partial denture. **H**, In a Class III arch with nonsupporting anterior teeth, the adjacent edentulous area is considered to be a free end, with a diagonal fulcrum line passing through the two principal abutments as in a Class II arch.

Fig. 125. The most common location for indirect retainers for a Kennedy Class I (bilateral free-end) partial denture. The greatest distance from the axis of rotation (fulcrum line) would fall on the incisor teeth, which are ill-suited to provide adequate support without tooth movement and/or slippage of the retainer. Dual occlusal rests on prepared rest seats at the mesial marginal ridge of the first premolars provide effective indirect retention with optimal tooth support. (**A**, From McCracken, W. L.: Contemporary Partial Denture Designs, J. Pros. Den. 8:71-84, 1958.)

Fig. 126. Two examples of indirect retention used in conjunction with a palatal plate. In either case, a secondary function of the auxiliary occlusal rests is to prevent settling of the anterior portion of the palatal plate.

The same principle applies to any maxillary Class I partial denture where indirect retainers are used. Bilateral rests on the mesial marginal ridge of the first premolars are almost always used in preference to rests on incisor teeth (Fig. 126). Not only are they effective without jeopardizing the weaker single-rooted teeth but also interference to the tongue is far less when the minor connector can be placed in the embrasure between canine and premolar instead of anterior to the canine teeth.

Maxillary Class I partial dentures with wide palatal coverage do not usually require indirect retainers. This will be discussed under *direct-indirect retention*.

Indirect retainers for Class II partial dentures are usually placed on the mesial marginal ridge of the first premolar tooth on the opposite side of the arch from the free end (Fig. 127). Bilateral rests are seldom indicated except where an auxiliary occlusal rest is needed for support of the major connector or where the prognosis of the distal abutment is poor and provision must be made for later conversion to a Class I partial denture should that tooth be lost.

Where full palatal coverage is used with a maxillary partial denture, an indirect retainer may not be needed, but, again, an auxiliary rest may be needed for support of a corner of the major connector. One must be able to differentiate, by its location in relation to the fulcrum line, whether or not an auxiliary rest is needed primarily as an indirect retainer or as auxiliary support.

Canine Extensions From Occlusal Rests. Occasionally, a finger extension from a premolar rest is placed on the unprepared lingual slope of the adjacent canine tooth (Fig. 128). The purpose of such an extension is to add to the effectiveness of the indirect retainer by increasing the distance from the fulcrum line. This is particularly applicable where a first premolar must serve both as a primary abutment and as support for an indirect retainer. The distance anterior to the ful-

Fig. 127. A lower Class II design utilizing embrasure clasping on the nonedentulous side. The indirect retainer on the distal marginal ridge of the rotated first premolar is favorably located in relation to the fulcrum line. Note the use of a wrought-wire retentive clasp arm on the buccal side of the free-end abutment.

Fig. 128. A lower Class I design utilizing continuous clasping for horizontal stabilization. The effective indirect retention is on the rest seat prepared on the mesial marginal ridge of each first premolar, made still more effective by a finger extension onto the canine. Continuous clasping is not necessary for indirect retention but is added usually where weak abutment teeth will benefit from its splinting effect.

crum line is only the distance between mesial and distal occlusal rests on the same tooth. This may be increased almost the width of one tooth by the canine extension. In this instance, although the extension rests on an inclined plane, it is used in conjunction with a terminal rest on the mesial marginal ridge of the premolar tooth. Tipping leverage on the canine tooth is thus avoided. *Even when not used as indirect retainers, canine extensions, secondary lingual bars, and lingual aprons should never be used without terminal rests because of the resultant forces effective when they are placed on inclined planes alone.*

Canine Rests. Where the mesial marginal ridge of the first premolar is too close to the fulcrum line or the teeth are lapped so that it is not accessible, a rest on the adjacent canine tooth may be used. Such a rest may be made more effective by placing the minor connector in the embrasure anterior to the canine, either curving back onto a prepared cingulum rest seat or extending to a mesioincisal rest as an embrasure hook. The same types of canine rests as previously outlined may be used, which are the cingulum rest, the circumferential lingual shoulder, or the incisal rest (see occlusal rests on canine teeth, Chapter 8).

Secondary Lingual Bars (Kennedy Bars; Continuous Clasps) and Lingual Aprons. Technically, these are not indirect retainers, since they rest on unprepared lingual inclines of anterior teeth. The indirect retainers are actually the terminal rests at either end, in the form of auxiliary occlusal rests or canine rests.

In Class I and Class II partial dentures, a secondary lingual bar or lingual apron may extend the effectiveness of the indirect retainer if used with a terminal rest at each end. In tooth-borne partial dentures, they are placed for other reasons but always with terminal rests. (See Major Connectors; the lingual apron, Chapter 7.)

In Class I and Class II partial dentures especially, a secondary lingual bar or the superior border of the lingual apron should never be placed above the middle third of the teeth, so as to avoid orthodontic movement during the rotation of a free-end denture. This is not so important where the six anterior teeth are in nearly a straight line, but when the arch is narrow and tapering, a bar or apron on anterior teeth extends well beyond the terminal rests, and orthodontic movement of those teeth is more likely. While these are intended primarily to stabilize weak anterior teeth, they may have the opposite effect if not used with discretion.

Modification Areas. Occasionally, the occlusal rest on a secondary abutment in a Class II partial denture may be used also as an indirect retainer. This will depend upon how far from the fulcrum line the secondary abutment is located.

The primary abutments in a Class II, modification 1, partial denture are the abutment adjacent to the free end and the most distal abutment on the tooth-borne side. The fulcrum line is a diagonal axis between the principal occlusal rest areas of these two abutments, disregarding any auxiliary occlusal rests which may be present on the same teeth.

The anterior abutment on the tooth-borne side is a secondary abutment, serving to support and retain one end of the tooth-borne segment, as well as adding horizontal stabilization to the denture. If the modification space were not present, as in an unmodified Class II arch, auxiliary occlusal rests and bracing

Fig. 129. An upper Class II, modification 1, partial denture. The fulcrum line is from the mesial rest on the second premolar to the mesioincisal rest on the canine on the free-end side. The only effective indirect retention is at the incisal rest on the mesial surface of the opposite canine. The auxiliary occlusal rest on the molar adds horizontal stabilization and prevents settling of the posterior palatal bar but cannot act as an indirect retainer because it lies posterior to the axis of rotation.

Fig. 130. An upper Class II partial denture design with indirect retainer located favorably in relation to the fulcrum line. An additional function of the auxiliary occlusal rest is to prevent tissueward movement of that portion of the palatal plate. Note the use of a bar clasp on the free-end abutment engaging an undercut adjacent to the free end. This design utilizes a full metal base with nailhead retention and an undercut finishing line all around.

components would still be essential to the design of the denture. But the presence of a modification space conveniently provides an abutment tooth for both retention and support—so much so, in fact, that a restorable but questionable tooth is sometimes removed to provide such a space in preference to embrasure clasping.

If the occlusal rest on the secondary abutment lies far enough from the fulcrum line, it may serve adequately as an indirect retainer. Its dual function, then, is both tooth support for one end of the modification area and support for an indirect retainer. The most typical example is a distal occlusal rest on a first premolar, where second premolar and first molar are missing and the second molar serves as one of the primary abutments. The longest perpendicular to the fulcrum line falls in the vicinity of the first premolar, making the location of the indirect retainer nearly ideal.

On the other hand, if only one tooth, such as a first molar, is missing on the modification side, the occlusal rest on the second premolar abutment is too close to the fulcrum line to be very effective. In such case, an auxiliary occlusal rest on the mesial marginal ridge of the first premolar is needed, both for indirect retention and as support for an otherwise unsupported major connector.

Support for a modification area extending anteriorly to a canine abutment is obtained by any one of the accepted canine rest forms, as previously outlined. In this case, the canine tooth provides nearly ideal indirect retention, and support for the major connector as well.

Rugae Support. Some authorities consider coverage of the rugae area of the maxillary arch as a form of indirect retainer, since the rugae area is firm and usually well situated to provide indirect retention for a Class I denture. While it is true that broad coverage over the rugae area can conceivably provide such support, the facts remain that tissue support is less effective than positive tooth support and that rugae coverage is undesirable if it can be avoided.

The use of rugae support for indirect retention is usually part of a palatal horseshoe design. Since posterior retention is usually inadequate in this case, the requirements for indirect retention are probably greater than can be satisfied by tissue support alone. On the other hand, if adequate palatal coverage posteriorly is used, there is no need for such indirect retention.

Direct-Indirect Retention. In the mandibular arch, retention from the free-end base alone is usually inadequate to prevent lifting of the base away from the tissues. Perhaps the only exception to this is where cast gold bases are used. Forces of gravity acting upon a heavy metal base may be sufficient to prevent lifting and thereby eliminate the need for indirect retention. It is questionable, however, whether or not such a constant weight against living tissues is physiologically acceptable.

In the maxillary arch, where only anterior teeth remain, full palatal coverage is always necessary. In fact, with any Class I partial denture extending distally from the premolar teeth, except where a maxillary torus prevents its use, palatal coverage may be used to advantage. While full coverage may be in the form of a resin base, the added retention and lesser bulk of the cast metal palate makes the latter preferable (see Major Connectors; the palatal strap or palatal plate, Chapter 7).

If retention from a cast palatal strap or palatal plate will provide sufficient direct retention to prevent movement of the base away from the tissues, despite forces of gravity and other dislodging forces, separate indirect retention may not be necessary (Figs. 68 and 72). This is called *direct-indirect retention.*

Reaction of Tissues to Metallic Coverage. The reaction of tissues to metallic coverage has been the subject of some controversy between oral pathologists and prosthodontists. Particular areas over which the controversy is concerned are gingival crossings and broad areas of metal contact with tissues.

From the prosthodontic viewpoint, if oral tissues may not be safely covered with the framework of removable partial dentures, then all parts of the partial denture resting on or crossing soft tissues jeopardize the health of those tissues. If this is true, it is because of several reasons, none of which is the fact of coverage alone.

First of these is *pressure due to lack of support.* If relief over gingival crossings and other areas of contact with tissues which are incapable of supporting the prosthesis is inadequate, then impingement of those tissues is inevitable. Impingement will likewise occur if the denture settles due to loss of tooth support. This may be due to failure of the occlusal rest areas as a result of improper design, caries involvement, or the flow of amalgam alloy restorations, or to intrusion of abutment teeth under occlusal loading. It is the responsibility of the prosthodontist to provide and maintain adequate relief and adequate occlusal support.

Settling of the denture may also result in pressure elsewhere in the arch, such as beneath major connectors. Again, the cause of settling must be prevented or corrected if it becomes manifest. Fisher has shown that pressure alone may cause a nonspecific effect on tissues, which has been mistaken for allergic response or the effect of coverage. Pressure then must be avoided whenever oral tissues must be covered or crossed by elements of the partial denture.

The second reason is *uncleanliness.* It is known that tissues respond unfavorably to an accumulation of food debris and to bacterial enzymes. Coverage of oral tissues with dentures that are not kept clean results in irritation of those tissues, not because of the fact that they are covered but because of the accumulation of irritating factors. This has lead to a misinterpretation of the effect of tissue coverage by prosthetic restorations.

A third explanation of unfavorable tissue response to coverage is the *amount of time the denture is worn.* It is apparent that mucous membrane reverts to connective tissue if isolated from the oral environment for a long enough period of time. Evidence of this is the appearance of tissue, once mucous membrane, beneath the pontics of fixed bridges. A raw, denuded surface is visible upon removal of the fixed restoration. The same thing can occur beneath removable prosthetic restorations if they are allowed to remain against the tissues long enough.

Some patients become so accustomed to wearing a removable restoration that they neglect to remove it often enough to give the tissues any respite from constant contact. This is frequently true where anterior teeth are replaced by the partial denture and the individual will not allow the restoration to be out of the mouth at any time except in the privacy of the bathroom during toothbrushing.

The fact remains that living tissue should not be covered all of the time or changes in those tissues will occur. Partial dentures should not be worn at night, so that the tissues may rest and be returned to a normal environment at least several hours in the twenty-four hours. Clinical experience with the use of lingual aprons, palatal straps, and palatal plates has shown conclusively that when factors of pressure, cleanliness, and time are controlled, tissue coverage is not in itself detrimental to the health of oral tissues.

Denture bases and stress breakers

DENTURE BASES

The purposes of the denture base is to support the supplied teeth and to effect the transfer of occlusal stresses to the supporting oral structures.

Although its primary purpose is related to masticatory function, the denture base may also add to the cosmetic effect of the replacement, particularly where modern techniques for tinting and the reproducing of natural-looking contours are used. Most of the modern techniques for creating naturalness in complete denture bases are applicable equally well to partial denture bases.

Still another function of the denture base is the stimulation, by massage, of the underlying tissues of the residual ridge. Some vertical movement occurs with any denture base, even those supported entirely by abutment teeth due to the physiologic movement of those teeth under function. It is clearly evident that oral tissues placed under functional stress within their toleration limits maintain their form and tone better than similar tissues suffering from disuse. The term *disuse atrophy* is applicable to both periodontal tissues and the tissues of a residual ridge.

Functions of the Tooth-Supported Partial Denture Base. Denture bases differ in functional purpose and in the material of which they are made. In a tooth-borne prosthesis, the denture base is primarily a span between two abutments supporting artificial occlusal surfaces. Thus, occlusal forces are transferred directly to the abutment teeth through occlusal rests. Also, the denture base and the supplied teeth serve to prevent horizontal migration of the teeth in the partially edentulous arch and vertical migration of teeth in the opposing arch.

Where only posterior teeth are being replaced, esthetics is usually a secondary consideration. On the other hand, where anterior teeth are replaced, esthetics may be of primary importance. But except for esthetic considerations, the tooth-borne partial denture base is essentially a framework supporting occlusal surfaces. Theoretically, occlusal surfaces alone would accomplish masticatory efficiency and maintain the relative position of the natural teeth but would lack desirable esthetics, create undesirable food traps, and deprive the tissues of the stimulation by a massage that they would receive from an accurate denture base. The reasons, then, for providing more than only the necessary support for occlusal surfaces in a tooth-borne denture are (1) esthetics, (2) cleanliness, and (3) stimulation of the underlying tissues.

Functions of the Free-End Partial Denture Base. In a free-end partial denture, the denture bases, other than those in tooth-supported modifications, must contribute to the support of the denture. Close to the free-end abutment, only a framework supporting occlusal surfaces is necessary. But farther from the abutment the support from the underlying ridge tissues becomes increasingly important. Maximum support from the residual ridge may be obtained only by using broad, accurate denture bases which spread the occlusal load equitably over the entire area available for such support. This is accomplished through the accuracy of the impression registration and the accuracy of fit of the denture base. It is a principle as old as the snowshoe—that broad coverage furnishes the best support with the least load per unit area. Support should therefore be the primary consideration in selecting, designing, and fabricating a free-end partial denture base. Of secondary importance, but to be considered nevertheless, are esthetics, stimulation of the underlying tissues, and oral cleanliness.

In addition to their difference in functional purpose, denture bases differ in material of construction. This is related to their function because of the need for future rebasing in one instance and not in the other.

Since the tooth-supported base has an abutment tooth at each end upon which an occlusal rest has been placed, future relining or rebasing will not be necessary to re-establish support. Relining is necessary only when tissue changes have occurred beneath the tooth-borne base to the point that poor esthetics and the accumulation of debris result. For these reasons alone, tooth-borne bases made soon after extractions should be made of a material that permits later relining. Such materials are the denture resins, the most common of which are copolymer methyl methacrylate resins. Other materials, such as styrene and vinyl-acrylic resins, may also be satisfactorily added to for the purpose of relining.

Resin bases are attached to the partial denture framework by means of a retentive framework so designed that a space exists between it and the underlying tissues of the residual ridge (Fig. 131). A blockout of at least 28-gauge thickness over the master cast is used to create a raised platform on the investment cast upon which the pattern for the retentive frame is formed. Thus, after casting, that portion of the retentive framework to which the resin base will be attached will stand away from the tissue surface sufficiently to permit a flow of resin base material beneath.

The retentive framework should be embedded in the base material with sufficient thickness of resin to allow for relieving, should this become necessary during denture adjustment over tender areas or during rebasing procedures. Thickness is also necessary to avoid weakness and subsequent fracture of the resin base material surrounding the metal framework.

The use of plastic mesh patterns in forming the retentive framework is gen-

Fig. 131. An upper Class II, modification 1, design utilizing a full metal base on the modification side and retention for a resin base on the free-end side. Note the design of the undercut finishing line on the free-end side, parallel to the crest of the edentulous ridge.

Fig. 132. The replaced lateral incisor and canine are abutted to the residual ridge for better esthetics. Occasionally the first premolar is treated similarly, depending on how visible this tooth is. Note that the cast has been scraped to assure close contact of the abutted teeth with the residual ridge.

erally less satisfactory than a more open framework. Less weakening of the resin by the embedded framework results from the use of the more open form. Pieces of 16- and 18-gauge round wax are therefore used to form a ladderlike framework rather than the finer latticework of the mesh pattern. The precise design of the retentive framework is not so important as its effective rigidity and strength when embedded in the resin base—free of interference to future adjustment and open enough to avoid weakening any portion of the attached resin.

The Ideal Denture Base. The requirements for an ideal denture base are as follows:

1. Accuracy of adaptation to the tissues, with low volume change.

2. Dense, nonirritating surface that is capable of receiving and maintaining a good finish.

3. Thermal conductivity.

4. Low specific gravity; lightness in the mouth.
5. Sufficient strength; resistance to fracture or distortion.
6. Self-cleansing factor, or easily kept clean.
7. Esthetic acceptability.
8. Potential for future relining.
9. Low initial cost.

Obviously such an ideal denture base material does not exist; nor is it likely to be developed in the future. However, any denture base—whether of resin or metal and regardless of the method of fabrication—should come as close to this ideal as possible.

Advantages of Metal Bases. Except for those edentulous ridges with recent extractions, metal is preferred to resin for tooth-supported bases because of the several advantages of the metal base. Its principal disadvantage is that it can be rebased only with difficulty, if at all. Nevertheless, the stimulation that it gives to the underlying tissues is so beneficial that it probably prevents some alveolar atrophy that would otherwise occur under a resin base and thereby prolongs the stability of the tissues supporting it. Some of the advantages of a metal base are as follows.

1. *Thermal conductivity.* Temperature changes are transmitted through the metal base to the underlying tissues, thereby helping to maintain the health of those tissues. Freedom of interchange of temperature between the tissues covered and the surrounding external influences (temperature of liquid and solid foods and inspired air) contributes much to the patient's acceptance of a denture and avoids the feeling of the presence of a foreign body. Denture resins, on the other hand, all have insulating properties which prevent interchange of temperature between the inside and the outside of the denture base. (Fig. 133.)

2. *Accuracy and permanence of form.* Cast metal bases, whether of gold or chrome alloys, not only may be cast more accurately than denture resins but also they maintain their accuracy of form without change in the mouth. Internal strains which may be released later to cause distortion are not present. While some resins and some processing techniques are superior to others in accuracy and

Fig. 133. Palatal view of a palatal strap major connector extended to form a partial metal base. Thermal conductivity and other advantages of a metal base are retained while permitting the buccal fullness and esthetic advantages of a resin base.

permanence of form, modern cast alloys are generally superior in this respect. Evidence of this fact is that an additional posterior palatal seal may be eliminated entirely where a cast palate is used, as compared with the need for a definite attempt in this regard when the palate is made of resin. Distortion of a resin base is manifest in the maxillary denture by a distortion away from the palate in the midline and toward the tuberosities on the buccal flanges. The greater the curvature of the tissues, the greater this distortion. Similar distortions occur in a mandibular denture but are less easily detected. Accurate metal castings are not subject to distortion by the release of internal stains as are most denture resins.

Because of its accuracy, the metal base provides an intimacy of contact which contributes considerably to the retention of a denture prosthesis. Sometimes called *interfacial surface tension,* direct retention from a cast denture base is significant in proportion to the area involved. This has been previously mentioned as an important factor in both direct and direct-indirect retention of maxillary appliances. Such intimacy of contact is not possible with resin bases.

Permanence of form of the cast base is also assured due to its resistance to abrasion from denture cleaning agents. Cleanliness of the denture base should be stressed, yet constant brushing of the tissue side of a resin denture base, if effective, inevitably causes some loss of accuracy by abrasion. Intimacy of contact, which was never as great with a resin base as with a metal base, is therefore further jeopardized by cleaning habits. The metal bases, particularly the harder chrome alloys, withstand repeated cleaning without significant changes in surface accuracy.

3. *Cleanliness.* This is listed apart from resistance to abrasion because the inherent cleanliness of the cast base contributes to the health of the tissues regardless of the patient's cleaning habits. Resin bases tend to accumulate mucinous deposits containing food particles, as well as calcareous deposits. Unfavorable tissue reaction to decomposing food particles and bacterial enzymes and to mechanical irritation from calculus results if the denture is not kept mechanically clean. While calculus which must be removed periodically does precipitate on a cast metal base, other deposits do not accumulate as they do on a resin base. For this reason, a metal base is naturally cleaner than a resin base.

4. *Weight and bulk.* Metal alloys may be cast much thinner than resin and still have adequate strength and rigidity. Still less weight and bulk are possible when the denture bases are made of chrome alloys. Cast gold must be given slightly more bulk to provide the same amount of rigidity but may still be made with less thickness than resin materials.

There are times, however, when both weight and thickness may be used to advantage in denture bases. In the mandibular arch, weight of the denture may be an asset in regards to retention, and for this reason a cast gold base may be preferred. On the other hand, extreme loss of residual alveolar bone may make it necessary to add fullness to the denture base to restore normal facial contours and to fill out the buccal pouch with a denture contour that will prevent food from being lost in the cheek and working beneath the denture. In these cases, a resin base may be preferred to the thinner metal base.

In the maxillary arch, a resin base may be preferred to the thinner metal base to provide fullness where needed, such as in buccal flanges or to fill a maxillary pouch buccal to the tuberosities. Resin may also be preferred over the thinner metal base for esthetic reasons. In these several instances, the thinness of the metal base may be of no advantage, but in areas where the tongue and cheek need maximum room, thinness may be desirable.

Denture contours for functional tongue and cheek contact can best be accomplished with resin. Whereas metal bases are usually made thin to minimize bulk and weight, resin bases may be contoured to provide ideal polished surfaces which contribute to the retention of the denture, restore facial contours, and avoid the accumulation of food at denture peripheries. Lingual surfaces are usually made concave, except in the distal palatal area. Buccal surfaces are made convex at gingival margins, over root prominences, and at the periphery to fill the area recorded in the impression. Between the periphery and the gingival contours, the base is made concave to aid in retention and to facilitate the food bolus being returned to the occlusal table during mastication. Such contours prevent food from being lost in the cheek and working under the denture. This cannot usually be accomplished with metal bases.

However, the advantages of a metal base need not necessarily be sacrificed for the sake of esthetics or desirable denture contours where the use of such a base is otherwise indicated. Denture bases may be designed to provide almost total metallic coverage, yet with resin peripheries to avoid a display of metal and to add buccal fullness where needed (Fig. 133). The advantages of thermal conductivity are not necessarily lost by covering a portion of the metal base as long as other parts of the denture are exposed to effect temperature changes through conduction.

Attaching Artificial Teeth to Metal Bases. Artificial teeth may be added to denture bases by several means. Some of these are as follows:

1. *Porcelain or resin denture teeth attached to a metal base with resin.* Retention of the resin to the metal base may be accomplished by nailhead retention, retention loops, or diagonal spurs placed at random. Nailheads should be so placed that they will not interfere with the placement of the teeth on the metal base.

Any junction of resin with metal should be at an undercut finishing line or associated with some retentive undercut. Since only a mechanical attachment exists between metal and resin, every attempt should be made to avoid separation and seepage which results in discoloration and uncleanliness. Denture odors are frequently caused by accretions at the junction of resin with metal where only mechanical union exists. Separation occurring between resin and metal leads eventually to some loosening of the resin base.

2. *Porcelain or resin tube teeth cemented directly to metal bases* (Fig. 45). Some of the disadvantages of this type of attachment are the difficulties in obtaining satisfactory occlusion, lack of adequate contours for functional tongue and cheek contact, and unesthetic display of metal at gingival margins. The latter is avoided when the tooth is butted directly to the ridge, but then the retention for the tooth frequently becomes inadequate.

A modification of this method is the attachment of ready-made resin teeth

Fig. 134. Partial metal bases used with a full palatal plate and "pressed-on" anterior teeth. Attachment of denture with resin is accomplished by diagonal spurs and lingual undercut finishing line. The visible buccal flange will be of resin, yet without sacrificing most of the advantages of a metal base. Support anteriorly is by a mesioincisal rest on a canine and by a lingual ledge prepared on all remaining anterior teeth.

Fig. 135. An upper Class I, modification 2, partial denture replacing four anterior teeth with Steele's facings. Although it is not as esthetically acceptable as "pressed-on" resin teeth, strength of bite and occlusion frequently dictate that this method of replacing anterior teeth be used. Note the occlusal support anteriorly by both occlusal rests on the premolars and lingual ledges prepared on the canine abutments.

to the metal base with acrylic resin of the same shade. This is called *pressing on* a resin tooth and is not the same as using resin for cementation. It is particularly applicable to anterior replacements, where it is desirable to know in advance of making the casting that the shade and contours of the selected tooth will be acceptable. (Fig. 134.) After making a labial index of the position of the teeth, the lingual portion of the tooth then is cut away to make room for retention on the casting. Subsequently, the tooth is attached to the denture with acrylic resin of the same shade. Being done under pressure, the acrylic attachment is comparable to the manufactured tooth in hardness and strength.

Tube or side-groove teeth must be selected in advance of waxing the denture

Fig. 136. An upper Class III, modification 2, partial denture with palatal plate supporting tubed teeth posteriorly and Steele's facings anteriorly. This design is actually an anatomic replica palatal plate extended anteriorly to support anterior replacements. The entire palatal plate should be as thin as mechanically feasible and of uniform thickness, made possible by the Tru-Rugae method. Esthetics dictated the spacing between the incisor teeth, which could not easily have been accomplished with a fixed bridge. Note also the clearance lingual to the premolar abutments. **A,** The wax and plastic pattern for this casting, with a plaster index for positioning anterior Steele's facings. The backings are plastic waxed to the anatomic replica palatal wafer. **B,** The completed casting.

framework. Yet, for best occlusal relationships, jaw relation records should always be made with the denture casting in the mouth. This problem may be solved by selecting tube teeth for width but with occlusal surfaces slightly higher than will be necessary. The teeth are ground to fit the ridge with sufficient clearance beneath for a thin metal base and beveled to accommodate a boxing of metal. If a plastic tube tooth is used, the diatoric hole should be made slightly larger than provided. The casting is completed and tried in, occlusal relationships are recorded, and then the teeth are ground in to harmonious occlusion with the opposing dentition. As will be discussed under occlusal relationships in Chapter 16, artificial posterior teeth on partial dentures should never be used unaltered but rather should be considered material from which occlusal forms may be created to function harmoniously with the remaining natural occlusion.

3. *Resin teeth processed directly to metal bases.* Modern cross-linked copolymers enable the dentist or technician to process acrylic teeth which have satisfactory hardness and abrasion resistance. Occlusion may thus be created without resorting to the modification of ready-made denture teeth (Fig. 137). Recesses in the denture pattern are either carved by hand or created around manufactured teeth which are used only for the purpose of forming the recess in the pattern. Occlusal relations are established in the mouth on the denture framework, and then the teeth are carved and processed in acrylic resin of the proper shade to fit the opposing occlusal record. Better attachment to the metal base than by cementation is thus possible. In addition, unusually long, short, wide, or narrow teeth may be created where necessary to fill spaces not easily filled by the limited selection of ready-made teeth.

Fig. 137. Direct attachment of resin teeth to metal bases. These are waxed to fit the space and opposing occlusion and processed to retention previously provided on the metal framework.

Fig. 138. Functional occlusal surfaces cast with inlay-type gold and cemented to the denture teeth.

Occlusion on resin teeth may be re-established to compensate for wear or settling by reprocessing new acrylic occlusal surfaces at a later date should this become necessary. Distinction should always be made between the need for relining to re-establish occlusion (on a free-end partial denture) or the need for rebuilding occlusal surfaces on an otherwise satisfactory base (on either a tooth-supported or a tooth-and-tissue-supported partial denture).

Re-establishment of occlusion may also be accomplished by placing gold inlays on existing resin teeth. While this may be done also on porcelain teeth, it is very difficult to cut inlay recesses in porcelain teeth, unless air abrasive methods are used. Therefore, if later additions to occlusal surfaces are anticipated, plastic teeth should be used, thereby facilitating the addition of new resin or cast gold surfaces (Fig. 138).

4. *Metal teeth.* Occasionally, a second molar tooth may be replaced as part of the partial denture casting. This is usually done where space is too limited for the attachment of a denture tooth and yet the addition of a second molar is desirable to prevent migration of an opposing second molar. Since the occlusal

surface must be waxed prior to casting, perfect occlusion is not possible. Since metal, particularly a chrome alloy, is abrasion resistant, the area of occlusal contact should be held to a minimum to avoid damage to the periodontium of the opposing tooth and the associated discomfort to the patient. While occlusal adjustment on gold occlusal surfaces is readily accomplished, metal teeth made of chrome alloys are difficult to adjust and are objectionably hard for use as occlusal surfaces. Therefore they should be used only to fill a space and to prevent tooth migration and no more.

Need for Relining. The free-end base differs from the tooth-borne base in several respects, one of which is that it must be made of a material that can be relined or rebased when it becomes necessary to re-establish tissue support for the free-end base. Therefore, resin denture base materials that can be re-lined are generally used.

While there are satisfactory techniques for making free-end partial denture bases of cast metal (see Chapter 15, Support for the Free-End Denture Base), the fact that metal bases are difficult if not impossible to reline limits their use to stable ridges that will change little over a long period of time.

Changes in ridge form over a period of time may not be visible. *Manifestations of change* may be seen, however. One of these is a *loss of occlusion* between the free-end denture base and the opposing dentition, increasing as the distance from the abutment increases. This is proved by having the patient bite on strips of 28-gauge green casting wax, or any similar wax, tapping in *centric occlusion* only. Indentations in a wax strip of known thickness are *quantitative,* whereas marks made with articulating ribbon are only qualitative. In other words, indentations in the wax may be interpreted as being light, medium, or heavy, whereas it is difficult if not impossible to interpret a mark made with articulating ribbon as being light or heavy. In fact, the heaviest occlusal contact may perforate paper articulating ribbon and make a lesser mark than areas of lighter contact. Therefore, the use of any articulating ribbon is of limited value in checking occlusion intraorally. In making occlusal adjustments, articulating ribbon should be used only to indicate *where* to relieve after the *need for relief* has been established by using wax strips of known thickness. Twenty-eight-gauge green or blue casting wax is usually used for this purpose, although the thinner 30-gauge or the thicker 26-gauge wax may also be used for the purpose of better evaluating the clearance between areas not in contact.

Loss of support for a free-end base will result in a loss of occlusal contact between the denture teeth and the opposing dentition and a return to heavy occlusal contact between the remaining natural teeth. Usually, this is an indication that relining is needed to re-establish the original occlusion by re-establishing supporting contact with the residual ridge. It must be remembered, however, that occlusion on a free-end base is sometimes maintained at the expense of migration of the opposing natural teeth. In such case, checking the occlusion alone will not show that settling of the free-end base due to changes in the supporting ridge has occurred. A second manifestation of change must also be observable to justify relining.

This second manifestation of change in the supporting ridge is evidence of rotation about the fulcrum line with the indirect retainers lifting from their seats as the free-end base is pressed against the ridge tissues. Originally, if the free-end base was made to fit the supporting form of the residual ridge (see Functional Impressions in Chapter 15), rotation about the fulcrum line is not visible. At the time the denture is delivered, no teeter-totter should exist when alternating finger pressure is applied to the indirect retainer and the distal end of a free-end base or bases. Following changes in the ridge form, which causes some loss of support, rotation occurs about the fulcrum axis when alternating finger pressure is applied. This is evidence of changes in the supporting ridge that must be compensated for by relining or rebasing.

If occlusal contact has been lost and rotation about the fulcrum line is evident, then relining is indicated. On the other hand, if occlusal contact has been lost without any evidence of denture rotation, and if stability of the denture base is otherwise satisfactory, then reocclusion is the remedy rather than relining. For the latter the original denture base may be used in much the same manner as the original trial base was used to record occlusal relations. Teeth may then be reoccluded to an opposing cast or to an occlusal template, using the original denture teeth, new denture teeth, cast gold occlusal surfaces, or new acrylic resin occlusal surfaces. In any case, new occlusion may be established on the existing bases. Relining in this instance would be the wrong solution to the problem.

More often, however, loss of occlusion is accompanied by settling of the denture base to the extent that rotation about the fulcrum line is manifest. Since relining is the only remedy short of making completely new bases, use of a resin base originally facilitates later relining. For this reason, resin bases are generally preferred for free-end partial dentures.

The question remains as to when, if ever, metal bases with their several advantages may be used for free-end partial dentures. It is debatable as to what type of ridge will be the most likely to remain stable under functional loading without apparent change. Certainly the age and general health of the patient will influence the ability of a residual ridge to support function. Minimal and harmonious occlusion and the accuracy with which the base fits the underlying tissues will influence the amount of trauma that will occur under function. Undoubtedly, the absence of trauma plays a big part in the ability of the ridge to maintain its original form.

The best risk for the use of metal free-end bases is a ridge that has supported a previous partial denture without having become soft, narrowed, or flat. Where such changes have occurred under a previous denture, further change may be anticipated because of the possibility that the oral tissues in question are not capable of supporting a denture base without retrogressive change. Despite every advantage in their favor, there are some such individuals whose ridges respond unfavorably to being called upon to support any denture base.

In other instances, such as where a new partial denture is to be made because of the loss of additional teeth, the ridges may still be firm and healthy. Having previously supported a denture base and having sustained occlusion, bony trabeculae will have become arranged so as to best support vertical and horizontal loading, cortical bone will have been formed, and tissue tone will have become favorable for continued support of a denture base.

Admittedly, there are relatively few instances where the need for future relining of a free-end base need not be considered and metal bases may be used. There are, however, many instances which may be considered borderline. In these, metal bases may be used with full understanding on the part of the patient that a new or rebuilt denture may become necessary in the future should unforeseen tissue changes occur. A technique is given in Chapter 15, which permits replacing metal free-end bases without having to remake the entire denture. This method should be seriously considered any time a free-end partial denture is to be made with a metal base or bases.

For reasons previously outlined, the possibility that tissues will remain healthier beneath a metal base than beneath a resin base may justify its wider use for free-end partial dentures. Through careful treatment planning, better patient education of the problems involved in making a free-end denture, and greater care in the fabrication of the denture bases, metal may be used to advantage in some situations where resin bases are ordinarily used.

STRESS BREAKERS

The previous chapters on component parts of a partial denture have presumed absolute rigidity of all parts of the partial denture framework except the direct retainer. All vertical and horizontal stresses applied to the supplied teeth are thus distributed throughout the supporting portions of the dental arch. Broad distribution of stress is accomplished through the rigidity of the major and minor connectors. The effect of the stabilizing components is also made possible by the rigidity of the connectors.

In a free-end appliance, strain on the abutment teeth is minimized through the use of functional basing, broad coverage, harmonious occlusion, and flexible direct retainers. Retentive clasp arms may be cast only if they engage undercuts on the abutment teeth in such a manner that tissueward movement of the free-end base cannot transmit leverage to the abutment. Otherwise wrought-wire retentive clasp arms should be used because of their greater flexibility. Because of its flexibility, the wrought-wire clasp arm may be said to act as a *stress breaker* between the denture base and the abutment tooth.

A concept of stress-breaking exists, however, which insists upon separating the action of the retaining elements from the movement of the free-end base. Thus, when the term *stress breaker* is used, it is generally applied to a device that allows some movement between the denture base or its supporting framework and the direct retainers, whether they are intracoronal or extracoronal in design.

A stress breaker is also sometimes referred to as an *amortizer*. The term *articulated prosthesis* is also frequently applied to a broken-stress partial denture.

More than thirty years ago Kennedy wrote as follows:

> Since the advent of the cast clasp and the removable bridge, a great number of men have advocated the use of "stress breakers" between their saddles and the clasps. These have been shown to be absolutely essential by dentists who had used

cast clasps for partial dentures. They found that in a short time the teeth to which such clasps were attached loosened, and that this was due mainly to the rigidity of the clasp.

A well-designed round wire clasp is, in itself, a stress breaker, and allows sufficient saddle movement to prevent excessive strain upon the abutment teeth. . . .

In my hands, stress breakers used on partial dentures have permitted so much movement of the saddles, that they produce excessive soreness, and, after many trials, especially after patients have worn them for some time, I found that a greater number of abutment teeth were loosened than where we used the double bar, . . . the "continuous clasp" [what is now known as the secondary lingual bar or Kennedy bar]. It is only where we have too few teeth in the mouth that it is necessary to use some form of specially designed stress breaker between the clasps and saddles.

. . . Clasps should not be made so rigid that they hold the denture in place. We must depend on the inherent stability of the saddles to prevent strain on the teeth. . . . If there are only one or two teeth present, we would not expect these teeth to do the work of fourteen, without excessive strain being placed upon them, and it is in such conditions that some form of stress breaker becomes useful.*

Several partial denture textbooks have little to say about stress breakers, as though to avoid a controversial subject. That the subject is controversial is evidenced by the rigid adherence to their use with apparent success by some, whereas properly designed rigid appliances are routinely used by others without harm to abutments. It is only the improperly designed or ineffectively fabricated rigid appliance that has proved to be harmful to abutment teeth. There is little question that some form of mechanical stress breaker is preferable to a poorly designed and ineffectively fabricated rigid appliance.

It is interesting and significant to note that the development and promotion of stress breaker designs in this country has been largely through the efforts of the commercial dental laboratory. In most instances this has been due to the failure of the dentist to furnish the laboratory with a master cast which provides for adequate denture base support. If the dentist is not inclined to employ carefully contoured abutment retainers that permit the use of proper clasp designs, and is not willing to take the steps necessary to provide maximum support for tissue-supported denture bases, then he probably should utilize one of the stress breaker designs offered by the commercial dental laboratory.

Types of Stress Breakers. Stress breakers may be divided into two groups. In the first group are those having a movable joint between the direct retainer and the denture base. Into this group fall the hinges, sleeves and cylinders, and ball-and-socket devices (some of which are spring-loaded). Being placed between the direct retainer and the denture base, they may permit both vertical movement and hinge action of the free-end base. This serves to prevent direct transmission of tipping forces to the abutment teeth as the base moves tissue-ward under function.

Examples of this group are the various hinges, the Swiss-made Dalbo attachment and the C & M 637 attachment, the ASC 52 attachment, and many others.

---

*From Kennedy, E.: Partial Denture Construction, Brooklyn, 1942, Dental Items of Interest Publishing Co., Inc.

Fig. 139. The D-E hinge-type stress breaker utilizing a vertical stop to limit movement of the denture base away from the tissues. Properly applied, this type of stress breaker permits the effective use of one or more indirect retainers located anterior to the fulcrum line. The trunnion design of the stress breaker also prevents lateral movement, thus assuring a degree of bilateral stability comparable to that of a one-piece framework. (Courtesy Austenal, Inc., Chicago, Ill.)

Fig. 140. The D-E hinge-type stress breaker before and after the resin denture base has been added. Hinge action is limited to tissueward movement only by the presence of a stop bar. (Courtesy Austenal, Inc., Chicago, Ill.)

Fig. 141. A lower Kennedy Class II, modification 1, partial denture utilizing a hinge stress breaker of Baca design. Hinge and vertical movements are permitted by the fact that the action is protected by a metal sleeve rather than being embedded in the resin base material. (Courtesy Ticonium Division of CMP Industries, Inc., Albany, N. Y.)

Most of these attachments are prefabricated, but the laboratory may utilize dual-casting techniques for fabricating the attachment. Due to the rapid wear likely to occur with gold, such attachments are usually made of a harder alloy and therefore are usually machine-made.

The student is referred to two excellent textbooks which describe in detail the use of stress breakers and articulated partial denture designs: (1) *Precision Work for Partial Dentures*, by Alfred A. Steiger and Raoul H. Boitel of Zurich, Switzerland, and (2) *Protesis Parcial Removible* by Adalberto D. Rebossio of Buenos Aires, Argentina. The latter is available in Spanish, only.

The second group includes those designs having a flexible connection between the direct retainer and the denture base. These include the use of wrought-wire connectors, divided major connectors, and other flexible devices for permitting movement of the free-end base (Fig. 142). Included also in this group are those utilizing a movable joint between two major connectors. These are generally fabricated by the laboratory with a dual-casting technique. The earliest of such connectors were double lingual bars of wrought metal, one supporting the clasps and other components and the other supporting and connecting the free-end bases. The two bars were usually but not always united at the midline by binding with fine wire and soldering.

The latter principle is still widely used in the form of split major connectors. Instead of using wrought metal, a single cast connector is made flexible by separating a portion of its length. This may be done by making a saw cut part way through a gold casting with a jeweler's saw or by casting to a thin shim which is then removed, leaving a separation. Although mica and other materials have been used for this purpose, stainless steel is usually used (.02 Truchrome band material), which is then removed by acid. The nature of chrome-cobalt al-

Fig. 142. The stress-breaking effect of a split bar major connector. Vertical and diagonal forces applied to the tissue-supported base must pass anteriorly along the lower bar and then back along the more rigid upper bar to reach the abutment tooth. Thus, tipping forces which would otherwise be transmitted directly to the abutment tooth are dissipated by the flexibility of the lower bar and the distance traveled.

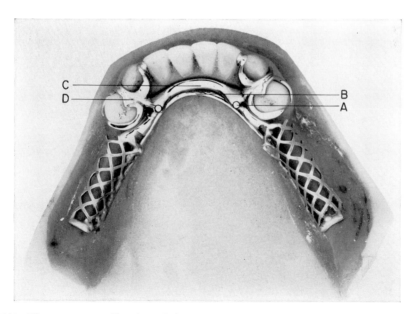

Fig. 143. The conventionally clasped lower partial denture framework with lingual bar connecting the rests and clasps. Circles indicate position of Ballard stress equalizer attachment (ball-and-socket joint). **A,** Location of the Ballard stress equalizers. **B,** 14-gauge round (wrought-wire) stabilizing bar. **C,** Rigid major connector. **D,** Casting which supports the anterior part by means of clasp attachments. (Courtesy Dr. Charles S. Ballard.)

loys permits the making of one casting first and then waxing and casting the second part to the first without union. This facilitates the making of split bars and movable joints with fine precision and nearly imperceptible junction lines. In any case, the resulting flexibility of the major connector acts to prevent direct transmission of forces to the abutment tooth.

Double major connectors must be coupled in some manner so that the two parts of the appliance cannot come apart in the mouth, yet will permit freedom of movement of the denture base. Many ingenious connections have been devised, such as a ball-and-socket device developed by Dr. Charles S. Ballard. This is a Vitallium acetabulum which is waxed into the denture in such a manner that a socket is cast around it which works freely yet prevents separation. (Figs. 143 and 144.)

The principal advantages claimed for partial dentures made with the Ballard stress equalizer attachment are as follows:

1. Occlusal pressures are distributed equally to the edentulous ridges and the supporting abutments.

2. Individual movement of saddle areas is permitted, both perpendicular and lateral, or a combination of both.

3. Torque is eliminated through the action of the universal joints connecting the saddle areas and the body of casting.

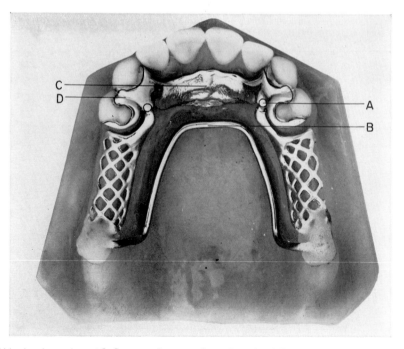

Fig. 144. An upper partial denture framework with palatal bar connecting the rests and clasps, both of which are set into routed portions of the crowns. Circles indicate position of the Ballard stress equalizer attachments. A, Location of the Ballard stress equalizers. B, 14-gauge round (wrought-wire) stabilizing bar. C, Rigid major connector. D, Casting which supports the anterior part by means of clasp attachments. (Courtesy Dr. Charles S. Ballard.)

A

B

Fig. 145. The Ticonium hidden-lock partial denture. **A,** The top half, consisting of a lingual plate, is cast first with a bi-bevel circle formed in the wax pattern. The bottom half is waxed to the upper half on a second investment cast. **B,** The second half is cast to the first. The hidden-lock and split bar are made possible because of the thin oxide shell which forms during the second casting, leaving an almost imperceptible junction line between the two sections. Hinge movement occurs at the circle in the midline. (Courtesy Ticonium, Division of CMP Industries, Inc., Albany, N. Y.)

The equalizer principle may be applied to both upper and lower arches in many different combinations of remaining teeth. It may be used with the conventional lingual bar design or in combination with the continuous or secondary (Kennedy) lingual bar.

Ideally, the Ballard stress equalizer attachment should be placed on a line between the principal abutments, but it may be placed distogingivally to the posterior abutments. Unlike the hinge, which presumably permits vertical movement only, the denture bases may move laterally also, controlled and stabilized by the presence of a 14-gauge wrought-wire functioning as a "second" bar.

Another design utilizing a dual-casting technique is the Ticonium hidden-lock design (Fig. 145). This is a two-piece casting. The top half, which is the major connector supporting the direct retainers and other rigid components, is cast first and the bottom half, which is the connector between the denture bases, is cast to the first. The latter is completely independent of the first except that it is locked in by a circle-type retention, prepared in the wax pattern.

The hidden-lock is created by mechanical means and the split between the two connectors is made possible by the thin oxide shell which forms during the making of the two sections. What appears to be a conventional lingual bar or plate actually is two bars connected by a movable joint at the midline.

Still other devices permit disassembly of the denture by the patient for the purpose of cleaning. All mechanical devices that are free to move in the mouth collect debris and become unclean; therefore, disassembly is a desirable feature whether done daily by the patient or periodically by the dentist (some hinged devices have small screws which may be removed for the purpose of cleaning or adjusting the action of the device).

In addition to the trapping of debris, some split connectors used as stress breakers have been known to pinch the underlying soft tissues on the tongue as they open and close under function. Further, such flexible connectors, especially those made of cast alloys, became fatigued through repeated flexing, resulting in permanent distortion of the denture framework and possible ultimate failure through fracture.

Regardless of their design, all stress breakers effectively dissipate vertical stresses, which is the purpose for which they are used. At the same time their very flexibility or mechanical movement eliminates the horizontal stability at the free-end base which is inherent in a rigid partial denture design. The effectiveness of minor connectors, stabilizing components, occlusal rests, and indirect retainers is either lost or dissipated by the action of the stress breaker. As a result, consideration for the abutments is at the expense of the tissues of the residual ridge. This is evidenced by the fact that the stress-broken denture will often require relief on the tissue side of the buccal flange. Since horizontal stresses cannot be resisted by rigid stabilizing components elsewhere in the arch, the residual ridge is forced to bear those horizontal forces alone. This and the added cost are the most obvious disadvantages to the use of stress breakers in free-end partial denture designs.

Advantages of Stress Breakers. Some of the advantages of the stress-breaking principle may be listed as follows:

1. Since the horizontal forces acting on the abutment teeth are minimized, the alveolar support of these teeth is preserved.

2. By careful choice of the type of flexible connector, it is possible to obtain a balance of stress between the abutment teeth and the residual ridge.

3. Intermittent pressure of the denture bases massages the mucosa, thus providing physiologic stimulation which prevents bone resorption and eliminates the need for rebasing.

4. Should relining be needed but not done, the abutment teeth are not necessarily damaged.

5. Splinting of weak teeth by the denture is made possible despite the movement of a free-end base.

Disadvantages of Stress Breakers. Some of the disadvantages of the stress-breaking principle are as follows:

1. The broken-stress denture is usually more difficult to construct and therefore more costly.

2. Vertical and horizontal forces are concentrated on the residual ridge, resulting in increased ridge resorption. Many stress breaker designs are not well stabilized against horizontal forces. Proponents of broken-stress dentures claim that this is avoided by the intermittent massage which stimulates and promotes better health of the residual ridge.

3. If relining is not done when needed, excessive resorption of the residual ridge may result. This is offset to some extent by the fact that such a denture base is no longer in occlusion and therefore resorption is not progressive.

4. The effectiveness of indirect retainers is reduced or eliminated althogether.

5. The more complicated the prosthesis, the less it may be tolerated by the patient. Spaces between components are sometimes opened up in function, thus trapping food and, occasionally, the tissues of the mouth.

6. Flexible connectors may be bent and distorted by careless handling. Even a slightly distorted connector may induce more stress on the abutment rather than less.

7. Repair and maintenance of any stress breaker is difficult and costly.

Advantages of a Rigid Design. Some of the advantages of the rigid partial denture design may be listed as follows:

1. Mechanically, the framework is easier and less costly to make.

2. Equitable distribution of stress between abutments and the residual ridge(s) is possible with a rigid design.

3. The need for relining the rigid prosthesis is less frequent since the residual ridge does not have to carry the functional load unaided.

4. Indirect retainers and other rigid components may act to prevent rotational movement of the denture and will provide horizontal stabilization not possible when stress breakers are used.

5. By reducing the number of flexible or movable parts, there is less danger of distortion by careless handling on the part of the patient.

6. Moving parts being absent, the prosthesis is more easily kept clean.

Disadvantages of a Rigid Design. Some of the possible disadvantages of the rigid denture design are as follows:

1. Objectionable torque may be applied to the abutment teeth.

2. Rigid continuous clasping may be hazardous where stress breakers are not used.

3. Intracoronal retainers may not be used at all without stress breakers, because they are locked within the abutment and tipping forces would be transmitted directly to the abutment tooth. The only exception is where multiple splinting of abutments, coupled with a minimum of occlusion on the free-end denture base, acts to reduce abutment torque.

4. The use of wrought-wire retentive clasp arms as stress breakers presents some technical difficulties, particularly where high-fusing chrome alloys are used. Wrought wire may be crystallized by improper application of heat during casting or soldering operations, resulting in early fracture. It may also be easily distorted by careless handling, leading to excessive or insufficient retention, or ultimate fracture due to repeated adjustment.

5. If relining is not done when needed, the abutment tooth may bee loosened and suffer permanent periodontal damage due to the repeated application of torque and tipping stresses.

Chapter **12**

Mouth preparations

SURGICAL TREATMENT

Following diagnosis and treatment planning, mouth preparations should be accomplished in a logical sequence. The ultimate goal of mouth preparations is to make the mouth ready for the impression that will produce a master cast upon which the denture will be constructed. Sometimes this involves only modifications to healthy abutment teeth. More often, a rather lengthy sequence of treatment is necessary to prepare the mouth adequately for the partial denture.

Surgical treatment should be done as early as possible to allow for healing while other time-consuming operations are being done. It may consist of one or several of the following procedures:

1. Extraction of teeth diagnosed as unrestorable or detrimental to the design of the partial denture. This includes nonvital teeth and extruded or malposed teeth which cannot be or for some reason are not to be treated by conservative means.

2. Removal of pathologic residual roots and other areas of pathology.

3. Removal of hyperplastic tissues, flabby ridge tissues, and any other treatment that will improve the quality of soft tissue support for the denture bases.

4. Elimination of bony spicules and knife-edge ridges so as to obtain the best possible bony support for the denture bases.

5. Removal of tori and other bony growths that cannot be relieved or bypassed by the design of the denture.

It is not within the scope of this book to discuss surgical or periodontal techniques. Any of the above procedures may be done by the dentist preparing the mouth for the partial denture. While in metropolitan practices many or all of the surgical procedures are frequently referred to the oral surgeon, the average general practitioner is competent to do whatever routine surgical procedures are necessary. Nevertheless, disinclination to do so or lack of confidence in one's ability should not deprive the patient of any treatment that would favor the success of the partial denture.

238

PERIODONTAL TREATMENT

Several phases of periodontal treatment may be necessary prior to beginning prosthetic treatment. It is doubtful, however, if any single phase of periodontal treatment is as important as subgingival scaling combined with adequate home care. Most failures following periodontal treatment are due to a lack of patient cooperation in performing daily massage and oral hygiene measures at home. On the subject of subgingival curettage, Schluger has said, "[subgingival curettage] is a basic technique, the only definitive cure for periodontal disease. It attacks directly the problem of calculus and suppuration which, of course, affects tissue, contour and color. . . . Surgery is a prophylactic, a plastic procedure. . . . But curettage eliminates the disease itself."*

While no attempt at outlining periodontal treatment or techniques is intended, several accepted periodontal measures to be accomplished by the dentist or referred to the periodontal specialist will be discussed briefly.

Periodontal Scaling (Odontexesis). It has been stated previously that a thorough oral prophylaxis should precede, or be done concurrently with, oral diagnosis. Perhaps the term *prophylaxis* is a misleading one, since it implies prophylactic treatment. Denton, in his manual on dental nomenclature, has suggested the use of the term *odontexesis,* which means literally tooth scraping, as a substitute for the broader term *prophylaxis,* which more accurately describes all prophylactic measures used in dentistry. While a thorough cleaning of the teeth does have prophylactic value, it is also therapeutic and, as such, comprises periodontal treatment. Such periodontal treatment is the responsibility of the dentist instigating definitive treatment. It is a poor dentist who is incapable of or disinterested in accomplishing a thorough subgingival scaling for his patient.

Not only is a thorough cleaning of the teeth vital to adequate examination, diagnosis, and prognosis but it is also a very necessary part of mouth preparations that must precede restorative and prosthetic treatment.

Undoubtedly, one of the deterrents to routine periodontal treatment has been the patient's reaction to the fee for "having his teeth cleaned." If, as is frequently the case, he has become accustomed to paying a relatively low fee for "cleaning," he may object strongly to the fee charged for periodontal treatment. This is due entirely to a lack of understanding of the service being rendered.

Experience shows that fee resistance to "oral prophylaxis," especially where it involves considerable time and several appointments, is greater than to any other dental service. At the same time, no phase of dentistry is as unprofitable to the dentist in proportion to the time and skill involved and the significance of the service rendered. This has caused many dentists to avoid doing one of the most valuable dental services he has to offer.

As long as a minimum fee for a routine oral prophylaxis is customary, whether done by dentist or hygienist, both patient education and terminology must make clear the broader service of subgingival curettage and other aspects of periodontal

---

*From Schluger, S. S.: Diagnosis and Treatment of Periodontal Disease, D. Times 1:7, 1958.

treatment. In the latter, the polishing of exposed tooth surfaces is only incidental, whereas polishing may be the major part of a routine prophylaxis.

The number of treatments necessary to complete the entire mouth will depend upon several factors. Among them are the length of the appointments, the edema present, hemorrhage encountered, and the patient's reaction to the trauma of deep scaling. The fee, therefore, must almost always be based upon an hourly rate for such service. If the dentist cannot feel free to charge a just fee for periodontal treatment, he should refer the patient to a periodontist who is in a position to charge for his specialized services. Just as with routine exodontia and minor oral surgery, it is frequently expedient that the services of a specialist be enlisted rather than treatment neglected because of the patient's reluctance to pay the general practitioner or prosthodontist a fair fee for such services.

Elimination of Local Irritating Factors Other Than Calculus. Overhanging margins of amalgam alloy and inlay restorations, overhanging crown margins, and open contacts leading to food impactions should be corrected prior to beginning definitive prosthetic treatment.

Elimination of Periodontal Pockets and Reshaping Gingival Architecture. Elimination of periodontal pockets and the reshaping of gingival architecture to prevent their recurrence may be done by chemical cautery, by cold surgery, or by electronic surgery.

Chemical cautery may be used effectively for smaller areas where epithelization needs to be eliminated without resorting to extensive gingivectomy. Gratzinger proposed the following formula[*] for chemical cauterization:

Potassium hydroxide	9.0 grams
Magnesium carbonate	0.3 gram
Thymol	0.3 gram
Oil of peppermint	0.3 gram
Glycerine	q.s. to make a stiff paste

Label: Poison, for external use only

Extreme care must be taken to avoid contact of the cauterizing agent with lips, tongue, cheek, or throat, or serious consequences may result. For this reason, it must be used in small amounts and applied specifically to the area to be cauterized. Cotton rolls should be used sparingly so as to avoid the possibility of chemicals being trapped and hidden, only to be discovered after damage has occurred. Chemical cauterization may be used to eliminate the pocket wall, thereby facilitating further scaling, oral hygiene, and massage. It does not permit reshaping gingival architecture as does surgical gingivectomy.

Periodontal surgery should accomplish more than just the elimination of periodontal pockets. In addition, gingival architecture should be so recontoured that recurrence is unlikely. Adequate home care and the elimination of factors contributing to the original condition are also essential to the success of surgical treatment of periodontal disease.

---

[*]From Gratzinger, M.: Elimination of Periodontal Pockets by Chemical Cautery, D. Digest **51**:120-124, 1945.

Infrabony and interdental pockets may be eliminated by the judicious use of surgical flap procedures. When properly done, such operations are most successful in the elimination of many periodontal conditions that are considered untreatable by more conservative means.

Correction of Traumatic Occlusion by Occlusal Adjustment. Not only has improvement in techniques for the elimination of periodontal pockets led to a much higher percentage of successful treatment but also the science of selective occlusal adjustment has contributed in a large way to the continued success of periodontal treatment.

Occlusal adjustment has been called *occlusal equilibration*. The *Glossary of Prosthodontic Terms* defines occlusal equilibration as: "The modification of occlusal form by grinding with the intent of equalizing occlusal stress or of producing simultaneous occlusal contacts or of harmonizing cuspal relations."

The term occlusal equilibration implies equalization of tooth contact in all centric and eccentric positions. The purpose of equilibration is to eliminate all cuspal interference which may be traumatic, either to the supporting periodontium or to the tissues underlying a denture base. While cuspal interference between natural teeth may cause damage to the periodontium, similar interference from an artificial tooth or a denture will cause shifting of the denture base which may be traumatic and destructive to the residual ridge. The cause is the same in either case, but the effect is entirely different.

It is theoretically possible to equilibrate artificial dentition on an articulating instrument *if* the casts are so mounted that they coincide with the jaw relations of the patient, the movements of the articulating instrument approximate the natural jaw movements, and the denture bases are accurate and supported by stable ridge tissues. It is doubtful if this perfection of occlusion is very often obtained, hence the trend toward the use of flatter occlusal surfaces in artificial dentures.

It is impossible to equilibrate natural occlusion in the same manner as prosthetic occlusion, because (1) the teeth are not accessible to visualization as they are on an articulating instrument, (2) unfavorable tooth position cannot be altered as can denture teeth set in wax, and (3) reduction of interfering cusps is limited by the vitality of the tooth.

Not only is balanced occlusion impossible to obtain on natural dentition but it is also apparently unnecessary in view of its absence in most normal healthy mouths. Occlusion on natural teeth needs to be perfected only to a point where cuspal interference within the patient's functional range is eliminated and normal physiologic wear can occur. For this reason, the term *occlusal adjustment* is preferred to the more misleading term *equilibration*.

Much harm may be done to natural occlusion by those inexperienced in the science of selective grinding. Occlusal adjustment is irrevocable and may do more harm than good. While occlusal adjustment is important to the success of periodontal treatment by eliminating occlusal trauma, it is not in itself a cure for periodontal disease. But selective grinding, properly done, is frequently necessary to the success of periodontal treatment. Both periodontal surgery and occlusal adjustment should be done only by those competent to do so. This does not mean that the general practitioner who is so inclined cannot learn the skills necessary to successful periodontal treatment.

Guide to Occlusal Adjustment. Schuyler has provided the following guide to occlusal adjustment by selective grinding:

> In the study or evaluation of occlusal disharmony of the natural dentition, accurately mounted study casts are extremely helpful, if not essential, in determining static cusp to fossae contacts of opposing teeth and as a guide in the correction of occlusal anomalies in both centric and eccentric functional relations. Occlusion can be coordinated only by selective spot grinding. Ground tooth surfaces should be subsequently smoothed and polished.
>
> 1. A static coordinated occlusal contact of the maximum number of teeth with the mandible in centric relation to the maxilla should be our first objective.
>
>   A. A prematurely contacting cusp should not be reduced or the sulcus deepened until the relation of the cusp in eccentric positions has been evaluated. If the cusp point is in premature contact in both centric and eccentric relations the cusp point should be reduced. If a cusp point is in premature contact in the centric relation only, the opposing sulcus should be deepened.
>
>   B. When anterior teeth are in premature contact in centric, or both centric and eccentric relations, corrections should be made by grinding the incisal edge of the lower teeth. If in premature contact only in the eccentric relation, correction must be made by grinding the lingual incline of the upper teeth.
>
>   C. In a vast majority of instances premature contacts in the centric relation are relieved by grinding the buccal cusps of the lower teeth, the lingual cusp of upper teeth, and the incisal edges of the lower anterior teeth. We must always be mindful of the fact that in deepening the sulcus of a posterior tooth or the lingual contact area in centric of an upper anterior tooth, we are changing and increasing the steepness of the eccentric guiding inclines of the tooth and while we are relieving trauma in the centric relation, we may be predisposing the tooth to trauma in eccentric relations.
>
> 2. After establishing a static, even distribution of stress over the maximum number of teeth in the centric relation, we are ready to evaluate opposing tooth contact or lack of contact in eccentric functional relations. Our attention should be directed first to balancing side contacts. In extreme cases of pathological balancing contacts, some relief might be indicated even before the corrective procedures in the centric relation. It must be recognized that where balancing contacts exist it is extremely difficult to differentiate the harmless from the destructive or the non-pathological from pathological as we can not visualize the influence of these fulcrum contacts upon the functional movements of the condyle in the glenoid fossae. Subluxation, pain, lack of normal functional movement of the joint, or loss of alveolar support of the teeth involved may be evidence of excessive balancing contacts. We should recognize that balancing side contacts receive less frictional wear than working side contacts and that premature contacts may develop progressively with wear. We must realize also that a reduction in the steepness of the guiding tooth inclines on the working side will increase the proximity of the teeth on the balancing side and may contribute to destructive prematurities. In all corrective grinding to relieve premature or excessive contacts in eccentric relations, care must be exercised to avoid the loss of a static supporting contact in the centric relation. This static support in centric may exist between the lower buccal cusp fitting into the central fossae of the upper tooth and/or the upper lingual cusp fitting into the central fossae of the lower tooth. While both the upper lingual cusp and the lower buccal cusp may have a static centric contact in the sulcus of the opposing tooth, often only one of these cusps has this static contact. In this case this cusp must be left untouched to maintain this essential support in centric, and all corrective grinding to relieve premature contacts in eccentric positions would be done on the opposing tooth inclines. We find the lower buccal cusp

in a static central contact in the upper sulcus more often than we find the upper lingual cusp in a static contact in its opposing lower sulcus. Therefore, corrective grinding to relieve premature balancing contacts is more often done on the upper lingual cusps. Reference should be made to mounted study casts to determine these static supports.

3. To obtain the maximum function and distribution of functional stress in eccentric positions on the working side, grinding must, where necessary, be done on the lingual surfaces of the upper anterior teeth. Corrective grinding on the posterior teeth at this time should always be done on the buccal cusp of the upper bicuspids and molars and on the lingual cusp of the lower bicuspids and molars, as the grinding of the lower buccal cusps or the upper lingual cusps at this time would rob these cusps of their desired static contact in the opposing central sulcus in the centric relation.

4. Corrective grinding to relieve premature protrusive contacts of one or more anterior teeth should be accomplished by grinding the lingual surface of the upper anterior teeth. Anterior teeth should never be ground to bring the posterior teeth into contact in either the protrusive position or on the balancing side. In the elimination of premature protrusive contacts of the posterior teeth neither the upper lingual cusps or the lower buccal cusps should be ground. Corrective grinding should be done upon the surface of the opposing tooth upon which these cusps function in the eccentric leaving the centric contact undisturbed.

5. Any sharp edges left by grinding should be rounded off, especially on the buccal cusps of the upper teeth and the lingual cusps of the lower teeth.

6. Place abrasive paste on the occlusal surfaces of all teeth and have the patient tap in centric, then in lateral, and last in protrusive, making *only a few strokes* in each position. Remember in the use of abrasive paste, cusp points wear more rapidly than the planes on which the points function. Its primary use is to smooth the tooth surfaces. Ground surfaces should then be polished with a fine abrasive wheel.[*]

Splinting. Teeth may be immobilized during periodontal treatment by interdental wiring, with acrylic resin splints, or with cast removable splints. Following periodontal treatment, splinting may be accomplished with cast removable appliances or cast cemented restorations. The most preferred form of permanent splinting is with two or more cast restorations soldered or cast together. They may be cemented with either permanent (zinc oxyphosphate or resin) cements or temporary (zinc oxide-eugenol) cements.

It is debatable whether or not splinting should be classified as periodontal treatment other than for immobilization during the healing and repair of the supporting tissues. Physiologic movement of the individual teeth is prevented by immobilization, and a healthy tooth is frequently tied to a weak tooth to the detriment of both. If a tooth is too weak after treatment to stand alone, little is gained by jeopardizing the health of the adjoining tooth by joining the two together. On this subject, Schluger has said: "Splinting is not a treatment for periodontal disease. It is merely a device for stabilizing mobile teeth. If these teeth are in periodontal health, the splint will be successful. It is possible to hold a dead horse up, but I shouldn't expect you could ride him very far. It is possible to save teeth from moving by splints but unless periodontal disease is cured, the teeth will exfoliate in time.[†]

---

[*]Courtesy Dr. C. H. Schuyler, Montclair, N. J.

[†]From Schluger, S. S.: Diagnosis and Treatment of Periodontal Disease, D. Times 1:7, 1958.

The term *splinting* will be used in a subsequent chapter to refer to doubling abutments for *multiple abutment support.* Splinting may be used to unite two or more weak abutments for the purpose of distributing stress loads over a greater area of root surface. While splinting of multirooted teeth is occasionally done, it is usually the single-rooted tooth that needs assistance from its neighbor to withstand the added stress of serving as a partial denture abutment.

The most frequent application of splinting for multiple abutment support is the use of united restorations on adjacent mandibular premolars. Because of their conical single roots, these teeth are more easily rotated and tipped than any other posterior abutment used for partial dentures. Where the crown-root ratio is unfavorable, a multirooted abutment is thus created by splinting two teeth together. The absence or presence of periodontal disease is not necessarily the primary factor in deciding to use multiple abutments. Rather, the root formation and the amount of alveolar support remaining will govern the need for the splinting of partial denture abutments.

MOUTH PREPARATIONS

Abutment Restorations. Equipped with the study casts upon which a tentative partial denture design has been drawn, the dentist is able to accomplish mouth preparations with some degree of accuracy. The information at hand should include the proposed path of insertion, the areas of teeth to be disked and tooth contours to be changed, and the location of occlusal rests.

During examination and subsequent treatment planning, in conjunction with a survey of study casts, each abutment tooth is considered individually as to whether or not full coverage is indicated. Abutment teeth presenting sound enamel surfaces in a mouth where good oral hygiene habits are evident may be considered a fair risk for use as partial denture abutments. One should not be misled, however, by a patient's promise to do better, so far as oral hygiene habits are concerned. Good or bad oral hygiene is a habit of long standing, and is not likely to be changed appreciably because a partial denture is being worn. Therefore, one must be conservative in evaluating the oral hygiene habits of the patient in the future. It is well to remember that clasps as such do not cause teeth to decay, and if the individual will keep the teeth and the partial denture clean, one need not condemn clasps from a cariogenic standpoint. On the other hand, more partial dentures have been condemned as cardiogenic because the dentist did not provide for the protection of abutment teeth then because of inadequate care on the part of the patient.

The full cast gold crown is objectionable from an esthetic standpoint and therefore the veneer-type of full crown must be resorted to where a canine or premolar abutment is to be restored or protected. Less frequently does the molar have to be treated in such a manner, and the full gold crown is usually acceptable.

Where there is proximal caries on abutment teeth with sound buccal and lingual enamel surfaces, in a mouth exhibiting average oral hygiene and low caries activity, a gold inlay is usually indicated. The amalgam filling for the restoration of proximal caries should not be condemned, however, although one must admit that an inlay cast of a hard-type gold will provide the best possible support for occlusal rests, at the same time giving an esthetically pleasing restoration. But an amalgam restoration, properly condensed, is capable of supporting an occlusal rest, without appreciable flow, over a long period of time.

The most vulnerable area on the abutment tooth is the proximal gingival area which lies beneath the minor connector of the partial denture framework and is therefore subject to the lodgment of debris in an area most susceptible to caries attack. Even when the partial denture is removed for purposes of cleaning the teeth, these areas, especially those on the distal surface of an anterior abutment, are often missed by the toothbrush, and bacterial plaques and debris are allowed to remain for long periods of time. Except in a caries-immune mouth or in a mouth where the teeth are subjected to meticulous brushing, decalcification and caries frequently occur in this region. It is necessary, therefore, that this area of the tooth be fully protected by whatever restoration is used. When an inlay restoration is used, the preparation should be carried to or beneath the gingival margin and well out onto the buccal and lingual surfaces to afford the best possible protection of the abutment tooth. Even the full crown can be deficient in this most vulnerable area, which lies at and just above the gingival margin. The full crown which is cast short of this area will not afford protection where it is most needed.

All proximal tooth surfaces which are to serve as guiding planes for the partial denture should be disked so as to be made as nearly as possible parallel to the path of insertion. This is accomplished on sound enamel or on existing restoration by disking those tooth surfaces parallel to the path of insertion, and the same can be done for the recently placed full crown or inlay.

Contouring Wax Patterns. Modern indirect techniques using hydrocolloid or rubber base impression materials permit the contouring of wax patterns on the stone abutments with the aid of the surveyor blade. All of the abutment teeth to be restored with castings can be prepared at one time and an impression made which will provide an accurate stone replica of the prepared arch. Wax patterns may then be refined on separate individual dies or removable dies. All tooth surfaces facing edentulous areas should be made parallel to the path of insertion by the use of the surveyor blade. This will provide proximal tooth surfaces which will be parallel without any further disking in the mouth, will permit the most positive seating of the partial denture along the path of insertion, and will provide the least amount of undesirable space beneath minor connectors for the lodgment of debris.

Occlusal Rests. After the proximal surfaces of the wax patterns have been made parallel, and buccal and lingual contours have been established which will satisfy the requirements of retention with the best possible esthetic placement of clasp arms, the occlusal rests should be prepared in the wax pattern rather than in the finished gold restoration. The placement of occlusal rests should be considered at the time the teeth are prepared to receive cast restorations, so that there will be sufficient clearance beneath the floor of the occlusal rest. Too many times we see a completed gold restoration cemented in the mouth for a partial denture abutment without any provision for the occlusal rest having been made in the wax pattern. The operator then proceeds to cut an occlusal rest in the gold restoration, being ever conscious of the fact that he may perforate the gold during the process of forming an occlusal rest. The unfortunate result is usually a poorly formed occlusal rest that is too shallow and one that does not incline toward the center of the tooth in the desired manner.

If tooth structure has been removed so as to provide for the placement of the occlusal rest, the occlusal rest may be ideally placed in the wax pattern by using a No. 8 round bur to lower the marginal ridge and establish the outline form of the occlusal rest, and then using a No. 6 round bur to deepen slightly the floor of the occlusal rest inside this lowered marginal ridge. This provides for an occlusal rest which best satisfies the requirements of an occlusal rest preparation, that is, that the rest be so placed that any occlusal force will be directed toward the center of the tooth and that there will be the least possible interference to occlusion with the opposing teeth.

Perhaps the most important function of the occlusal rest is the division of stress loads coming upon the partial denture so as to provide for greatest efficiency with the least damaging effect to the abutment teeth. For a free-end partial denture, the occlusal rest must be able to transmit occlusal forces to the abutment teeth in an occlusal direction only, thereby permitting the least possible lateral stresses to be transmitted to the abutment tooth.

For this reason, the floor of the occlusal rest should incline toward the center of the tooth so that the occlusal forces, in so far as possible, are centered over the root apex. Any other form but that of a spoon shape permits a locking of the occlusal rest and the transmission of tipping forces to the abutment tooth. A ball-and-socket type of relationship between occlusal rest and abutment tooth is the most desirable. At the same time, the marginal ridge must be lowered so that the angle formed by the occlusal rest with the minor connector will stand above the occlusal surface of the abutment tooth as little as possible and avoid interference with the opposing teeth. At the same time, sufficient bulk must be provided for, in order to prevent a weakness in the occlusal rest at the marginal ridge. The marginal ridge must be lowered and yet not be the deepest part of the rest preparation. To permit occlusal stresses to be directed toward the center of the abutment tooth, the angle formed by the floor of the occlusal rest with the minor connector should be less than 90 degrees. In other words, the floor of the occlusal rest should incline slightly from the lowered marginal ridge toward the center of the tooth.

This proper form can be readily accomplished in the wax pattern if care is taken during crown or inlay preparation to provide for the location of the occlusal rest. If an amalgam restoration is used, there must be sufficient bulk in this area to allow proper occlusal rest form without weakening the restoration. When the occlusal rest is placed in sound enamel, it is best accomplished by the use of round diamond points of approximately Nos. 4 and 6 sizes in the following sequence: first, the larger of the two diamonds is used to lower the marginal ridge and at the same time create the outline form of the occlusal rest. The result is an occlusal rest preparation with marginal ridge lowered and gross outline form established but without sufficient deepening of the rest preparation toward the center of the tooth. The smaller diamond point or a carbide bur of approximately No. 4 size may then be used to deepen the floor of the occlusal rest to a gradual incline toward the center of the tooth. Enamel rods are then smoothed by the planing action of a round bur revolving with little pressure. This is all the polishing of the enamel surface that is usually needed.

Occlusal rest preparations in existing restorations, or on abutment teeth where no restorations are to be placed, should always follow, not precede, the disking of proximal tooth surfaces. The disking of proximal tooth surfaces should be done first, for if the occlusal rest is placed first and the proximal tooth surface is disked later, the outline form of the occlusal rest is sometimes irreparably altered.

The success or failure of a partial denture may well depend upon how well the mouth preparations were accomplished. It is only through intelligent planning and competent execution of mouth preparations that the partial denture can satisfactorily restore lost dental functions and contribute to the health of the remaining oral tissues.

Chapter 13

Preparation of abutment teeth

Following surgery, periodontal treatment, and any endodontic treatment of the arch involved, the abutment teeth may then be prepared to provide support, stabilization, bracing, and retention for the partial denture.

Endodontic treatment of any teeth elsewhere in the arch, as well as abutment teeth, should precede the making of the partial denture, so that the success of treatment can be reasonably well established before proceeding. Similarly, favorable response to any deep restorations and the results of periodontal treatment should be established prior to construction of the denture, for if the prognosis of a tooth under treatment becomes unfavorable, its loss can be compensated for by a change in the denture design. The condemned tooth or teeth may then be included in the original denture design, whereas if they are lost subsequently, the partial denture must be added to, remade, or replaced. Many partial denture designs do not lend themselves well to later additions, although this eventuality should be kept in mind when designing the denture.

Particularly where the tooth in question will be used as an abutment, every diagnostic aid should be used to determine the success of previous treatment. It is usually not so difficult to add a tooth or teeth to a partial denture as it is to add a retaining unit when the original abutment is lost and the next adjacent tooth must be used for that purpose.

It is sometimes possible to so design a partial denture that a single posterior abutment about which there is some doubt can be retained and utilized as one end of a tooth-supported base. Then, should that posterior abutment be lost, it can be replaced with a free-end base. Such a design will include provision for future indirect retention and flexible clasping on the future free-end abutment. Anterior abutments which are considered to be poor risks may not be so freely used because of the problems involved in adding a new abutment retainer when the original one is lost. It is better that such questionable teeth be condemned in favor of a better abutment, even though the original treatment plan must be modified accordingly.

CLASSIFICATION OF ABUTMENT TEETH

The subject of abutment preparations may be grouped thus: (1) those abutment teeth that are to be used in their present state; (2) those that are to have cast inlays; and (3) those that are to have cast crowns. The latter group includes abutments for fixed bridges, since inlay retainers are not commonly used as bridge abutments.

Abutment teeth to be used in their present state include teeth with sound enamel, those having small restorations not involved in the denture design, those having acceptable restorations which will be involved in the denture design, and those having existing crown restorations. The latter may exist either as an individual crown or as the abutment of a fixed bridge restoration.

The use of unprotected abutments has been discussed previously. Although full protection of all abutments is desirable, it is not always possible nor practical to do so. The decision to use unprotected abutments involves certain risks of which the patient must be advised, including his own responsibility for maintaining oral hygiene and caries control. The making of crown restorations to fit existing denture clasps is an art in itself which will be covered later in this chapter, but the fact that it is possible to do so may influence the decision to use uncrowned but otherwise sound teeth as abutments.

Preferably, amalgam alloy should not be used for the support of occlusal rests because of its tendency to flow. Although cast gold will provide the best possible support for occlusal rests, an amalgam alloy restoration, properly condensed, is capable of supporting an occlusal rest without appreciable flow over a long period of time. Should the patient's economic status or other factors beyond the control of the dentist prevent the use of cast restorations, any existing amalgam alloy fillings about which there is any doubt should be replaced with new amalgam restorations. This should be done far enough in advance of disking and the preparation of occlusal rest seats to permit aging and polishing of the restoration.

SEQUENCE OF ABUTMENT PREPARATIONS ON SOUND ENAMEL OR EXISTING RESTORATIONS

Abutment preparations on either sound enamel or existing restorations should be done in the following order:

1. The disking or slicing of proximal surfaces parallel to the path of insertion so as to provide guiding planes (Fig. 146, A). The term disking is used in a broad sense and refers to the paralleling of proximal surfaces by the use of abrasive instruments. With ultra speeds parallelism can frequently be accomplished as well or better by the use of cylindrical diamond points moved buccolingually across the proximal surface. The term disking may ultimately be replaced by terminology descriptive of modern cutting methods.

2. The reduction of excessive tooth contours (Fig. 146, B and C), thereby lowering the height of contours so that (a) the origin of circumferential clasp arms may be placed well below the occlusal surface, preferably at the junction of the occlusal and middle thirds; (b) retentive clasp terminals may be placed in the gingival third of the crown, for better esthetics and better mechanical ad-

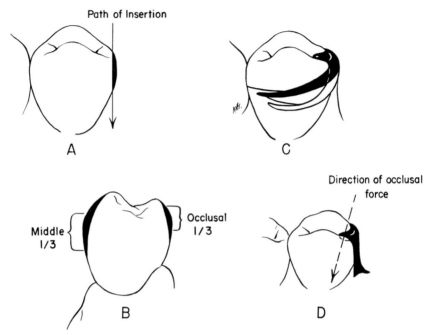

Fig. 146. Abutment contours should be altered during mouth preparations in the following sequence. **A,** The proximal surface is disked parallel to the path of insertion to create a guiding plane. **B,** The height of contours on the buccal and lingual surface is lowered where necessary to permit the retentive clasp terminus to be located within the gingival third of the crown and the reciprocal clasp arm on the opposite side of the tooth to be placed no higher than the junction of the occlusal and middle thirds. **C,** The area of the tooth where a retentive clasp arm originates should be altered if necessary to permit more direct approach to the gingival third of the tooth. **D,** An occlusal rest preparation which will direct occlusal forces toward the long axis of the tooth should be the final step in mouth preparations.

vantage; and (c) reciprocal clasp arms may be placed on and above a height of contour no higher than the junction of the occlusal and middle thirds.

3. The preparation of occlusal rest areas which will direct occlusal forces toward the long axis of the abutment tooth (Fig. 146, *D*).

Mouth preparation should follow a plan previously outlined on the study cast in red pencil at the time the study cast was surveyed and the design of the partial denture outlined. Better still, as discussed in Chapter 3, Diagnosis and Treatment Planning, proposed changes to abutment teeth may be actually made on the study cast and *outlined* in red pencil to indicate not only the area but also the *amount* and angulation of the disking to be done. Although occlusal rests may also be prepared on the study cast, indication of their *location* in red pencil is usually sufficient for the experienced operator, since rest preparations follow a definite pattern, as covered in Chapter 8, Occlusal Rests.

ABUTMENT PREPARATIONS USING CAST INLAYS

Inlay preparations on teeth to be used as partial denture abutments differ from conventional inlay preparations in the amount of protection afforded the tooth, the width of the preparation at the occlusal rest, and the depth of the preparation beneath the occlusal rest.

Conventional inlay preparations are permissible on the proximal surface of the tooth not to be contacted by a minor connector of the partial denture. On the other hand, proximal and occlusal surfaces supporting minor connectors and occlusal rests require somewhat different treatment than the conventional inlay preparation. The extent of occlusal coverage (that is, whether or not cusps are capped) will be governed by the usual factors, such as the extent of caries, the presence of unsupported enamel walls, and the extent of occlusal abrasion and attrition.

Of primary consideration in the preparation of proximal inlays which will lie beneath minor connectors is the amount of protection afforded vulnerable areas by the inlay. The most vulnerable area on the abutment tooth is the proximal gingival area lying beneath the minor connector of the partial denture, because of accumulation of debris and the difficulty of keeping this area clean.

Except in a caries-immune mouth or in a mouth where the teeth are kept meticulously clean there is inevitably some decalcification and caries attack in this region. Even the most conscientious toothbrushing may miss the distal surfaces of abutments because they cannot be seen. It is always important that the patient be instructed, with study casts and before a mirror, in the importance of brushing these areas.

It is necessary that these areas be fully protected by the cast restoration, whether it be an inlay or a partial or full crown. Even the full crown can be deficient in this most vulnerable area which lies at or just above the gingival margin. A full crown that is short or becomes short due to gingival recession does not afford protection where it is most needed.

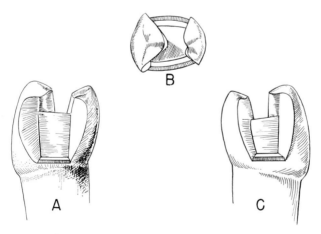

Fig. 147. An MOD inlay preparation for a lower left second premolar to be used as a partial denture abutment. **A,** A view of the distal surface showing the broad extension of the box, well beyond the area that will be covered by the minor connector of the partial denture. **B,** An occlusal view showing that the axial wall is curved to conform with the external proximal curvature of the tooth. **C,** A view of the mesial surface where normal tooth contact occurs, being extended into a free cleansing area but not as broadly as the distal surface.

When an inlay is the restoration of choice for an abutment tooth, certain modifications of the outline form are necessary. In order to prevent the buccal and lingual proximal margins from lying at or near the minor connector or the occlusal rest, these margins must be extended well beyond the line angles of the tooth. This additional extension may be accomplished by slicing the conventional box preparation. However, the gold margin produced by such a preparation may be quite thin and may be damaged by the clasp during insertion or removal of the partial denture. This hazard may be avoided by extending the outline of the box beyond the line angle, thus producing a strong gold-to-tooth junction. (Fig. 147.)

In this type of preparation the pulp is particularly vulnerable unless the axial wall is curved to conform with the external proximal curvature of the tooth. Where caries is of minimal depth, the gingival seat should have an axial depth at all points about the width of a No. 559 fissure bur. It is of utmost importance that the gingival seat be placed below the free tissue margin. The proximal contour necessary to produce proper guiding plane surface and the close proximity of the minor connector render this area particularly vulnerable to future caries attack. Every effort should be made to provide the restoration with maximum resistance and retention as well as clinically imperceptible gold margins. The first requisite can be satisfied by preparing opposing cavity walls 5 degrees or less from parallel and producing flat floors and sharp, clean line angles. Through the use of modern impression materials and casting technique, the second requisite is not nearly as difficult as it was a few years ago.

The extended box provides the broad occlusoproximal area necessary to accommodate an occlusal rest. Care should be exercised to place the rest area in

Fig. 148. An MO inlay preparation on a lower left first premolar to be used for the support of a mesially placed occlusal rest. The weak lingual cusp is protected by an extension of the inlay margin lingually.

such a manner as to allow an adequate amount of gold in both buccal and lingual directions. The proposed depth of the rest must be determined prior to preparing the tooth in order to ensure an adequate thickness of gold in the axiopulpal area. Additional depth in this area may be obtained by rounding the axiopulpal line angle of the preparation. In most cases, if the preparation is well into dentin at this point, adequate thickness of gold will be ensured. However, in problem cases, a careful study of the roentgenogram will give some indication regarding the depth to which the pulpal floor can be carried with safety.

It is sometimes necessary to use an inlay on a lower first premolar for the support of an indirect retainer. The narrow occlusal width buccolingually and the lingual inclination of the occlusal surface of such a tooth often complicates the two-surface inlay preparation. Even the most exacting occlusal cavity preparation often results in a thin and weak lingual cusp remaining.

Fig. 148 illustrates a modification of the two-surface extended-box inlay preparation which lends support to a weak lingual cusp. Enough of the tip of the lingual cusp must be removed to allow for sufficient thickness of gold to withstand occlusal forces. Tooth structure should be removed in the direction of the enamel rods, and the cut is terminated with a bevel just lingual to the proximal embrasure. A short bevel is then placed along the lingual surface of the reduced cusp. A modified inlay preparation such as this permits adequate coverage of a potentially weak cusp and eliminates the necessity of resorting to some type of more extensive restoration such as an MOD inlay or three-quarter crown.

An inlay preparation should be wide enough that the margins will be well beyond the occlusal rest area (Fig. 149). Since the rest seat will be carved in the wax pattern with round burs, the margins of the inlay should not be jeopardized by their proximity to the rest seat. Generally, there should be at least 1 to 1.5 mm. of gold between the occlusal rest and the inlay margin. Nor should the refinement of the margins, which is the final step in creating an inlay wax pattern, infringe upon the outline form of the rest seat. The depth of the occlusal rest seat should be provided for in the preparation. If there is any doubt, the axiopulpal line angle should be beveled or made concave to accommodate the occlusal rest.

One of the advantages of making cast restorations for abutment teeth is that mouth preparations which would otherwise have to be done in the mouth may be done on the surveyor with far greater accuracy. It is extremely difficult,

Fig. 149. An occlusal view of a Class II inlay properly designed to support an occlusal rest. The inlay preparation has been made with sufficient width to accommodate the occlusal rest without jeopardizing the inlay margins.

Fig. 150. A full arch with removable dies for five abutment crowns. Note the depressions in the preparations to accommodate occlusal rests.

and many times impossible, to make several proximal surfaces parallel to one another by disking them intraorally. No device has ever been invented, nor likely will be, which will permit such precision cutting in the mouth. The opportunity of paralleling and contouring wax patterns on the surveyor in relation to a path of insertion should be utilized to the fullest advantage whenever cast restorations are being made.

Although it is not always possible, it is best that all wax patterns be made at the same time. A cast of the arch with removable dies may be used if they are sufficiently keyed for accuracy (Fig. 150). If preferred, the paralleling and contouring of wax patterns may be done on a solid cast of the arch, using supplementary individual dies for the purpose of refining margins. Modern impression materials and indirect techniques make either method equally satisfactory.

The same sequence for preparing teeth in the mouth applies to the contouring of wax patterns, differing only in that it may be done with greater accuracy and precision when indirect methods are used. After the cast has been placed on the surveyor so as to conform to the selected path of insertion, and the wax patterns have been carved for occlusion and contact, proximal surfaces which are to act as guiding planes may then be carved parallel to the path of insertion with a surveyor blade. This will usually be extended to the junction of the middle and gingival thirds of the tooth surface involved but not to the gingival margin, since the minor connector must be relieved where it crosses the gingivae. A guiding plane which includes the occlusal two thirds or even one half of the proximal area is usually adequate without endangering gingival tissues.

Following the paralleling of guiding planes and any other contouring, occlusal rests seats are carved in the wax pattern with suitable round burs, thus lowering the marginal ridge and inclining the floor of the rest preparation toward the center of the tooth. This has been outlined under occlusal rests in Chapter 8.

It should be pointed out that critical areas thus prepared in wax should not be destroyed by careless spruing or polishing. The wax pattern should be sprued so as to preserve paralleled surfaces and rest areas. Polishing should consist of little more than burnishing. Rest areas should need only refining with round finishing burs of the same sizes that were used to carve the rest seat originally. Should some interference by spruing be unavoidable, the casting should be returned to the surveyor for the refinement of proximal surfaces. However, this can only be done accurately with the aid of a handpiece holder attached to the vertical arm of the surveyor or some similar machining device. Need for later corrections to the casting can be avoided by carving the wax pattern with care and spruing and polishing with equal care.

ABUTMENT PREPARATIONS USING CAST CROWNS

Much that has been said in the preceding paragraphs about the preparation of inlays for partial denture abutments applies equally to cast-crown restorations. These may be in the form of three-quarter or full cast gold crowns or resin or porcelain veneer crowns. The latter are, of course, used for esthetic reasons only, but consideration for esthetics must not be allowed to jeopardize the success of the partial denture design. Retentive contours, therefore, must be provided on veneer crowns the same as on full cast crowns.

The ideal crown restoration for a partial denture abutment is the full cast gold crown, which can be carved to satisfy ideally all of the requirements for support, stabilization, and retention without compromise for cosmetic reasons. Porcelain and resin veneer crowns can be made equally satisfactory but only by the added step of contouring the veneered surface on the surveyor. If this is not done, retentive contours may be excessive or inadequate. The full cast crown is preferable as an ideal abutment piece whenever esthetics will allow its use.

The three-quarter crown does not permit the creating of retentive areas as does the full crown. But, if buccal or labial surfaces are sound and retentive areas are acceptable or can be made so by slight modification of tooth surfaces,

Fig. 151. A close-up view of a full crown abutment preparation with depression to accommodate the depth of the occlusal rest.

the three-quarter crown is a conservative restoration of merit. The same criteria apply in the decision to leave a portion of an abutment unprotected, as in the decision to leave any tooth unprotected which is to serve a partial denture abutment.

Regardless of the type of crown used, the preparation should be made to accommodate the depth of the occlusal rest seat. This is best accomplished by creating a depression in the prepared tooth at the occlusal rest area (Fig. 151). Since the location of any occlusal rests will have been established previously during treatment planning, this will be known in advance of any crown preparations. If, for example, double occlusal rests are to be used, this will be known so that the tooth can be prepared to accommodate the depth of both rests. It is almost as bad to find, when waxing a pattern, that a rest seat has to be made more shallow than is desirable because of lack of foresight as it is to have to make a rest seat shallow in an existing crown or inlay because its thickness is not known. Here, the opportunity for creating an ideal rest seat depends only upon the few seconds it takes to create space for it.

LEDGES ON ABUTMENT CROWNS

In addition to providing abutment protection, more nearly ideal retentive contours, definite guiding planes, and optimal occlusal rest support, crown restorations on teeth used as partial denture abutments offer still another advantage not obtainable on natural teeth. This is the crown ledge or shoulder for the purpose of providing effective reciprocation and stabilization.

The functions of the reciprocal clasp arm have been stated in Chapter 9, Direct Retainers. Briefly, these are reciprocation, stabilization, and auxiliary indirect retention. Any rigid reciprocal arm may provide horizontal stabilization.

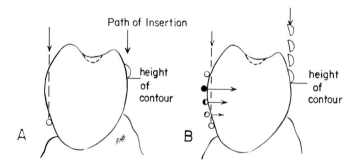

Fig. 152. A, The relationship of a retentive and a reciprocal clasp arm to each other when the partial denture framework is fully seated. As the retentive clasp arm flexes over the height of contour during insertion and removal, the reciprocal clasp arm cannot be effective because it is not in contact with the tooth until the denture framework is fully seated. B, The horizontal forces which are applied to an abutment tooth as a retentive clasp flexes over the height of contour during insertion and removal. The open circle at the top and bottom illustrates that the retentive clasp is only passive at its first contact with the tooth during insertion and when in its terminal position with the denture fully seated. During insertion and removal a rigid clasp arm placed on the opposite side of the tooth cannot provide resistance against these horizontal forces.

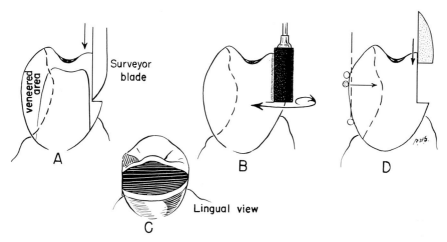

Fig. 153. A, The preparation of a ledge on a wax pattern with the surveyor blade parallel to the path of insertion. B, The refinement of the ledge on a gold casting, using a suitable carborundum stone in a handpiece attached to a dental surveyor or a specialized drill press for the purpose. C, The approximate width and depth of the ledge formed on an abutment crown, which will permit a reciprocal clasp arm to be inlayed within the normal contours of the tooth. D, The true reciprocation throughout the full path of insertion and removal that is possible when a reciprocal clasp arm is inlayed onto a ledge on an abutment crown.

To a large extent, since it is placed above the height of convexity, a rigid reciprocal arm may also act as an auxiliary indirect retainer. But its function as a reciprocating arm against the action of the retentive clasp arm is limited only to stabilization against possible orthodontic movement when the denture framework is in its terminal position. Only when the retentive clasp becomes an active orthodontic force, due to accidental distortion or improper design, is such reciprocation needed. Reciprocation is most needed when the appliance is being inserted or when a dislodging force is applied, to prevent transient horizontal forces which may be detrimental to abutment stability. Perhaps the term orthodontic force is incorrect, since the term signifies a slight but continuous influence which would logically reach equilibrium as soon as the tooth is orthodontically moved. Instead, the transient forces of insertion and removal lead to periodontal destruction and eventual instability rather than to orthodontic movement followed by consolidation.

True reciprocation is not possible with a clasp arm that is placed upon an occlusally inclined tooth surface, because it does not become effective until the prosthesis is fully seated. Immediately, when a dislodging force is applied, the reciprocal clasp arm, along with the occlusal rest, breaks contact with the supporting tooth surfaces and they are no longer effective. Thus, as the retentive clasp flexes over the height of contour, thereby exerting a horizontal force on the abutment, reciprocation is nonexistent just when it is needed most. (Fig. 152.)

True reciprocation can only be obtained by creating a path of insertion for the reciprocal clasp arm which is parallel to other guiding planes. In this manner, the inferior border of the reciprocal clasp makes contact with its guiding surface before the retentive clasp on the other side of the tooth begins to flex (Fig. 153). Thus, reciprocation exists during the entire path of insertion and removal. The presence of a ledge on the abutment crown acts as a terminal stop for the reciprocal clasp arm, as well as augmenting the occlusal rest and providing some indirect retention for a free-end partial denture.

There is still another advantage to a ledge on an abutment crown. While

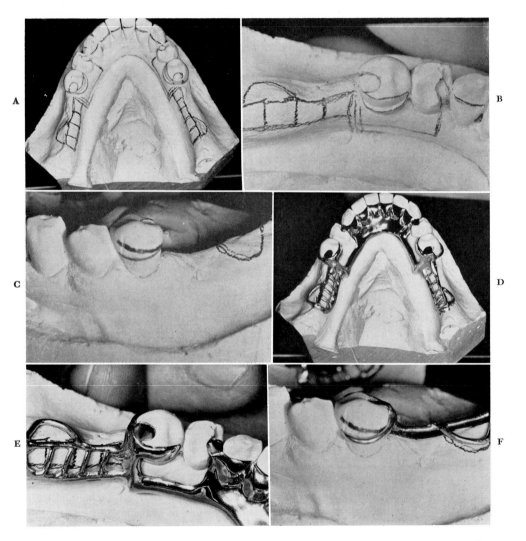

Fig. 154. Mandibular Class I partial denture utilizing lingual crown ledges on premolar abutments. **A,** The penciled design on the master cast. Note the occlusal rests at each end of the lingual plate, which serve also as indirect retainers. **B,** Close occlusal view of penciled design on the left side. **C,** Close buccal view of red pencil line indicating the location of the 18-gauge wrought-wire retentive clasp in relation to the surveyed height of contour. Note the path of insertion scored on the base of the cast. **D,** Finished cast framework following precisely the penciled design. **E,** Close occlusal view of the left side. A reciprocal clasp arm "inlayed" into a lingual ledge avoids objectionable bulk by restoring a smooth lingual contour.

the usual reciprocal clasp arm is half-round, and therefore convex, and is super-imposed upon an already convex surface, a reciprocal clasp arm built on a crown ledge is actually inlayed into the crown and reproduces more nearly normal crown contours (Fig. 154). The patient's tongue then contacts a continuously convex surface rather than the projection of a clasp arm. Unfortunately, the enamel cap is not thick enough nor the tooth so shaped that an effective ledge can be created on an uncrowned tooth. Narrow enamel shoulders are sometimes used in selected cases for occlusal rests on anterior teeth, but these do not provide the parallelism which is essential to reciprocation during insertion and removal.

The crown ledge may be used on any full or three-quarter crown restoration which covers the nonretentive side of an abutment tooth. It is used most frequently on premolars and molars but may also be used on canine restorations. It is not ordinarily used on buccal surfaces for reciprocation against lingual retention because of the excessive display of metal, but it may be so used just as effectively on posterior abutments where esthetics is not a factor.

Fig. 155. **A,** A Faro laboratory handpiece attached to a Ney surveyor by means of a handpiece holder. With the use of a bur or stone, the lingual surface and ledge are machined in relation to the previously established path of insertion. **B,** The Austenal Micro-Drill used to mill precision rest seats and lingual grooves and ledges in cast gold restorations. Such a device permits more precise milling than is possible with a dental handpiece attached to a dental surveyor. To be effective, the cast must be positioned on the Micro-Drill in such a manner that the previously established path of insertion is maintained. The movable stage or base, therefore, should be adjustable until the relation of the cast to the axis of the drill has been made the same as that obtained when the cast was on the dental surveyor. (**B,** Courtesy Austenal, Inc., Chicago, Ill.)

The fact that a crown ledge is to be used should be known in advance of crown preparation to assure sufficient removal of tooth structure in this area. Although a shoulder or ledge is not included in the preparation itself, adequate space must be provided so that the ledge may be made sufficiently wide and the surface above it may be made parallel to the path of insertion. The ledge should be placed at about the middle third of the tooth, curving slightly to follow the curvature of the gingival tissues. On the side of the tooth where the clasp arm will originate, the ledge must be kept low enough to allow the origin of the clasp arm to be wide enough for sufficient strength and rigidity.

In forming the crown ledge, which is usually located on the lingual surface, the wax pattern of the crown is completed except for refinement of the margins before the ledge is carved. After the proximal guiding planes and the occlusal rests and retentive contours are formed, the ledge is so carved with the surveyor blade that the surface above is parallel to the path of insertion. Thus, a continuous guiding plane surface will exist from the proximal around the lingual surface, the difference being only that the lingual portion ends in a definite ledge and the proximal does not.

The full effectiveness of the crown ledge cannot be had with a crown that is not returned to the surveyor for refinement after casting. To afford true reciprocation, the crown casting must have a surface above the ledge that is parallel to the path of insertion. This can be accomplished with precision only by machining the casting parallel to the path of insertion with a handpiece holder in the surveyor or some other suitable machining device (Fig. 155). Similarly, the parallelism of proximal guiding planes needs to be perfected after casting and polishing. While it is possible to *approximate* parallelism and, at the same time, form the crown ledge on the wax pattern with a surveyor blade, some of

Fig. 156. Lingual ledges on cast gold crowns are machined, using a No. 558 dental bur. Experience has shown that in the absence of a rigid jig for holding the cast, a bur is difficult to use. Therefore, it is best that the ledge be formed as accurately as possible on the wax pattern and that machining of the finished casting be done with a cylindrical carborundum point. Note the scratch line on the left heel of the cast, indicating the path of insertion.

Fig. 157. Lingual ledges after machining and polishing. Note that embrasures for clasping are also machined parallel to the path of insertion and that occlusal rests are used in addition to the supporting ledges. These are to prevent tooth separation and to shunt food away from interproximal areas.

Fig. 158. Buccal and lingual views of abutment crowns designed to accept embrasure clasps and lingual reciprocal arms resting on prepared ledges. All surfaces above the ledges are made parallel with the path of insertion. Note the size and form of the occlusal rests on either side of the embrasure ledges.

its accuracy is lost in casting and polishing. The use of suitable burs, such as Nos. 557, 558, and 559 fissure burs, and true cylindrical carborundum stones in the handpiece holder permits the paralleling of all guiding planes on the finished casting with the accuracy necessary to the effectiveness of those guiding plane surfaces (Figs. 156, 157, and 158).

The reciprocal clasp arm is ultimately waxed on the investment cast so as to be continuous with the ledge inferiorly and contoured superiorly to restore the crown contour including the tip of the cusp. It is obvious that polishing must not be allowed to destroy the form of the shoulder that was prepared in wax nor destroy the parallelism of the guiding plane surface. It is equally vital that the denture casting must be polished with great care so as not to destroy the accuracy of the counterpart. Modern investments, casting alloys, and polishing techniques make this degree of accuracy possible. Only the human element, by carelessness or lack of understanding, may fail to produce a crown and counterpart with the desired accuracy. It is just as necessary that the technician understand the purpose of the crown ledge as the dentist who designs and plans for its use.

VENEER CROWNS FOR THE SUPPORT OF CLASP ARMS

Resin and porcelain veneer crowns are used for cosmetic reasons on abutment teeth that would otherwise display an objectionable amount of metal. They may be in the form of porcelain veneers retained by pins and cemented to the crown, porcelain fused directly to a cast crown, or acrylic resin processed directly to a cast crown.

Perhaps the ideal veneer crown is one that provides for the retentive clasp terminal to rest on metal rather than on the veneer itself (Fig. 159). In such case, the crown is contoured to be retentive in the desired area, and that area is not included in carving the space for the veneer. While the suprabulge portion of the clasp arm crosses the surface of the veneer, that portion which crosses the height of contour and engages an undercut where abrasion could occur is

Fig. 159. A close-up view of the relation of the surveyor blade to the distal surface of an abutment crown. Note that this guiding plane is made parallel to the path of insertion as indicated by the scratch line on the base of the cast. Note also the gold surface on the veneer crown where the retentive terminus of the clasp arm will rest.

supported by the metal of the crown itself. The only disadvantage of a veneer crown so prepared is the display of metal which, more often than not, is on the mesial side of the abutment tooth and therefore is cosmetically objectionable.

If the veneer crown is not contoured to provide retention on metal, suitable retention does not exist until the veneer has been added. This means that the veneer must be slightly overcontoured and then shaped to provide the desired undercut for the location of the retentive clasp arm. If the veneer is of porcelain, this procedure must precede glazing, and if of resin, before final polishing. If this most important step in the making of veneered abutments is neglected or omitted, excessive or inadequate retentive contours may result, to the detriment of effective clasp design.

The flat underside of a cast clasp makes sufficient contact with the surface of the veneer so that abrasion of a resin veneer may result. While the underside of the clasp may be polished (with some loss in accuracy of fit), abrasion results from the trapping and holding of food debris against the tooth surface as the clasp moves during function. Therefore, unless the retentive clasp terminal rests on metal, glazed porcelain should be used to assure the future retentiveness of the veneered surface. Present-day acrylic resins, being cross-linked copolymers, are much harder than formerly and will withstand abrasion for considerable time but not to the same degree as porcelain. Acrylic resin veneers are therefore best used in conjunction with exposed metal supporting the half-round clasp terminal.

On the other hand, the round, wrought-wire clasp, since it makes only a line contact with the tooth surface, is much less capable of abrading the surface of a resin veneer. Experience has shown that it may be placed on acrylic resin veneers if the veneer material is made with a cross-linked monomer giving sufficient hardness and the wrought wire has a smooth polished surface. Under such conditions, the retentive undercut may be made in the gingival one third of the veneered surface without exposing any of the crown metal. As explained previously, the round surface of an 18-gauge wrought wire, tapered to still lesser diameter at its terminal end, is the least visible of any clasp. When placed in the gingival third of a veneered surface, the retentive terminal is still less noticeable and is cosmetically acceptable in the majority of mouths.

SPLINTING OF ABUTMENT TEETH

Frequently a tooth is deemed too weak to use alone as a partial denture abutment due to the short length and/or excessive taper of a single root or to bone loss resulting in an unfavorable crown-root ratio. In such cases, splinting of weak abutment teeth to the adjacent tooth or teeth is utilized as a means of gaining *multiple abutment support*. Two single-rooted teeth may thus be used as a multirooted abutment.

Splinting should not be used for the purpose of retaining a tooth that would otherwise be condemned for periodontal reasons, in the futile hope that by doing so the tooth may be retained. Such a gamble may be justified where, if successful, the need for a prosthetic appliance would be avoided. But where the length of service of a prosthetic appliance may depend upon the serviceability of an abutment, any periodontally questionable tooth should be condemned in favor of using an adjacent healthy tooth as the abutment, even though the span is increased one tooth by doing so.

The most frequent application of the use of multiple abutments is the splinting of two premolars or a first premolar and a canine. Mandibular premolars generally have round and tapered roots which are easily loosened by rotation as well as by tipping. They are the weakest of posterior abutments. But maxillary premolars also often have tapered roots which make them also poor risks as abutments, particularly where they will be called upon to resist the leverage of a free-end base. Such teeth are best splinted by casting or soldering two crowns or inlays together. When a first premolar to be used as an abutment has poor root form or support, it is best that it be splinted to the stronger canine in a similar manner.

Anterior teeth upon which cingulum rests are to be placed frequently need to be splinted together to avoid orthodontic movement of individual teeth. Mandibular anterior teeth are seldom so used, but if so, splinting of the teeth involved is advisable. Where such splinting is impossible for one reason or another, individual cingulum rests on cast restorations may be inclined slightly toward the center of the tooth to avoid possible tooth displacement, or cingulum rests may be used in conjunction with incisal hooks, engaging slightly the labial surface of the teeth.

Cingulum rests should always be placed as low on the cingulum as possible, and single anterior teeth, other than canines, should not ordinarily be used for occlusal support. Where cingulum rests are employed on central and lateral incisors, as many teeth as possible should be included so as to distribute the load over several teeth, thereby minimizing the force on any one tooth. Even so, some movement of individual teeth is likely to occur, particularly where they are subjected to the forces of indirect retention. This is best avoided by splinting several teeth with united cast restorations. The condition of the teeth and cosmetic considerations will dictate whether full veneer crowns, three-quarter crowns, or pinledge inlays will be used for this purpose.

Splinting of molar teeth for the purpose of multiple abutment support is less frequently used, because they are generally multirooted teeth to begin with and a two- or three-rooted tooth that is not strong enough alone is probably a poor abutment risk. There may be exceptions, however, notable where because of fused and conical roots the abutment would benefit from the effect of splinting.

USE OF ISOLATED TEETH AS ABUTMENTS

While splinting is advocated for any abutment teeth that are considered too weak to risk using alone, a single anterior abutment standing alone in the dental arch almost always requires the splinting effect of a fixed bridge if a free-end base will extend distally from it. Even though the form and length of the root and the supporting bone seem to be adequate for an ordinary abutment, the fact that the tooth lacks proximal contact endangers the tooth when it is used to support a free-end base.

The average abutment tooth is subjected to some distal tipping, to rotation, and to horizontal movement, all of which must be held to a minimum by the design of the denture and the quality of tissue support for the free-end base. The isolated abutment tooth, however, is subjected also to mesial tipping due to lack of proximal contact. Despite indirect retention, some lifting of the free-end base is inevitable, causing torque to the abutment as the fulcrum of a teeter-totter.

In a tooth-borne prosthesis an isolated tooth may be used as an abutment by using a fifth abutment for additional support. Thus, rotational and horizontal forces are resisted by the additional stabilization obtained from the fifth abutment. Where two such isolated abutments exist, e.g., two second premolars with first premolars missing, the sixth abutment should be used. Thus, the two canines, the two isolated premolars, and two posterior teeth are used as abutments.

In contrast, an isolated anterior abutment adjacent to a free-end base should almost always be splinted to the nearest tooth by means of a fixed bridge. The effect is twofold: (1) the anterior edentulous segment is eliminated, thereby creating an intact dental arch anterior to the free-end space; (2) the isolated tooth is splinted to the other abutment of the fixed bridge, thereby providing multiple abutment support. Here, also, splinting should be used only to gain multiple abutment support rather than to hold up an otherwise weak abutment tooth.

The economic aspect of using fixed bridges as part of the mouth preparations for a partial denture is essentially the same as that for any other splinting procedure: the best design of the partial denture which will assure the longevity of its service makes the additional procedure and expense necessary. While it must be recognized that economic considerations, combined with a particularly favorable prognosis of an isolated tooth, may influence the decision to forego the advantages of using a fixed bridge, the original treatment plan should include this precautionary measure even though the alternative method is accepted for economic reasons.

A second factor may also influence the decision to use an isolated tooth as an abutment; this is the esthetic consideration for an otherwise sound anterior tooth which would have to be used as an abutment for a fixed bridge. But neither esthetics nor economics should deter the dentist from recommending to the patient that an isolated tooth which will be used as a free-end abutment be given the advantage of splinting by means of a fixed bridge. Then, should compromises be necessary, the patient must share a measure of the responsibility for using the isolated tooth as an abutment.

MISSING ANTERIOR TEETH

When a partial denture is to replace missing posterior teeth, especially in the absence of distal abutments, any additional missing teeth anteriorly are best replaced by means of fixed bridgework rather than by being added to the denture. In any posterior free-end situation, some teeter-totter action will inevitably result from the adding of an anterior segment to the denture. Here again, the ideal treatment plan which treats the anterior edentulous space separately comes in conflict with economic and esthetic considerations. Each situation must be treated according to its own merits. Frequently, the best esthetic result can be obtained by replacing missing anterior teeth with the partial denture rather than with a fixed bridge. From a biomechanical standpoint, however, a partial denture should replace only the missing posterior teeth, *after* the remainder of the arch has been made intact by means of fixed restorations.

Although the occasional need for compromises is recognized, the decision to include an anterior segment on the denture will depend largely upon the support available for that part of the denture. The greater the number of natural anterior teeth remaining, the better the support that will be available for the edentulous segment.

If definite tooth rests are obtainable, the anterior segment may be treated as any other tooth-bounded modification space. Sound principles of occlusal rest support apply just as much as elsewhere in the arch. Inclined tooth surfaces should not be used for occlusal support, nor should finger rests be placed upon unprepared lingual surfaces. The best possible support for an anterior segment is multiple support extending, if possible, posteriorly across prepared cingulum rests on the canine teeth to mesial occlusal rests on the first premolars. Such support will permit the missing anterior teeth to be included in the denture, frequently with some cosmetic advantages over fixed bridgework.

There are instances where the replacement of anterior teeth by means of a partial denture cannot be avoided. But without adequate tooth support, any such prosthesis will lack the stability that would exist from replacing only the posterior teeth with the partial denture and the anterior teeth with fixed restorations. However, where anterior teeth have been lost through accident or have been missing for some time, resorption of the anterior ridge may have progressed to the point that neither bridge nor denture replacements may be butted to the residual ridge. In such case, for esthetic reasons, the missing teeth must be replaced with a denture base supporting teeth that are more nearly in their original position, considerably forward from the residual ridge. While such teeth may be positioned to better cosmetic advantage, the contouring and coloring of a denture base to be esthetically pleasing requires the maximum artistic effort of both the dentist and the technician. Such a partial denture, both from an esthetic and a biomechanical standpoint, is one of the most difficult of all prosthetic restorations.

TEMPORARY CROWNS AND BRIDGES

Each time a tooth is prepared for a full crown, a temporary crown must be placed for the protection and comfort of the exposed dentin. Ideally, this crown will restore occlusion and contact, although not necessarily so.

Most inlay preparations may be filled with a thick mix of white WondrPak cement. Occasionally, this may suffice also for a three-quarter crown preparation where only the deeper grooves need to be filled. However, for most three-quarter crown preparations and for large inlay preparations, a modified aluminum crown is used in preference to the WondrPak alone. In any case, WondrPak is the preferred cementing medium.

Individual full crown preparations, where esthetics does not prevent their use, may be satisfactorily covered with fitted aluminum crowns. Contact and

Fig. 160. The making of a single anterior resin temporary crown. **A,** A contoured copper band that has been flattened labiolingually is filled with resin of the correct shade and pressed onto the prepared tooth that has been coated with petrolatum. **B,** When the resin has reached a leathery consistency, the copper band is removed from the tooth momentarily and then re-seated onto the tooth until the resin has hardened. This is necessary to assure the withdrawal of the hardened resin without difficulty. **C,** As soon as the resin has hardened, the copper band is slit longitudinally with a carborundum disk and peeled off. **D,** The resin coping, which will be shaped in the form of a temporary crown, is placed back onto the tooth and marked with a pencil where excess thickness and occlusal interference is to be reduced. This is repeated until a temporary crown of acceptable contours has been formed. At the same time, any flash extending beyond abutment shoulders must be removed. **E,** The resin crown is then polished and temporarily cemented to the abutment tooth.

occlusion may be less than ideal, but the length of time the crown will be worn is usually short. Aluminum temporary crowns should be trimmed short of the gingival tissues and should be smoothed and contoured to eliminate rough edges. The temporary crown should protect the tooth, yet should not interfere with gingival healing nor induce inflammation which might cause gingival pathology or recession.

For esthetic reasons, anterior temporary crowns should be made of a rapid-curing acrylic resin of a matching tooth shade. Anterior temporary bridges may also be made of resin, and even posterior bridges where better esthetics or occlusion is desirable. Single resin crowns may be made by filling a contoured copper band with the tooth-shade resin and pressing onto the prepared tooth that has been coated with petrolatum (Fig. 160). On anterior teeth, the copper band may be pinched labiolingually to form a more natural tooth contour. *In any direct ap-*

plication of tooth-shade resin for temporary purposes, the crown must be removed and reseated while the material is still plastic, to make sure that the hardened crown will withdraw. After hardening, the crown is removed and the copper band is slit on the lingual side and stripped away. The crown may then be ground to resemble the tooth being restored, polished, and cemented with temporary cement. Such a temporary crown provides excellent esthetics and fit and will serve for an indefinite period if necessary.

Individual resin crowns may also be made by the same methods as those for making a temporary bridge. Once a technique has been adopted, resin temporary crowns are quickly made and are preferable because of their appearance and the fact that their natural contours are much more comfortable to the patient. Several methods for making resin temporary crowns and bridges are outlined as follows:

1. (a) An impression is made of the mouth before the tooth or teeth are prepared. This impression may be made in alginate hydrocolloid or with baseplate wax in a crown and bridge impression tray. The use of baseplate wax for this purpose is expedient, inexpensive, does not require special handling during the interlude, and is rigid enough to permit compression molding. It is easily carved to create teeth to be added and is easily trimmed to increase the thickness of temporary crowns where little tooth structure has been removed, such as in the gingival one third.

Prior to making this impression, missing tooth contours should be restored with inlay wax so that an impression of intact tooth surfaces can be made. If missing teeth are to be replaced, they may be waxed into the space or a denture tooth may be fitted into each space before the impression is made. An alternate method is to carve the tooth form of the tooth or teeth to be replaced into the impression, which is then filled and shaped along with adjacent crowns. By placing some of the impression material on the opposite side of the tray and having the patient close into it, a means of stabilizing the tray in the mouth later is established. The patient may then close into the impression, thus making it unnecessary for the dentist to hold it while the plastic resin material is setting.

(b) Instead of making an impression of the mouth before the preparations are begun, the dentist or assistant may make an impression of a previous study cast, after artificial tooth replacements have been waxed in to form the bridge span.

Whether method (a) or (b) is used, the impression should be trimmed to eliminate undercut areas and projections into interproximal spaces which would interfere with reseating. If the impression is of alginate hydrocolloid, it must be wrapped in a wet towel and set aside while the teeth are being prepared. A baseplate wax impression may be set aside without any special precautions.

2. (a) After the preparations are completed and impressions for working casts and jaw relations have been made, the prepared teeth are dried and coated with petroleum jelly. If the original impression was made with alginate, it is now removed from the wet towel and dried with compressed air.

That portion of the impression involving the crowns or bridge is now filled with a self-curing resin of the desired shade. Although powder and liquid may be mixed to form a dough, a sprinkling method is preferred. At the time of this writing, a material known as Jet repair acrylic is available in new-hue shades and has proved to be a nearly ideal material for making temporary crowns and bridges. The powder is packaged in a flexible container which permits dispensing without waste and is therefore both economical and convenient to use for filling tooth molds by sprinkling. Some powder is sprinkled into the mold first and then wet with liquid from a medicine dropper. This is repeated until the mold is filled, tapping the impression on the bench each time to facilitate absorption. After the crown or bridge area is filled, any excess that has flowed into other areas should be removed with a pledget of cotton. The material must then be allowed to reach a soft, rubbery state before it is seated onto the petrolatum-coated teeth.

Using the unprepared teeth as a guide, the impression is reseated into the mouth and held until sufficient time has elapsed for the material to reach a stiff rubbery consistency. Unfortunately, this must come from experience with the particular resin material being used. It is necessary that the crowns be removed once before the material has hardened, to assure their withdrawal. Preferably, the rubbery plastic will remain in the impression at this time. It may then be removed from the impression, excess material trimmed away with fine scissors, and reseated in the impression. The impression is then reseated in the mouth to finish compression molding of the plastic resin while it hardens. After time has elapsed for hardening, the impression is removed. This time the hardened resin will remain on the teeth, but having been removed once, it may easily be tapped off, trimmed, and polished. Parallelism of abutment teeth is an absolute necessity where temporary bridges are made by this method. Otherwise, serious difficulty may be encountered in attempting to remove the rigid resin appliance. To avoid this hazard, the rubbery plastic resin may be allowed to harden in the impression out of the mouth. If the material has reached a stiff rubbery state before removal from the mouth, this does not seem to materially affect its accuracy. (Even a well-fitting temporary crown should be reamed slightly to accommodate the temporary cement and make its subsequent removal less difficult.) After the material has hardened, it is removed from the impression, the excess trimmed away, and then polished, taking care to preserve the accuracy of the gingival margins.

(b) Instead of forming the temporary crowns or bridge in the mouth, the following alternate method may be used: As soon as the preparations are completed, an alginate hydrocolloid impression of the prepared teeth is made and poured immediately in stone. The making of this impression should precede the making of other impressions, which may then be made while the stone cast is hardening. Retraction of tissues is not necessary for this impression, and if some of the alginate is first smeared onto the prepared teeth with the finger, the impression will be relatively free of defects.

As soon as the cast can be separated from the hydrocolloid impression of the prepared teeth, any small air bubbles are removed and the cast is then painted with a tin-foil substitute. The original impression is filled with tooth-shade resin as in 2 (a), but instead of being placed back into the mouth, it is seated onto the cast of the prepared teeth. It is removed while rubbery, as before, the excess trimmed with scissors, and then reseated until it hardens. This method differs from method 2 (a) only in that the prepared teeth are made more accessible and the danger of damage to the mouth during removal of the hardened resin is avoided. Should the stone teeth fracture during removal, no harm has been done, and the stone may be picked out of the hardened resin crowns.

The alginate hydrocolloid impression of the prepared teeth may be poured in low-fusing metal instead of stone and thus separated immediately instead of waiting for the stone to set. While some cooling shrinkage of the metal occurs, temporary crowns made on such a die can be reamed slightly if necessary. This should usually be done anyway to allow for the thickness of the temporary cement and to make removal of the crowns easier. The impression should be dried thoroughly with compressed air before pouring the low-fusing metal (such as Dialoy) into it. The molten metal should be poured from the ladle when just slightly above the congealing point rather than immediately after removal from the flame. This avoids sizzling and results in a more accurate cast.

Low-fusing metal may also be used to advantage in other ways where an immediate cast is desired. For example, during the preparation of abutment teeth there may be some question as to the parallelism of the preparation or of two or more bridge abutments. An alginate hydrocolloid impression of the prepared and adjacent teeth may be poured in low-fusing metal and separated immediately. In this way the operator may see what further modifications are necessary before proceeding. Since the low-fusing metal is reusable, little time and material are used, and the possibility of taking final impressions of inadequate preparations is thus eliminated.

TEMPORARY CROWNS WHERE A PARTIAL DENTURE IS BEING WORN

Occasionally, an existing partial denture must remain serviceable while the mouth is being prepared for a new denture. In such cases, temporary crowns must be made which will support the old denture and not interfere with its insertion and removal. Only rarely can an aluminum crown be made to serve this purpose. Instead, a resin temporary crown must be made which duplicates the original form of the abutment tooth (Fig. 161).

The technique for making temporary crowns to fit the inside of denture clasps is similar to that given for other types of resin temporary crowns. The principal difference is that an alginate impression must be made of the entire arch with the old partial denture in place. This is wrapped in a wet towel and set aside while the tooth or teeth are being prepared for new crowns.

After the preparations are completed and the impressions and jaw relation records have been made, the prepared teeth are dried and coated with petroleum jelly. The original alginate impression is trimmed to eliminate any excess, undercuts, and interproximal projections that would interfere with reinsertion.

The tooth-shade resin is sprinkled into the impression in those areas that are to be temporary crowns, and any excess is removed with a pledget of cotton. When the material reaches a soft rubbery state, the impression is seated into

Fig. 161. A sequence of mouth preparations with temporary crowns formed so as to support an old partial denture while a new one is being made. **A,** Several abutment teeth have been prepared to receive full coverage. **B,** Acrylic resin temporary crowns duplicating the original tooth contour. An impression of the teeth before preparation was begun was used to establish the shape of the temporary crowns. **C,** The old partial denture, seated onto the temporary crowns. These are then removed as often as necessary during succeeding appointments. **D,** Gold castings are tried in, prior to soldering and adding veneers. The temporary crowns and old partial denture are then returned to the mouth until the abutment pieces are ready for cementation.

the mouth, where it is held by the dentist until time has elapsed for it to reach a stiff rubbery stage. This must be based on experience with the particular plastic material being used. At this time, the impression is removed, the crowns remaining in the impression. These are then stripped out of the impression; all excess is trimmed away with scissors and the crowns are reseated on the prepared abutments. The partial denture is then removed from the alginate impression and reseated in the mouth onto the plastic crowns which are at this time in a stiff rubbery state. The patient may bring the teeth into occlusion to re-establish the former position and occlusal relationship of the old partial denture.

After the plastic crown or crowns have hardened, the partial denture is removed, the crowns remaining on the teeth. These are then tapped off, trimmed, polished, and temporarily cemented. The result is a temporary crown which restores the original abutment contours and allows the partial denture to be inserted and removed without interference, at the same time providing the same support to the denture that existed before the teeth were prepared. This service, made possible by modern materials, should be routine in all such cases.

Cementation of Temporary Crowns. Cementation of resin temporary crowns differs from the cementation of aluminum crowns in that the plastic crowns fit closely and do not require cementation for retention. Since little or no space exists for the temporary cement, the crowns may need to be reamed slightly to accommodate the temporary cement and to facilitate removal. The temporary cement should be thin and applied only to the inside rim of the crowns to assure complete seating. As soon as the temporary cement has hardened, the occlusion may be checked and relieved accordingly.

Regardless of the type of temporary cement used, any excess which might be irritating to the gingivae should be removed. Too frequently, the final act before dismissing the patient is the cementation of the temporary crowns. Instead, two considerations are necessary. One is the removal of excess cement after it has hardened. The second is the application of some medication to the lacerated gingivae to facilitate healing and to prevent discomfort to the patient. Topical application of some antibacterial agent is, at best, a very transient treatment that does little to prevent discomfort. Hydrocortisone acetate, 0.5 per cent, in a denture adhesive powder, when applied topically to a freshly lacerated surface, both facilitates healing and prevents after-pain. It should be applied to the lacerated gingivae around each temporary crown and the patient dismissed without further rinsing of the mouth. Tissue response to this treatment has been so favorable that it is included here as a specific treatment. Apparently, it is effective only on fresh wounds and is of little value as a follow-up treatment.

THE MAKING OF CROWNS AND INLAYS
TO FIT EXISTING DENTURE CLASPS

It is frequently necessary that an abutment tooth be restored with a full crown (and occasionally with an inlay) which will fit the inside of the clasp of an otherwise serviceable partial denture. The technique for doing so is simple enough but requires that an indirect-direct-indirect pattern be made and therefore justifies a fee for service above that for the usual full crown.

The technique for making a crown to fit the inside of a denture clasp is as follows: An alginate impression of the mouth is made with the partial denture in place. This impression, which is for the purpose of making the plastic temporary crown, is wrapped in a wet towel and set aside while the tooth is being prepared. Even though several abutment teeth are to be restored, it is usually necessary that each one be completed before beginning the next. This is necessary so that the original support and occlusal relationship of the partial denture can be maintained as each new crown is being made.

The abutment tooth is then prepared, during which time the partial denture is reinserted frequently enough to ascertain that sufficient tooth structure is being removed to allow for the thickness of the gold casting. When the preparation is completed, a copper band impression of the tooth is obtained, from which a stone die is made.

A resin temporary crown is then made in the original alginate impression as outlined in the preceding paragraphs. It is trimmed, polished, and temporarily cemented, and the denture is returned to the mouth. The patient is dismissed

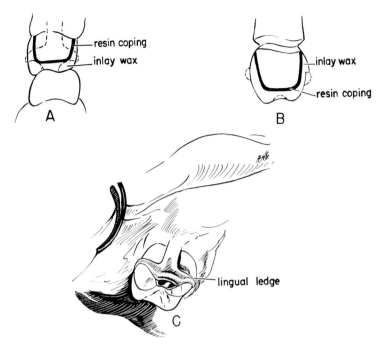

Fig. 162. The making of a cast crown to fit an existing partial denture clasp. **A,** A thin resin coping is first made on an individual die of the prepared tooth. Inlay wax is then added and the coping placed onto the prepared tooth where occlusal surfaces and contact relations are established directly in the mouth. The clasp assembly is warmed with a needle-point flame only enough to soften the inlay wax, and the partial denture is placed in the mouth where it is guided gently to place by the opposing occlusion. This step must be repeated several times and excess wax removed or wax added until full supporting contact with the underside of the clasp assembly has been established, with the denture fully seated. Usually the wax pattern withdraws with the denture and must be gently teased out of the clasp each time. **B,** The wax pattern is then placed back onto the individual die for the purpose of completing occlusal anatomy and refining the margins. Excess wax remaining below the impression of the retentive clasp arm must be removed, but a wax ledge may be left below the reciprocal clasp arm. **C,** The finished casting in the mouth. The terminus of the retentive clasp is then readapted to engage an undercut. It is frequently necessary to remove some interference from the casting, as indicated by articulating paper placed between the clasp and the crown, until the clasp is fully seated.

after removing excess cement and treating the traumatized gingiva as mentioned previously.

Upon the stone die made from the copper band impression, a very thin self-curing resin coping will be formed with a brush technique. The stone die should first be trimmed to the finishing line of the preparation, which is then delineated with a pencil, and the die painted with a tin-foil substitute. A material such as Al-Cote tin-foil substitute must be used which will form a thin film on a cold, dry surface. Not all tin-foil substitutes are suitable for this purpose.

With self-curing acrylic resin powder and liquid in separate dappen dishes and a fine sable brush, a coping of acrylic resin of uniform thickness is painted onto the die. This should extend not quite to the pencil line representing the limit of the crown preparation. After hardening, the resin coping may be re-moved, inspected, and trimmed if necessary. The thin film of foil substitute should be removed before reseating the coping onto the die.

The wax pattern is usually not begun until the patient returns, at which time it is built up at the chair. First, the occlusal portion of the wax pattern is established by having the patient close and carve excursive paths in the wax (Fig. 162, *A*). Dull areas are added to until a smooth occlusal registration has been obtained. Except for narrowing the occlusal surface and the carving of grooves and spillways, this will be the occlusal anatomy of the finished restoration.

The second step is the adding of sufficient wax to establish contact relations with the adjoining tooth. At this time, the occlusal relation of the marginal ridges must also be established.

Next, wax is added to buccal and lingual surfaces where the clasp arms will contact the crown, and the pattern is again reseated in the mouth. The clasp arms, minor connectors, and occlusal rests involved on the partial denture are warmed with a needle-point flame, being careful to avoid flaming any adjacent resin, and the denture is inserted onto the wax pattern (Fig. 162, *B*). Several attempts may be necessary until the denture is fully seated and the components of the clasp clearly recorded in the wax pattern. Each time the denture is re-moved, the pattern will draw with it and must be teased out of the clasp.

When contact with the clasp arms and the occlusal relation of the denture has been established satisfactorily, the temporary crown may be replaced and the patient dismissed. The crown pattern is completed on the die by narrowing the occlusal surface buccolingually, adding grooves and spillways and refining the margins.* Any wax ledge remaining below the reciprocal clasp arm may be left to provide some of the advantages of a crown ledge described earlier in this chapter. Excess wax remaining below the retentive clasp arm, however, must be removed so as to permit the adding of a retentive undercut later (Fig. 162, *C*).

If an acrylic veneer is to be added, the veneer space must now be carved in the wax pattern. In such case, the contour of the veneer may be recorded by making a stone matrix of the buccal surface, which can later be replaced onto the completed casting for the purpose of waxing in the veneer. This stone matrix is then invested with the casting when the acrylic veneer is being processed.

The wax pattern must be sprued with care so as not to destroy essential areas on the pattern. After casting, the crown should be subjected to a minimum of polishing, since the exact form of the vertical and occlusal surfaces must be maintained.

Since it is impossible to withdraw a clasp arm from a retentive undercut on the wax pattern, the casting must be made without any provision for clasp retention. After trying the crown in the mouth, with the denture in place, the location of the retentive clasp terminal is identified by scoring the crown with

---

*Margins on all crown and inlay wax patterns are refined with S. S. White red casting wax, which contrasts with the blue or green wax used for the pattern and permits the carving of delicate margins with accuracy. The preferred wax for the body of crown and inlay patterns is Maves inlay wax. This wax is available in both cone and stick form and has excellent carving properties and color.

a sharp instrument. The crown may then be ground and polished slightly in this area to create a retentive undercut. The clasp terminal may then be adapted into this undercut, thereby creating clasp retention on the new crown.

The technique for making inlay patterns to fit the inside of denture clasps is essentially the same as for full crowns, except that it may be done entirely in wax. However, patterns for larger inlays that might be distorted during insertion of the denture are best supported also by an acrylic resin foundation. In such cases, the pattern is started by brushing in the acrylic resin until a supporting frame has been established. The wax pattern is then completed in the mouth as for a full crown.

Ideally, all abutment teeth would best be protected with full crowns before the partial denture is constructed. Except for the possibility of recurrent caries due to defective crown margins or gingival recession, abutment teeth so protected may be expected to give many years of satisfactory service in the support and retention of the partial denture. Economically, a policy of insisting on full coverage for all abutment teeth may well be justified from the long-term viewpoint. It must be recognized, however, that in practice full coverage of all abutment teeth is not always possible nor at the time indicated. Many factors act to influence the future health status of an abutment tooth, some of which cannot be foreseen. It is necessary, therefore, that the dentist be able to treat abutment teeth which become defective at some later date in such a manner that their service as abutments may be restored and the serviceability of the partial denture maintained. Although it is not part of the original mouth preparations, this service accomplishes much the same purpose by providing the denture with support, stability, and retention, and the dentist must be technically equipped to provide this service when it becomes necessary.

CEMENTATION FOR FIXED RESTORATIONS

Final cementation of fixed restorations should be deferred until evidence of the success of the restoration can be evaluated. Single crowns may be cemented permanently more often than bridge restorations. It seems that nonpermanent cementation of fixed restorations has many advantages and very few disadvantages. Zinc oxide and eugenol temporary cements will adequately retain the restoration and protect the abutment teeth, yet may be removed without difficulty for future inspection of the abutments and the adjacent tissues. The restoration may then be cemented permanently or again only semipermanently. Restorations have been removed after intervals as long as three and five years without evidence of leakage or deterioration of zinc oxide-eugenol cements.

Advantages of Semipermanent Cementation of Fixed Restorations. Some of the advantages of semipermanent cementation are as follows:

1. By cementing the restoration temporarily at first, the dentist can be sure that the crowns are fully seated and that the margins are satisfactory.

2. Less postoperative discomfort generally results from cementation with a temporary cement. Temporary cements are sedative, while zinc oxyphosphate cements are irritating to a pulp suffering already from trauma caused by operative procedures.

3. Restorations may be removed for the purpose of inspecting the tooth beneath and for taking roentgenograms. The hazard of a single leaking abutment piece causing destruction of the tooth before it is detected can thus be eliminated.

4. Restorations may be removed for the purpose of inspecting and treating gingival and subjacent tissues. Future periodontal treatment is thus facilitated.

5. Should root canal therapy become necessary, treatment may be accomplished without cutting through a cemented restoration.

6. Porcelain or resin pontics may be extended where needed to compensate for changes in the residual ridge.

7. Resin veneers may be replaced if they are lost or if they have become discolored or the shade no longer matches the ageing enamel on adjacent teeth.

8. Fractured porcelain veneers or pontics may be more satisfactorily replaced.

9. Solder joints may be reinforced if they become weakened by attrition.

10. The future addition of another abutment for increased support is made possible.

11. The patient is encouraged to return at recommended intervals for inspection and maintenance. In this way the dentist has an opportunity at reasonable intervals to inspect both the fixed restorations and any partial dentures present and to recommend relining or the re-establishment of occlusion on the latter when needed. Oral hygiene habits may also be noted and the patient advised accordingly.

Patients seem quick to appreciate the value of semipermanent cementation, particularly for fixed bridgework, and are prone to request a continuation of the practice. To the patient, as to the dentist, permanent cementation appears to be an irrevocable act that has fewer advantages than cementation with a reliable, semipermanent material.

Chapter **14**

Impression materials and procedures for partial dentures

Impression materials used in the various phases of partial denture construction may be classified as being rigid, thermoplastic, or elastic substances. Rigid impression materials are those that set to a rigid consistency. Thermoplastic impression materials are those that become plastic at higher temperatures and resume their original form when the temperature has again been lowered. Elastic impression materials are those that remain in an elastic or flexible state after removal from the mouth.

All impression materials used in prosthetic dentistry may be included in this classification as follows:

Rigid materials
    Plaster of Paris
    Metallic oxide pastes
Thermoplastic materials
    Modeling plastic
    Impression waxes and resins
Elastic materials
    Reversible hydrocolloid (agar-agar)
    Irreversible hydrocolloid (alginate)
    Mercaptan rubber-base materials (Thiokol)
    Silicone materials
    Thermoplastic elastic materials

While rigid impression materials may be capable of recording tooth and tissue details accurately, they cannot be removed from the mouth without fracture and reassembly. Thermoplastic materials cannot record minute details accurately because they undergo distortion during withdrawal from tooth and tissue undercuts. Elastic materials are the only ones that can be withdrawn from tooth and tissue undercuts without permanent deformation and are therefore the only ones that are suitable for impressions of irregular contours of oral tissues. Whereas the rigid and thermoplastic impression materials are most frequently used in various combinations in the making of impressions for complete dentures, the elastic impression materials are most generally used for the making of impressions for partial dentures, immediate dentures, and crowns and bridges, where tooth and tissue undercuts and surface detail must be recorded with accuracy.

RIGID MATERIALS*

Plaster of Paris. One type of rigid impression material is plaster of Paris, which has been used in dentistry for over 200 years. Although all plaster-of-Paris impression materials are handled in approximately the same manner, the setting and flow characteristics of each manufacturer's product will vary. Some are pure, finely ground plaster of Paris with only an accelerator added for the purpose of expediting setting within reasonable working limits. Others are modified impression plaster in which binders and plasticizers have been added to permit limited muscle molding while the material is setting. These do not set as hard or fracture as clean as pure plaster of Paris and therefore cannot be reassembled with as much accuracy if fracture occurs. However, they are preferred by some operators because of their setting characteristics.

Plaster of Paris was once the only material that could be used for partial denture impressions, but now elastic materials have completely replaced the impression plasters in this phase of prosthetic dentistry. It is still widely used for making accurate transfers of abutment castings or copings in the fabrication of fixed bridges and precision attachment dentures and for making rigid indexes and matrices for various purposes in prosthetic dentistry.

Metallic Oxide Pastes. A second type of "rigid impression materials is that classified as metallic oxide pastes, these usually being some form of a zinc oxide-eugenol combination. A number of these pastes are available today and they are probably more widely used than any other secondary impression material." They are not used as primary impression materials and are not used in stock impression trays.

"Metallic oxide pastes are manufactured with a wide variation of consistencies and setting characteristics. For convenience, most of them are dispensed from two tubes, an arrangement which enables the operator to mix the correct proportion from each tube onto a glass or paper mixing slab. The previously prepared tray is loaded and the impression is inserted with or without any attempt at muscle-molding. Generally, muscle-molding of metallic oxide impression pastes is not advisable, as wrinkles will occur if movement is permitted at the time the material reaches its setting state. Therefore, as in most modern impression techniques, the accuracy of the primary impression and of the impression tray has a great influence upon the final impression. Some metallic oxide pastes remain fluid for a longer period of time than others, and some manufacturers claim that muscle-molding is possible. In general, however, all metallic oxide pastes have one thing in common with plaster of Paris impression materials; this is that they all have a setting time during which they should not be disturbed and after which no further muscle-molding is effective."

---

*Much of this discussion has been quoted or paraphrased from McCracken, W. L.: Impression Materials in Prosthetic Dentistry, D. Clin. North America, pp. 671-684, Nov., 1958.

Although metallic oxide pastes, being rigid substances, are widely used as secondary impression materials for complete dentures, they are also used for secondary impressions in partial denture techniques. One widely used partial denture impression technique utilizes a paste impression of the edentulous ridge made in a resin or shellac impression tray which is then finger-loaded through an opening in a stock perforated tray while an over-all alginate impression is taken of the entire arch. This technique attempts to relate the zinc oxide impression of the edentulous ridge to the rest of the arch in a relationship similar to that which will be assumed when an occlusal load is applied. (See recording of functional or supporting ridge form, Chapter 15.)

Metallic oxide pastes are also used as an impression material for denture relining and may be used successfully for this purpose if the original denture base has been relieved sufficiently to allow the material to flow without displacement of either the denture or the underlying tissues.

THERMOPLASTIC MATERIALS*

Modeling Plastic. Like plaster of Paris, modeling plastic is among the oldest of the impression materials used in prosthetic dentistry. It is manufactured "in several different colors, each color being an indication of the temperature range at which the material is plastic and workable. A common error in the use of modeling plastic is that it is subjected to higher temperatures than intended by the manufacturer. It then becomes too soft and loses [some of] its favorable working characteristics. If a controlled water bath is not used, a thermometer should be used routinely to maintain a temperature within limits that will not cause a weakening of the material or influence its working characteristics. If modeling plastic is softened at a temperature above that intended by the manufacturer, the material becomes brittle and unpredictable. Also, there is the ever-present danger of burning the patient when the temperature used in softening the modeling plastic is too high."

The most commonly used modeling plastic is the red material which, in cake form, softens at about 132° F. It should never be softened at temperatures much above this. "Neither should it, nor any other modeling plastic, be immersed in the water bath for an indefinite period of time. Rather, it should not leave the operator's fingers during the softening period. It should be dipped and kneaded until soft, and it should be subjected to no more heat than necessary before inserting the material into the tray and into the mouth. It may then be flamed with an alcohol torch for the purpose of muscle-molding, but should always be dipped back into the water bath before returning to the mouth in order to avoid burning the patient. The modeling plastic may then be chilled before removal from the mouth [although this is not necessary]. During sectional flaming and muscle-molding, it should be chilled after each insertion. It may then be trimmed with a sharp knife without danger of fracture or distortion."

The red, gray, and green modeling plastics are obtainable in stick form,

*Much of this discussion has been quoted or paraphrased from McCracken, W. L.: Impression Materials in Prosthetic Dentistry, D. Clin. North America, pp. 671-684, Nov., 1958.

for use in muscle-trimming an impression or an impression tray. The green material is the lowest fusing of the modeling plastics. The red and gray sticks have a higher and broader working range than the cakes of like color so that they may be flamed without harming the material. Because of its contrasting lighter color, the gray material in stick form is preferred by some operators for muscle-trimming. The choice between the use of green and gray sticks is purely optional and entirely up to the operator or the operator may prefer to use the higher fusing red sticks for muscle-trimming the peripheries of a red modeling plastic impression.

Although modeling plastic has been used in past years as an impression material for study casts, it has now been replaced by the elastic materials for this purpose. Some dentists still prefer to use modeling plastic as a secondary impression material for the recording of edentulous ridges in partial denture construction, but when this is done the limitations and disadvantages are the same as for making a full modeling plastic impression for complete dentures. Similarly, modeling plastic is sometimes used as a reline impression material for partial denture bases. It is generally used, however, only as a means of building up the underside of the denture prior to recording the tissues with some secondary impression material. (See functional relining method, Chapter 15.)

Impression Waxes and Resins. "A second group of thermoplastic impression materials is those impression waxes and resins commonly spoken of as 'mouth-temperature waxes.' The most familiar of these are the Korecta waxes and the Iowa wax, both of which were developed for specific techniques. One must be cognizant of the characteristics of mouth-temperature waxes and use them knowingly.

"The Iowa impression wax, for example, was designed to be used as a wax impression over a modeling plastic correction in an acrylic tray. . . . The Korecta waxes were also developed for a specific purpose, this being to record the supporting form of the edentulous areas which provide support for a free-end partial denture base. Although four Korecta waxes are available, the No. 4 wax is the most fluid and is quite similar to the Iowa formula in most respects. In fact, the two waxes may be used interchangeably without any detectable difference in results. The No. 1 Korecta wax is not an impression wax, but is instead a supporting wax that is unaffected by mouth temperature. Therefore, it is used as a means for supporting the impression of the periphery during the making of fluid wax impressions." (The No. 2 and No. 3 Korecta waxes, although developed to provide a broader range of flow characteristics, are not generally used today as impression waxes.)

The No. 4 Korecta wax was developed to be used for the purpose of recording the functional or supporting form of an edentulous ridge beneath a free-end partial denture base. It may be used either as a secondary impression material or as an impression material for rebasing the finished partial denture to obtain support from the underlying tissues. "The mouth-temperature waxes lend themselves well to all rebasing techniques as they will flow sufficiently in the mouth to avoid overdisplacement of tissues. As with any rebasing technique, it is necessary that sufficient relief be provided. In addition, escapement slots or holes in the original base must be used, to avoid locking the impression material against the tissues without opportunity for escape." Given an opportunity to flow, the fluid waxes record the tissues without overdisplacement and assure uniformity of support for the partial denture base.

The difference between impression wax and modeling plastic is that the impression waxes have the ability to flow as long as they are in the mouth and thereby permit equalization of pressure and prevent overdisplacement, whereas the modeling plastics flow only in proportion to the amount of flaming and tempering which can be done out of the mouth, and this does not continue after the plastic has approached mouth temperature. The principal advantage of mouth-temperature waxes is that they displace tissues which are not themselves capable of rendering support to the denture, but given sufficient time, they permit a rebound of those tissues which have been overdisplaced.

"The impression waxes may also be used to correct the periphery of impressions made of more rigid materials, thereby establishing firmer contact at the periphery of the denture. All mouth-temperature wax impressions have the ability to record peripheral detail accurately and at the same time establish better than any other material the correct width of the denture periphery. They have the advantage of being correctible, and if the operator will take sufficient time in the making of the correction, he may record accurately not only surface detail but all peripheral areas that are available for support and retention of the denture."

Some mouth-temperature waxes vary in their working characteristics from those mentioned above. Among these are the Jelenko Adaptol impression material and the Stalite impression material. Both of these seem to have a more resinous base. They are designed primarily for impression techniques that attempt to record the tissues under an occlusal load. In such techniques the occlusion rim or the denture setup is completed first. Mouth-temperature wax is then applied to the tissue side of the denture base, and the final impression is made under functional loading, using various muscle movements approximating functional activity. However, these mouth-temperature materials may also be used successfully in open-mouth impression techniques.

The Iowa wax and the Korecta wax will not distort after removal from the mouth at ordinary room temperatures, but the more resinous waxes must be stored at much lower temperatures to avoid flow out of the mouth. Resinous waxes are not ordinarily used in partial denture impression techniques, their use being limited to specific techniques for complete denture impressions.

ELASTIC MATERIALS*

Reversible Hydrocolloids. Reversible (agar) hydrocolloids, which are fluid at higher temperatures and gel upon a reduction in temperature, are used primarily as impression materials for fixed and removable bridge prostheses. They are unsurpassed for accuracy when properly used. However, the reversible

---

*Much of this discussion has been quoted or paraphrased from McCracken, W. L.: Impression Materials in Prosthetic Dentistry, D. Clin. North America, pp. 671-684, Nov., 1958.

hydrocolloid impression materials offer few advantages over the irreversible, or alginate, hydrocolloids when used as a partial denture impression material. Present-day alginate hydrocolloids are sufficiently accurate for the making of master casts for partial dentures

Irreversible Hydrocolloids. The irreversible (alginate) hydrocolloids are used for the making of study casts, orthodontic treatment casts, and master casts for crown and bridge and partial denture procedures. When properly handled, they are sufficiently accurate for the making of partial denture master casts. Since they are a colloidal materal, an alginate hydrocolloid impression cannot be stored for any length of time but must be poured immediately. The same precautions in handling apply equally to both the reversible and irreversible hydrocolloid impression materials.

Mercaptan Rubber-Base Impression Materials. The mercaptan rubber-base (Thiokol) impression materials are not as widely used for partial denture impressions as in crown and bridge procedures because of their cost and because an individual impression tray is required To be accurate, the impression must have a uniform thickness not exceeding $\frac{1}{4}$ inch. This necessitates the use of a carefully made individual impression tray of resin or some other material possessing adequate rigidity and stability. It is doubtful that the accuracy of a mercaptan rubber-base impression exceeds that of a properly made alginate hydrocolloid impression, and as with the hydrocolloid impression materials, certain precautions must be taken to avoid distortion of the impression. The mercaptan rubber-base impression materials do have an advantage over the hydrocolloid materials in that the surface of a Hydrocal poured against them is of a smoother texture and therefore appear to be smoother and harder than one poured against a hydrocolloid material. This is probably due to the fact that the rubber material does not have the ability to retard or etch the surface of the setting stone. Despite their accuracy, this has always been a disadvantage of all hydrocolloid impression materials. A cast made from a mercaptan rubber or silicone impression possesses a smoother surface which may possibly lead to a more accurate dental casting. The fact that a smoother surface results does not, however, preclude the possibility of a grossly inaccurate impression and stone cast resulting from other causes.

Another use of the mercaptan rubber-base impression materials is in the making of stabilized bases for recording jaw relations. The elasticity of the rubber material offers comfort to the patient during the recording of jaw relations. However, there is some question as to how accurately this jaw relation record may then be transferred back onto a rigid cast.

Silicone Impression Materials. The silicone impression materials are similar in their accuracy and convenience to the rubber-base impression materials. They are used primarily as impression materials for crown and bridge procedures and require the same precautions as the rubber-base materials. However, they are more delicate to handle in the laboratory, and because of their cost and delicate nature, they are not widely used as impression materials for partial denture master casts. They require the same precautions as the mercaptan rubber materials. They are somewhat more delicate to handle in the laboratory and at the present time are a little more costly than Thiokol materials. In general, however, they possess many of the same advantages and disadvantages and may be similarly used when handled with care.

IMPRESSIONS OF THE PARTIALLY EDENTULOUS ARCH

An impression of the partially edentulous arch must record accurately the anatomic form of the teeth and surrounding tissues. This is necessary so that the prosthesis may be designed to follow a definite path of insertion and removal and also that support and retention on the abutment teeth may be precise and accurate.

Materials that could be permanently deformed by removal from tissue undercuts may not be used for this purpose. This excludes the use of the thermoplastic impression materials for recording the anatomic form of the dental arch. The rigid materials, such as plaster of Paris, are capable of recording tissue detail accurately, but they must be sectioned for removal and subsequently reassembled.

Before the advent of the elastic hydrocolloid materials, plaster of Paris and modeling plastic were the only impression materials available for impressions of the partially edentulous arch. Modeling plastic was used for making preliminary impressions for study casts, despite its distortion upon removal from undercuts. Such study casts were grossly inaccurate and permitted only approximate evaluation of tooth contours. Impressions for master casts were made of plaster of Paris, which was scored and sectioned for removal and then reassembled. This was time-consuming and discomforting to the patient.

Plaster of Paris is accurate and dimensionally stable, is inexpensive, and requires no special equipment for its use. Its main disadvantages are its inflexibility and the fact that some separating medium must be used prior to pouring the cast to prevent the cast material, which is usually also a gypsum product, from adhering to it. Damage to the resulting cast can easily occur during removal of the impression from the cast. Since it must be removed from the mouth sectionally, small pieces from essential areas may be lost, and reassembly of the pieces may take considerable time.

The introduction of hydrocolloids as impression materials was a long step forward in dentistry. For the first time impressions could be made of undercut areas with a material that was elastic enough to be withdrawn from those undercuts without permanent distortion. It permits the making of a one-piece impression which does not require the use of a separating medium, and it is an extremely accurate material when handled properly.

Phillips has reduced the complicated chemistry of the hydrocolloid impression materials to its simplest form in the following paragraphs:

> Hydrocolloids can be classified into two general types: reversible and irreversible. These materials are suspensions of aggregates of molecules in a dispersing medium of water, the water being held by capillary action. Gelation of the reversible hydrocolloids is primarily a physical change in which a latticework of fibrils forms as the temperature is lowered. This gel can be readily dispersed by merely heating the material—thus the term reversible. An example of a reversible hydrocolloid is ordinary gelatin. When gelatin is dissolved in boiling water, it forms a colloidal sol which gels

upon cooling. This gel can be returned to the liquid sol by heating, formed again by cooling, etc.

The base for dental reversible hydrocolloids is agar-agar, a material that can be liquefied at temperatures compatible to oral tissues and then solidified to a firm, yet elastic, gel at temperatures slightly above 100° F. This gelation is accomplished by means of water-cooled impression trays. Such factors as ability to secure routinely accurate reproductions of cavity preparation with one impression, reproductions of minor undercuts without rupture or distortion, and actual saving in chair time have been instrumental in the successful adaptation of this material for use in the indirect inlay technique. It is unexcelled when used in this procedure.

The irreversible hydrocolloids, or alginates, are not thermally reversible and their gelation is induced by an actual chemical reaction rather than by physical means. The powder is essentially sodium alginate and calcium sulphate which when mixed with water react to form a latticework of fibrils of insoluble calcium alginate. These materials have been used extensively in prosthetics and orthodontia. . . .

In general it can be said that the alginates approach the accuracy of reversible hydrocolloid but, due to the greater number of variables both in their manufacture and use, they are not routinely quite as accurate.*

The principal differences between agar and alginate hydrocolloids are as follows:

1. Agar converts from the gel form to a sol by the application of heat. It may be reverted to gel form by a reduction in temperature. This physical change is reversible.

2. Alginate hydrocolloid becomes a gel via a chemical reaction as a result of mixing alginate powder with water. This physical change is irreversible.

Agar hydrocolloid does have some disadvantages. It must be introduced into the mouth while warm enough to be a sol, converting to an elastic gel upon cooling. Therefore, there is an ever-present danger of burning the tissues of the mouth, a burn that is very painful and slow to heal. It requires warming and tempering equipment which is thermostatically controlled and necessitates the use of water-jacketed impression trays for cooling.

All hydrocolloids are dimensionally stable only during a brief period following removal from the mouth. If exposed to the air they rapidly lose water content, with a resulting shrinkage and other dimensional changes. If immersed in water, they imbibe water, with an accompanying swelling and dimensional changes. All hydrocolloid impressions should be poured immediately, but if they must be stored for a brief period of time, it should be in a saturated atmosphere rather than in water. This is accomplished simply by wrapping the impression in a wet towel.

All hydrocolloids also exhibit a phenomenon known as syneresis, which is associated with the giving off of a mucinous exudate. This mucinous exudate has a retarding effect on any gypsum material, which results in a soft or chalky cast surface. Sometimes this is less obvious and only detected by a close examination of the impression after removal from the cast. Nevertheless, such a cast surface is inaccurate and an inaccurate denture casting ultimately results in

---

*From Phillips, R. W.: The Physical Properties of Hydrocolloids and Alginates and Factors Influencing Their Work Qualities and Accuracy, Fort. Rev. Chicago D. Soc. **26**:9-12, 1953.

proportion to the inaccuracy of the master cast. This can only be prevented by (1) pouring the impression immediately and (2) using some chemical accelerator such as potassium sulfate to counteract the retarding effect of the hydrocolloid.

Agar hydrocolloid impressions should be immersed in a 2 per cent solution of potassium sulfate for five to ten minutes prior to pouring the cast even though some accelerator may have been incorporated by the manufacturer. Most all modern alginate hydrocolloid impression materials have an accelerator incorporated into the powder and no longer need to be treated with a "fixing solution" unless it is supplied by the manufacturer. However, an alginate hydrocolloid impression material that is compounded to require a "fixing solution" consistently gives a smoother cast surface than those that do not require immersion in such a solution. It is probably because of the popular demand for alginate impression materials that do not require fixing that the suppliers have all but abandoned the manufacture of those requiring a "fixing solution."

Since no heat is employed in the preparation of alginate hydrocolloid, there is no danger of burning the patient. For this reason, the patient will be more relaxed and cooperative during the positioning of the tray. There are some disadvantages, however, associated with the use of alginate hydrocolloid. This material gels by means of a chemical reaction which is accelerated by the warmth of the tissues, whereas agar hydrocolloid gels from the tray in toward the tissues, due to the cooling action of the water circulating through the tray. In the former, gelation takes place first next to the tissues, and any movement of the tray during gelation of the remote portions results in internal stresses which are released upon removal of the impression from the mouth. A distorted and therefore inaccurate impression results from an alginate hydrocolloid impression that is not held immobile during gelation.

Another disadvantage of alginate hydrocolloid is that it must be introduced into the mouth at approximately 70° F., which causes an immediate increase in the viscosity and surface tension of the saliva. Air bubbles are therefore harder to dispel and it is inevitable that more air will be trapped in an alginate impression than in an agar impression. Every precaution must be taken to avoid the entrapment of air in critical areas.

Important Precautions to Be Observed in the Handling of Hydrocolloid. Some important precautions to be observed in the handling of hydrocolloid are as follows:

1. The impression should not be exposed to air because some dehydration will inevitably occur, resulting in shrinkage.

2. The impression should not be immersed in water for long periods because some imbibition will inevitably result, with an accompanying expansion.

3. The impression should be protected from dehydration by placing it in a humid atmosphere or wrapping it in a wet towel until it can be poured up. To avoid volume change, this should be within fifteen minutes after removal from the mouth.

4. The exudate from hydrocolloid has a retarding effect on the chemical reaction of gypsum products and results in a chalky cast surface. This can be

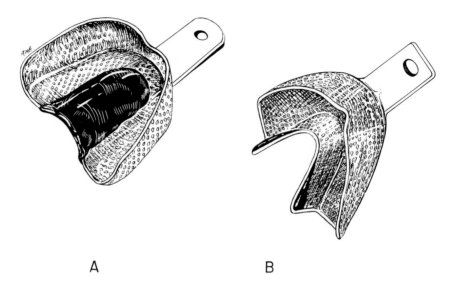

A　　　　　　　　　B

Fig. 163. **A,** A maxillary impression tray with the vault built up with utility wax to prevent impression material from sagging away from the palatal surface. **B,** A mandibular impression tray with utility wax added *inside* the distolingual flange to prevent the tissues of the floor of the mouth from rising inside the tray.

prevented by pouring the cast immediately and by first immersing the impression in a solution of accelerator.

Step-by-Step Procedure for Making a Hydrocolloid Impression. The step-by-step procedure and important points to observe in the making of a hydrocolloid impression are as follows:

1. Select a suitable impression tray that is large enough to provide adequate thickness of the impression material.

2. If the maxillary arch has a high vault, build up the tray with utility wax to prevent the hydrocolloid from sagging away from the palatal surface (Fig. 163, *A*). If gelation occurs next to the tissues while the deeper portion is still fluid, a distorted impression of the palate may result which cannot be detected in the finished impression. This may result in the major connector of the finished casting not being in contact with the underlying tissues.

3. The mandibular tray may need to be lengthened with utility wax in the retromylohyoid area but rarely ever needs to be lengthened elsewhere. Utility wax may need to be added *inside* the distolingual flange to prevent the tissues of the floor of the mouth from rising inside the tray (Fig. 163, *B*). It is advantageous to have stoned away the tissue side of the metal bead on the distal aspect of the mandibular tray to prevent a distortion of the retromolar pad. (For similar reasons, the metal bead which would contact the post-tuberosity area of the maxillary arch should also be removed.)

4. Place the patient in an upright position, with the involved arch nearly parallel to the floor.

5. When using alginate hydrocolloid, place the measured amount of powder

in a clean, dry rubber mixing bowl (600 ml. capacity). Add the measure of water at a temperature between 65° and 70° F. Spatulate rapidly against the side of the bowl with a short, *stiff* spatula (Kerr laboratory spatula No. 1 or Buffalo dental spatula No. 11R). This should be accomplished in less than one minute.

6. In placing the material in the tray, try to avoid entrapping air. Have the first layer of material lock through the perforations of the tray to prevent any possible dislodgment after gelation.

7. After loading the tray, quickly place some material with the finger on any critical areas such as rest preparations and abutment teeth. If an upper impression, place material in the palatal vault and into any deep buccal and labial pouches.

8. Use a mouth mirror to retract the cheek on the side away from you as the tray is being rotated into the mouth from the near side.

9. Seat the tray first on the side away from you, then the anterior area while reflecting the lip, and then the near side, using the mouth mirror or finger for cheek retraction. Finally, make sure that the lip is draping naturally over the tray.

10. Be careful not to seat the tray too deeply, leaving room for a thickness of material over the occlusal and incisal surfaces.

11. Hold the tray immobile for three minutes with light finger pressure over left and right premolar areas. Do not allow the tray to move during gelation so as to avoid internal stresses in the finished impression.

12. After releasing the surface tension, remove the impression quickly in line with the long axis of the teeth to avoid tearing or other distortion.

13. Rinse the impression free of saliva with running tap water and examine critically. Cover the impression immediately with a wet towel.

Any hydrocolloid impression should be poured immediately to avoid dimensional changes and syneresis. Circumstances often necessitate some delay, but this time lapse should be kept to a minimum. A fifteen- or thirty-minute delay is not deleterious if the impression is kept in a humid atmosphere.

Step-by-Step Procedure for Making a Stone Cast From a Hydrocolloid Impression. The step-by-step procedure for making the stone cast from the impression is as follows:

1. Have the measured dental stone at hand, along with a measured quantity of water, as recommended by the manufacturer. For most laboratory stones, 28 ml. of water for each 100 grams is recommended; for Duroc and similar improved stones the proportion is 24 ml. of water for each 100 grams. A clean 600 ml. mixing bowl and stiff spatula, a 4 x 4 inch glass slab or a bathroom tile, and a vibrator complete the preparations. A No. 7 spatula should also be within reach.

2. First pour the measure of water into the mixing bowl and then add the measure of stone. Spatulate thoroughly for one minute, remembering that a weak and porous stone cast may result from insufficient spatulation. Mechanical spatulation may be used to advantage, or vacuum spatulation if such facilities are available. Following any spatulation other than in a vacuum, place the mixing

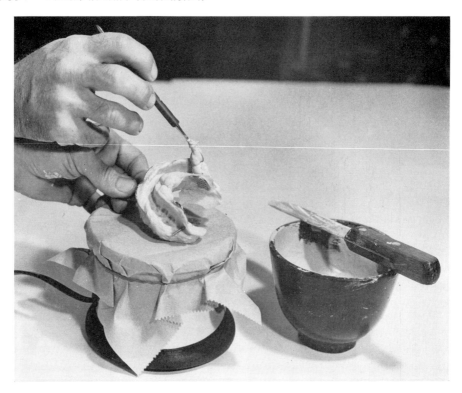

Fig. 164. After thoroughly mixing the stone in a 600 ml. plaster bowl with a stiff spatula, the material is kneaded on the vibrator to expel entrapped air bubbles. The impression is dried with compressed air and filled, in the manner illustrated. Small portions of stone are applied to one heel of the impression and vibrated around the arch, pushing moisture and diluted stone ahead of the mass. Stone is applied at this point only until the impressions of the teeth are filled and the diluted stone is discarded at the opposite heel. Only then is the remainder of the impression filled with larger portions, using the larger spatula. (Note that the vibrator is protected with a paper towel as the impression is being filled.)

bowl on the vibrator and knead the material, to permit the escape of any trapped air.

3. The hydrocolloid impression material used may require a fixing solution. If so, follow the manufacturer's instructions. Any fixing is done just prior to pouring the impression and is not meant to be used as a storing medium. After removing the impression from the damp towel or fixing solution, blow out surplus moisture with compressed air and hold it in the left hand over the vibrator, impression side up.

4. With the No. 7 spatula, add the first cast material to the distal area away from you. Allow this first material to be vibrated around the arch from tooth to tooth toward the anterior part of the impression (Fig. 164). Continue to add small increments of material at this same distal area, each additional portion of added stone pushing the mass ahead of it. This avoids the entrapment of air. The weight of the material causes any excess water to be pushed around the arch

where it is ultimately expelled at the opposite end of the impression. Discard this fluid material. When the impressions of all the teeth have been filled, continue to add cast material in larger portions until the impression is completely filled.

5. Place the material remaining in the mixing bowl on the glass slab and then gently invert the filled impression onto it. The material should have enough body to prevent settling. For the upper impression, lightly rake the material upward around the sides. For the lower impression, in addition to raking upward around the sides, rake the material in the tongue space and level it with the No. 7 spatula so that it does not extend above the lower border of the impression tray. If this is done carefully there will be no need for trimming the tongue space later. (Fig. 165.)

6. As soon as the cast material has developed sufficient body, trim the gross excess from the sides of the cast. The glass slab may then be gently immersed in still water during the initial setting period. The impression thus is prevented from losing water by evaporation, which might in turn deprive the cast material of sufficient water for crystallization. Chalky cast surfaces around the teeth are often the result of the hydrocolloid acting as a sponge and robbing the cast material of its necessary water for crystallization.

7. After the cast and impression have been immersed in still water for thirty minutes, separate the impression from the case. Thirty minutes is sufficient for initial setting, whereas more than an hour may cause a rough cast surface, due to the etching effect of the water. Any stone interfering with separation must be trimmed away with a knife.

8. Clean the impression tray immediately while the used impression material is still elastic.

Fig. 165. After filling the remainder of the impression, stone is piled onto a glass slab or ceramic tile and brought up around the sides and heels of the impression. It may be immersed in still water at this time, or the excess may first be trimmed away with a thin-bladed spatula as the stone reaches a consistency that permits such trimming. It may then be covered with a wet towel or immersed until the final set has occurred.

9. The trimming of the cast should be deferred until final setting has occurred. The sides and base of the cast may then be trimmed so as to be parallel and any blebs or defects due to air bubbles in the impression may be removed. If this is to be a study cast or a cast for permanent record, it may be trimmed to orthodontic specifications so as to present a neat appearance for demonstration purposes. Master casts and other working casts are ordinarily trimmed only to remove excess stone.

Possible Causes of an Inaccurate Cast of a Dental Arch. The possible causes of an inaccurate cast are as follows:

1. Distortion of the hydrocolloid impression (a) by partial dislodgement from tray; (b) by shrinkage due to dehydration; (c) by expansion due to imbibition (this will be toward the teeth and will result in an undersize rather than an oversize cast); (d) by pressing the impression into stone that is too resistant.

2. A ratio of water to powder that is too high. While this may not cause volumetric changes in the size of the cast, it will result in a weak cast.

3. Improper mixing. This also results in a weak cast or one with a chalky surface.

4. Trapping of air, either in the mix or in pouring, due to insufficient vibration.

5. Soft or chalky cast surface due to (a) the retarding action of the hydrocolloid or (b) the absorption of necessary water of crystallization by the dehydrating hydrocolloid.

6. Premature separation of the cast from the impression.

7. Leaving the cast immersed in water too long. The surface of the cast may be etched by the action of the water. This may be minimized by immersing the cast in water that has been deactivated, such as slush water from the model trimmer which has been allowed to stand or water in which pieces of plaster or stone have been placed for twenty-four hours or longer. Such water will have lost its ability to etch a gypsum surface. Even so, the cast should not be left immersed in water for long periods, such as overnight.

Pouring of Working Casts Upon Which Abutment Restorations Are to Be Fabricated. The pouring of hydrocolloid, mercaptan rubber, or silicone impressions for the purpose of making removable dies is adequately covered in crown and bridge textbooks. However, five methods will be given here for the making of working casts upon which the contours of wax patterns may be refined to satisfy the requirements of *noninterference to insertion, parallelism, and retention* for the partial denture. These are as follows:

1. The use of a double-pour technique, with separation of removable dies by means of a fine (No. 2) jeweler's saw blade (such as a Herkules saw for hard metals No. 2). The removable portion of the die must have keyed dowel pins for handling and for accuracy in seating back in the cast (Fig. 166). If a metal die surface is preferred, mercaptan and silicone impressions may be electroplated prior to pouring dies, which are then separated by sawing (Fig. 166).

2. The use of thin stainless steel separators in hydrocolloid impressions. Keyed dowel pins are placed in each removable segment. This method accomplishes the same purpose as the previous method without the necessity of

Fig. 166. A, Placement of dowel pins in an impression of prepared teeth is guided by indelible pencil or pen lines previously drawn buccally and lingually at the center of the long axis of those teeth. After the impression is filled above the level of the prepared teeth, it is supported between two pieces of clay and the dowel pins are placed between and parallel to the pencil lines. Lock washers may then be partially embedded into portions where separation is not desired. If the impression is of prepared bridge abutments, a lock washer is also placed in the edentulous space between the abutments. After the stone has set, areas to be separated are treated with a solution of sodium silicate or a commercial separating fluid such as Super-Sep. The impression may be boxed with wax if desired, and the ends of the dowel pins should be covered with a piece of utility wax so that they may be located after pouring the remainder of the cast. **B,** After the remainder of the impression is poured, preferably in stone of a different color, the sides of the cast should be trimmed and then allowed to dry overnight. With a No. 2 jeweler's saw blade in a saw frame, the cast is cut throughout the interproximal spaces, down to the junction with the second pour of stone. The saw cuts are made vertical unless a single die is involved; in such case, they are made converging. The dowel pin will not be encountered if it was placed perpendicular in the center of the prepared tooth. The utility wax is removed from the ends of the dowel pins, and each die is gently tapped out of its seat. **C,** The dies are now removed and are trimmed so as to expose precise gingival margins. The margins are lightly marked with pencil to facilitate accurate waxing and later finishing operations. The gingival thickness below the margins should be as in the die on the left rather than too close to the margin as on the right. (Courtesy Kerr Manufacturing Co., Detroit, Mich.)

sawing the cast and may provide greater accuracy in reseating the dies. By re-moving the separators prior to pouring the remainder of the cast and by using a suitable liquid separator, removable dies may be made which will seat ac-curately without any space for possible rotation such as is caused by a saw cut. This method may only be used with hydrocolloid impressions, and extreme care must be taken to avoid distortion of gingival margins in the placement of the thin metal separators. Two metal strips acting as coffer dams must be so placed for each tooth involved that a tapered die seat results.

3. The pouring of the impression as a solid cast without provision for sep-arating individual dies. The margins of each prepared tooth are then exposed by carefully trimming away the surrounding stone in much the same manner as the trimming of an individual or removable die. Interproximally this is a particularly meticulous procedure since these areas are not readily accessible. A sharp knife, such as a No. 11 Bard-Parker surgical blade, and some means of working under magnification facilitates accurate trimming of fixed dies.

After all margins of prepared teeth have been exposed, the cast is duplicated, following the duplication procedure outlined in Chapter 17, Laboratory Pro-cedures. A second stone cast is thus obtained, which is used as a solid working cast to be mounted on the articulator. (In this method a cast of the entire arch is always used instead of a unilateral or anterior segment. This facilitates the transfer of jaw relations with greater accuracy and permits the utilization of incisal and canine guidance in creating functional occlusal anatomy.)

The original cast is then cut into segments, using separating disks applied to the base of the cast between each prepared tooth. Individual dies are thus obtained upon which final waxing and finishing may be done. Wax patterns and finished castings may then be transferred to the fixed dies on the articulator for perfecting the occlusion and contact. This method demands precise technical skill but has the advantage of eliminating the possibility of removable stone dies becoming inaccurate due to abrasion of the die or its seat.

4. The replacement of electroformed dies into the original mercaptan rubber or silicone impression before pouring the remainder of the cast. Although this may not be done with hydrocolloid impressions, if the careful operator believes that he can reseat electroformed dies with accuracy, it is an acceptable method for making removable dies.

The method for making an electroformed die is as follows: After electroplat-ing the impression with silver or copper, the inside of the plated impression of each tooth involved is painted with a flux made of equal parts of concentrated hydrochloric acid, water, and glycerine. Into this fluxed concavity low-fusing metal alloy (Dialoy or Cerrosafe metal) is poured to the top of each impression. A keyed dowel pin for each tooth is fluxed and dipped into the ladle of low-fusing alloy to tin the portion to be embedded in the impression. The metal in the im-pression is then melted on the surface with a needle-point frame and the tinned dowel pin inserted and held until the metal has solidified. Each die may then be removed and trimmed without fear of separation of the electroformed surface from the core of the die.

5. The use of individual dies from copper band impressions combined with

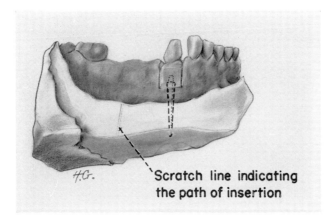

Scratch line indicating
the path of insertion

Fig. 167. A trimmed removable die for an abutment crown. The working cast is placed on the surveyor in relation to the path of insertion and the wax pattern formed with proximal guiding plane and with retentive and nonretentive contours in conformity with this path of insertion.

an accurate solid cast for the purpose of surveying and contouring the wax patterns. The stone at the gingival margin on the solid cast must be cut away to expose the full length of the preparation. The wax pattern is begun on the individual die, then placed on the solid cast where critical areas are carved with the surveyor blade, retentive contours are established, and contact and occlusion are perfected. The pattern is then returned to the individual die to finish the margins. It is always sprued from the individual die and returned to it for polishing. If marginal interference has been cut away on the solid cast, the casting may be returned to it for the purpose of checking and refining contours or for the purpose of establishing the contours of veneered surfaces.

Regardless of the method used, the individual die, whether or not it is a removable die, must be trimmed to expose all margins of the preparation (Fig. 167). This is done as illustrated, thereby facilitating both the waxing and polishing of precise gingival margins. If the die is not so trimmed, the location of gingival margins will be less exact, resulting in an overextended or, more often, an underextended restoration.

Copper Band Impressions. While it is possible to record subgingival portions of a prepared tooth with hydrocolloid, mercaptan, or silicone impression materials, there are times when those areas are not as sharply defined as might be desired. Unquestionably, a copper band impression is capable of recording subgingival areas better than any technique that calls for the injection of the impression material and subsequent removal from subgingival areas. For this reason, the use of copper band impressions continues to have a place in restorative dentistry.

The object of the copper band impression is to make an individual die for use with, or in place of, a removable die. It is used frequently to supplement the latter where subgingival areas are not sharply defined. In this application, modeling plastic may not be used because of its lack of flexibility. Withdrawal of such an impression from undercut areas apical to the preparation inevitably

Fig. 168. The steps in making an individual stone die from a copper band impression, using Dietrich's elastic impression material.

results in fracture of the impression. Therefore, some elastic material must be used. Mercaptan rubber or silicone may be used for this purpose, or the older but respected Dietrich's impression material. Believing that this is a dependable material for copper band impressions of prepared teeth, the step-by-step procedure for its use is included here, as follows (Fig. 168):

1. Select a copper band one size larger than would be used for a modeling plastic impression. Score it on the buccal side with a sharp instrument to identify its position, contouring it so that it extends beneath the gingivae in all areas except where buccal or lingual surfaces have not been prepared, as in a three-quarter crown or inlay preparation. Here the band is contoured above the height of convexity of the unprepared tooth surfaces.

2. With a carborundum disk, make two slots in the upper portion of the band at right angles to the long axis of the band. This is for the purpose of securing the chilled impression in the copper band.

3. Place sufficient Dietrich's material in a small amount of water in a test tube and bring to a boil. Dump this into a plaster bowl containing hot water. Fill the contoured copper band with the soft material, taking care to avoid wrinkles and voids. Again place the filled band in the test tube with a small amount

of water and again bring to a boil. Again dump the material into the bowl containing hot water and immediately remove it and carry it to the mouth.

4. Place the filled band on the tooth, using the scratch line on its buccal aspect to identify its original position. Seat it beneath the gingivae and then use the butt end of an instrument as a plunger to force the impression material beneath the gingivae and out the slots in the band which were placed there for retention. Then hold the band securely with a finger on the open end while three or more syringefuls of *iced* water are emptied slowly upon it. (Chilling is essential to the accuracy of such an impression. After removal from the mouth, it remains stable at room temperature but should be poured as soon as possible.)

5. Remove the chilled band by applying the edge of a chisel blade to one side of the band while stabilizing with the finger on the other. Since it is an elastic material, squeezing during removal must be avoided. Then check the impression for accuracy. A portion of the tooth below the preparation must be recorded, clearly identifying the margin of the preparation. The copper band should not be visible at any point.

6. Being elastic, gingival excess may not safely be trimmed away for fear thin areas may pull away and distort. The impression band may be boxed lightly with lead backing from an x-ray film, wax, or gummed paper. However, the preferred method is to slightly overfill the unboxed band with the die stone, place it on a ball of clay, and then add a dowel pin. After the stone has set, any excess is cut back to the limits of the copper band with a stone or arbor band which simplifies removal and trimming. Separation of the die from the impression is then accomplished under hot water.

This technique has been given as a respected and time-proved method of obtaining individual dies. Other elastic materials may be used if preferred, the only difference being the method of preparing the impression material and the use of heavier-gauge band materials and of adhesives for securing the material to the band.

An alternate method of using a copper band is the use of a loosely fitted band which is filled with rubber-base impression material and seated subgingivally before making an over-all impression with a mass of the same material. In this method, the band is trimmed almost to the height of the prepared tooth and must be formed with a rim that is crimped outward to ensure its being engaged by the over-all impression. This method recognizes the need for a subgingival record of crown preparations beyond that ordinarily obtained by the usual retraction and injection techniques and may serve to eliminate the necessity for individual impressions in difficult cases.

A modification of this method is to make an acrylic resin coping of each abutment tooth upon a cast made in quick-setting stone from a wax impression of the prepared teeth. If bridge abutments are involved, the resin copings are connected by a span of resin which is relieved of any tissue contact. The copings are reamed slightly, and after the gingiva has been retracted and the teeth dried, the copings are filled with the rubber-base or silicone impression material and seated on the teeth, thus forcing the impression material subgingivally. An over-all impression is then made of the same material, using a suitable metal or resin tray which had been treated with adhesive. A syringe for applying the impression material subgingivally is ordinarily not necessary when the impression is made in this manner. Upon removal, the copings are not visible, being embedded in the over-all impression, but they will have served the purpose of carrying the impression material beneath the gingivae without the use of a syringe, thus eliminating the need for a second mix of injectable material.

INDIVIDUAL IMPRESSION TRAYS

This chapter has dealt previously with the making of an impression in a stock tray of the anatomic form of a dental arch for the purpose of making either a study cast, a working cast for restorations, or a master cast. There are times, however, when a stock tray is not suitable for the making of the final anatomic impression of the dental arch. Most tooth-borne partial dentures may be made upon a master cast from such an impression. Some maxillary free-end partial dentures with broad palatal coverage, particularily those for a Kennedy Class I arch, may also be made upon an anatomic cast, but usually these necessitate the use of an individually made tray.

Unless a stock tray can be found that will fit the mouth with about a quarter of an inch of clearance for the impression material, yet without interference with bordering tissues, an individual tray made of some resin tray material should be used for the final anatomic impression.

Most partial denture trays are either of the rim-lock or perforated variety. Both are made in a limited selection of sizes and shapes. One manufacturer in particular has gone to considerable length to provide a wide selection of perforated trays, including trays for both bilateral and unilateral edentulous areas, trays with built-in occlusal stops, and trays for particular techniques.* (Fig 169.)

All of these trays have reinforced peripheries. While a full denture impression tray is, or should be, made of material that permits trimming and shaping to fit the mouth, the existence of a beaded periphery and the rigidity of a stock partial denture tray allows no trimming and very little shaping. The resulting impression is often a record of peripheral tissues distorted by an ill-fitting tray rather than an impression of tissues draping naturally over a slightly underextended impression tray. The technician must then do his best to interpret the limits of those distended tissues upon which the denture periphery must rest.

In individual resin tray, on the other hand, can be made with sufficient clearance for the impression material and can be trimmed just short of the mucous membrane reflection area so as to allow the tissues to drape naturally without distortion. The partial denture periphery may then be made with as accurate a periphery as a complete denture with equal advantages.

Although techniques have been proposed for the making of individual impression trays which incorporate plastic tubing for the purpose of water-cooling agar hydrocolloid impressions, the final anatomic impression will usually be made with alginate hydrocolloid, mercaptan rubber, or silicone impression materials.

---

*Nevin, J. J.: Tray Selection for Partial Denture Impressions, CAL Magazine, Coe Laboratories, Inc., Chicago, Ill., July, 1963.

Fig. 169. Impression tray cabinet with doors open, exposing a wide selection of perforated impression trays for alginate hydrocolloid impressions. Beginning at the top can be seen trays for completely edentulous mouths, depressed anterior trays, trays with unilateral occlusal stops, Hindels trays for use with a double impression technique, and the more commonly and regularly used perforated trays.

Technique for Making an Individual Resin Impression Tray. The technique for making an individual resin impression tray is as follows:

1. Adapt two thicknesses of wet strip asbestos onto the study cast. While this will usually provide adequate clearance, supply additional relief to the areas of prominence and deep undercut areas. By using wet asbestos instead of wax or clay, the surface of the study cast is not affected, since the asbestos will peel off easily. It usually comes off when the tray is lifted. Shape the wet asbestos to the desired peripheral limits rather than carry it indiscriminately beyond. This will serve as a definite guide to the trimming of the tray, thereby avoiding all but minor adjustments to the tray periphery in the mouth.

2. Paint the asbestos and adjacent cast surface with a tin-foil substitute which is used as a separator. This will give a smooth inner surface to the impression tray. This step, however, is not absolutely necessary. Although asbestos that is not treated with a separator is not easily removed from the tray, it leaves a rough sur-

Fig. 170. Bi-beveled drill used for making holes in resin impression trays. Such a drill will not clog and facilitates the making of a perforated impression tray for use with alginate hydrocolloid, mercaptan rubber, or silicone impression materials.

face which may possibly aid in securing the impression material to the tray. However, this alone does not afford sufficient retention for alginate, and perforations are still necessary.

3. Adapt plastic tray material to the asbestos blockout or form the resin tray by sprinkling. I prefer the latter, and the technique is given in Chapter 18, Laboratory Procedures.

4. Attach a handle to the tray, using a ball of plastic, a loop of wire, any suitable piece of metal, or a piece of tongue blade. The handle must be rigid and must not interfere with a normal drape of the lip.

5. Lift the hardened resin tray from the cast and trim away the excess to the limits of the asbestos spacer. If an alginate hydrocolloid impression material is to be used, perforate the tray freely.

Perforations in a resin tray are not easily made with a round bur, for after a few revolutions the bur becomes clogged. Instead, a bi-beveled surgical drill is used which will make the holes rapidly without clogging (Fig. 170). These are available in various sizes, Nos. 100 through 106, the higher number being the smaller size. The size of the perforations should be slightly larger than those in a stock tray, and only about one third as many are used. This will be sufficient to lock the impression material in the tray and thereby avoid distortion of the impression on removal from the mouth.

If mercaptan rubber or silicone is to be used, perforations are not necessary and probably not desirable, as the adhesive provided by the manufacturer provides reliable retention, and some confinement of these materials is desirable. With the use of adhesives the impression material is not easily removed from the tray should a faulty impression have to be done over, but this is an inconvenience common to all of the newer elastic materials and does not prevent reuse of the impression tray.

The pouring of an alginate impression made in an individual tray presents a minor problem, since it is usually covered with the elastic material and is delicate to handle. Some of the excess material must be cut away to expose enough of the rigid tray to make contact with the vibrator. The impression may then be vibrated while being filled and inverted on a glass or ceramic slab as any other hydrocolloid impression.

Master casts made from impressions in individual resin trays are generally more accurate than those made in ill-fitting stock trays. The use of individual trays should be considered a necessary step in the making of the majority of partial dentures where a secondary impression technique is not to be used. Reasons and methods for the making of a secondary impression will be considered in the following chapter.

Support for the free-end
denture base

In a tooth-supported partial denture, a metal base or the framework supporting a resin base is connected to and is part of a rigid framework which permits the direct transfer of occlusal forces to the abutment teeth through the occlusal rests. This is a *bridge* prosthesis, even though it is removable and is bilateral in design. The only differences between a unilateral and a bilateral removable bridge are that in the former, each clasp arm must provide both bracing and retention, whereas in the latter, cross-arch stabilization is made possible through the use of rigid connectors.

Even though the base of a tooth-supported (Kennedy Class III) partial denture supports the supplied teeth, the residual ridge beneath that base is not called upon to aid in the support of the denture. Therefore, the resiliency of the ridge tissues is not a factor in denture support. Regardless of the length of the span, if the framework is rigid, the abutment teeth are sound enough to carry the additional load, and the occlusal rests are properly formed, support comes entirely from the abutment teeth at either end of that span. Support may be augmented by splinting and by the use of additional abutments, but in any case, the abutments are the sole support of the removable bridge prosthesis.

An impression (and resulting reproduction in stone) which records faithfully the anatomic form of the teeth and their surrounding structures and the residual ridges of a dental arch is the only impression needed in the making of a tooth-borne partial denture. The impression should also record the moving tissues which will border the denture in an unstrained position so that the relationship of the denture base to those tissues may be as accurate as possible, being neither overextended nor underextended. Although underextension of the denture base in a tooth-supported prosthesis is the lesser of two evils, an underextended base may lead to food impaction and inadequate contours, particularly on the buccal and labial sides. For this reason, and also in order to record faithfully the moving tissues of the floor of the mouth in the mandibular arch, an individual impression tray should be used rather than an ill-fitting or overextended stock tray. This has been discussed at length in the previous chapter.

THE TRUE PARTIAL DENTURE

The true partial denture does not have the advantage of total tooth support, since one or more bases are extensions onto the residual ridge from the last available abutment. This is spoken of as a *free-end* or *distal-extension* prosthesis and is technically the only true *partial denture,* since it derives a major part of its support from the residual ridge. The proportion of ridge support will depend upon its distance from the occlusal rest on the last abutment tooth (sometimes called the *free-end abutment*).

Factors Influencing the Support of a Free-End Base. Support from the residual ridge becomes greater as the distance from the last abutment increases and will depend upon several factors:

1. The *quality of the residual ridge.*
2. The *extent of coverage* of the denture base. The broader the coverage, the greater the distribution of the load, thereby resulting in less load per unit area.
3. The *type and accuracy of the impression registration.*
4. The *accuracy of the denture base.*
5. The *total occlusal load applied.* This will be influenced by the number of supplied teeth, the width of their occlusal surfaces, and their occlusal efficiency.

In a series of experiments, Kaires has shown that "maximum coverage of denture-bearing areas with large, wide denture bases is of the utmost importance in withstanding both vertical and horizontal stresses." A second conclusion reached from a continuation of this investigation was that "the reduction of the size of the occlusal table reduces the vertical and horizontal forces acting on the partial denture and lessens the stress on the abutment teeth and supporting tissues."

Not only must the free-end partial denture base depend upon the tissues of the residual ridge for *support* but it must also obtain *retention* from that base, aided by *indirect retention* to prevent its lifting away from the tissues. Whereas the tooth-supported base is secured at either end by the action of a direct retainer and supported at either end by an occlusal rest, both support and direct retention are lacking in the free-end prosthesis. For this reason, a distal abutment should be preserved whenever possible. In event of the loss or absence of a distal abutment tooth, the patient must be made aware of the movements to be expected with a free-end partial denture and the limitations imposed upon the dentist when the residual ridge must be used for both support and retention for that part of the prosthesis.

The residual ridge consists of the elastic, fibrous connective tissue overlying the residual alveolar bone. In some areas, the overlying tissues are thin, with a dense cortical bone beneath; in others, they are firm and fibrous, overlying a relatively dense residual alveolar bone; in still other areas, they are soft and flabby, overlying a badly resorbed residual alveolar bone. Some areas will be firm with limited displaceability, while others will be soft and very easily displaced by

Fig. 171. A comparison of anatomic and functional ridge forms. **A,** The original master cast with edentulous area recorded in its anatomic form using an elastic impression material. **B,** The same cast after the edentulous area has been repoured to its functional form as recorded by a fluid-wax impression.

Fig. 172. **A,** A comparison of the functional and anatomic forms of the same edentulous ridge. On the right is the master cast with the edentulous area reproduced in its anatomic form from a hydrocolloid impression. On the left is the same master cast after the edentulous area has been repoured in its functional, or supporting, form as recorded with a fluid impression wax. Note not only the difference in surface anatomy but also that the functional impression has recorded the width available for the support of the denture base. **B,** The corrected master cast with the denture framework reseated upon it after the impression base has been removed from the framework. A new resin base may now be made by a sprinkling method for the purpose of establishing occlusal relationship on a base identical with that of the finished denture.

the lightest finger contact. This will depend upon the thickness and the structure of the tissues covering the residual bone.

This residual ridge may be said to have two forms (Figs. 171 and 172). One is the *anatomic form,* which is the surface contour of the ridge when not supporting an occlusal load. It is this resting or mucostatic form that is recorded by a soft impression material such as plaster of Paris or a metallic oxide impression paste. Depending upon the viscosity of the particular impression material used, it is also the form recorded by mercaptan rubber and silicone

Fig. 173. **A,** Fluid-wax functional impression, mandibular Class I, distal to canine abutments. **B,** Corrected master cast. **C,** Comparison of corrected master cast with original segment. **D,** Casting returned to master cast prior to forming sprinkled acrylic resin jaw relation record bases.

impression materials. It is also the form of the ridge recorded by a hydrocolloid impression material. Distortion and muco-compression by hydraulic pressure may result from confinement of the impression material within the tray and by insufficient thickness of impression material between the tray and the tissues, as well as by the viscosity of the impression material, but none of these factors are selective or physiologic in their action. These are accidental distortions of the tissues occurring through faulty technique.

It is the anatomic form of the residual ridge that is utilized for the support of most complete dentures. Such dentures are said to be made from mucostatic impressions. This is not only acceptable, but in the opinion of many prosthodontists, it is also the most physiologic form for the support of the complete denture.

Since there is no tooth support with which the denture base must be made compatible, and since the tissues are or should be in this form except during mastication, the complete denture may be made to fit the resting form of those tissues. Presuming that there is harmony of occlusion throughout the dental arch, the complete denture may move tissueward under function until the tissues beneath assume a supporting form or a compactness which will support an occlusal load. The same principle would apply to a partial denture made without abutment support, differing only in that the area of tissue support is less and the tissues adjacent to the remaining teeth would be impinged by tissueward movement of the denture. Without occlusal support from the natural teeth, occlusion on the tissue-supported partial denture would be negative, leaving only the remaining natural teeth to carry the masticatory load.

RECORDING OF FUNCTIONAL OR SUPPORTING RIDGE FORM

A number of years ago, McLean and others recognized the need for recording the tissues supporting a free-end partial denture base in their displaced or supporting state and then relating them to the remainder of the arch by means of a secondary impression. This was called a "functional impression" because it recorded the ridge relation under simulated function.

The technique consisted of taking an impression of the edentulous areas in a vulcanite or denture base tray which was provided with modeling plastic occlusion rims. Impression paste was used to record the ridge areas while under biting stress. This impression was then related to the remainder of the arch by taking a hydrocolloid impression with the original impression seated in the mouth. Upon removal from the mouth, the composite impression was poured to provide a master cast, with the edentulous areas recorded under functional loading. Although the tray used for the over-all impression was in contact with the occlusion rims, finger pressure was necessary to hold the original impression in its functional position while the hydrocolloid material gelled. Finger pressure thus applied could at best be only an approximation of the occlusal loading under which the original impression was recorded. This variable tended to nullify the advantage of making the original impression under occlusal loading.

A variation of this technique eliminated the occlusion rims as such but provided stops of modeling plastic against the underside of the hydrocolloid impression tray for the purpose of finger loading the original impression. In this method, also, the impression of the edentulous areas was made with impression paste but with the tissues in their resting form. A finger load was then applied to the hydrocolloid tray for the purpose of relating the edentulous areas under some loading to the remainder of the arch as the hydrocolloid gelled. The resulting master cast recorded the anatomic, or resting, form of the ridge in a pseudo-functional relationship to the rest of the arch.

More recently, Hindels and others have used with apparent success a method of finger loading the anatomic impression through a hole in the hydrocolloid impression tray. These trays are available for use with the technique and eliminate the possibility of error arising from ineffective or incorrectly placed modeling plastic stops. It does not eliminate the variable of the dentist's individual interpretation of what constitutes functional loading. The occlusal loading of McLean was unquesionably a more accurate and less variable method of recording the residual ridge beneath a free-end base, but it became a variable finger-loading relationship in the final impression. That such methods are better than making a partial denture from a one-piece anatomic impression cannot be denied, for they recognize the need for adequate support of the free-end base.

Any method, whether it accomplishes the recording of the *functional rela-tionship* of the ridge to the remainder of the arch or the recording of the *func-tional form* of the ridge itself may provide acceptable support for the partial denture. On the other hand, those who use the static ridge form or ridge relation-ship for the partial denture should seriously consider the need for some mechan-ical stress breaker to avoid the cantilever action of the free-end base against the abutment teeth.

Hindels has the following to say about support for the partial denture base:

> The one-piece colloidal or plaster impression will produce a cast which cannot possibly represent a functional relationship between the various supporting structures of the mouth. All that may be obtained from such an impression is a cast of the hard and soft tissues at rest. With the partial denture in position in the dental arch, the occlusal rest will fit the rest seat of the abutment tooth, while the denture base will fit the surface of the mucosa at rest. When a masticatory load is applied to the extension saddle, the rest will act as a definite stop, which will prevent the part of the saddle near the abutment tooth from transmitting the load to the underly-ing anatomic structures. The distal end of the saddle, however, being able to move freely, will transmit the full masticatory load.
>
> It is obvious that the soft tissues covering the alveolar bone cannot by themselves carry any load applied to them. They act as a protective padding for the bone which, in the final analysis, is the structure that receives and carries the masticatory load. Distribution of this load over a maximum area of bone is a prime requisite in prevent-ing trauma.
>
> In a partial denture constructed from a one-piece impression, the masticatory load will be carried only by the abutment teeth and that part of the bone which underlies the distal end of the free-end saddle. The balance of the bony alveolar ridge will not function in carrying the load. The result will be a traumatic load to the bone underlying the distal end of the saddle and to the abutment tooth, which, in turn, will result in bone loss and loosening of the abutment tooth.
>
> There are many who believe that every partial denture should be rebased before its final insertion in the mouth. One group believes in tissue displacement and uses impression materials of heavy consistency. They thereby introduce traumatic stresses to the underlying tissues, as previously discussed. Another group uses easy-flowing pastes which produce a rebase impression of the soft tissues at rest. During the functioning of such a partial denture, the sequence of events will be similar to that of a partial denture constructed from a one-piece impression. The occlusal rest will act as a stop, preventing an even distribution of the masticatory load by the saddle to the edentulous ridge.*

The technique as given by Hindels is as follows:

> An acrylic tray is processed on a cast made from an impression which should include all areas of future tissue support of the partial denture. The tray is selec-tively relieved and, when checked in the mouth, should cover the edentulous areas up to the border tissue attachments and should include the retromolar pads. The saddles of the tray should be connected with each other by means of an acrylic lingual bar. The bar should cover the area between the muscle attachments of the floor of the mouth and the lingual gingivae of the anterior teeth. The tray should clear the free gingivae around the abutment teeth to prevent future impingement and stripping.

*From Hindels, G. W.: Load Distribution in Extension Saddle Partial Dentures, J. Pros. Den. **2:**92-100, 1952.

This tray is loaded with an easy-flowing zinc oxide-eugenol paste and brought into position in the mouth, care being taken that the soft tissues are left in their passive state. After the material has hardened, the tray is removed and the impression examined. In a successful impression, the tissue side of the tray should be fully covered with impression material, and no part of the tray itself should be visible. The material that has flowed from the tray onto the abutment teeth should now be cut away and the tray reinserted in the mouth and tested for stability.

The next step is to make an impression of the teeth and to establish a relationship between the teeth and the mucosa in a displaced state. For this purpose, a perforated tray which has been provided with two circular openings of approximately ¾-inch diameter in the region of the first molars is used. The impression of the soft tissue areas is placed in the mouth. Then, while the tray is being loaded with an alginate impression material, some of this material is used to fill in the space between the soft tissue impression and the remaining teeth. The loaded metal tray is then inserted into position over both the teeth and the acrylic tray. The index fingers are passed through the openings in the perforated tray until they contact the underlying acrylic tray; then positive pressure is exerted upon it. This pressure should be maintained until the alginate impression material has hardened. The completed impression is then removed as one unit. The cast made in this impression will be a reproduction of both the surface of the teeth and the undistorted surface of the mucosa, but the two will be *related* to each other with the mucosa in a functional state as it would be found under the partial denture saddle during mastication. While the saddle is *related* to the occlusal rest with the mucosa in a functional state, the tissue surface of the saddle is actually a reproduction of the passive and undistorted mucosa as obtained with zinc oxide-eugenol paste in the individual impression tray.*

USE OF MOUTH-TEMPERATURE WAX TO RECORD TISSUE FORM

When a mouth-temperature wax is used to record the form of the tissues that will support a complete denture, it is done on the theory that it is better to record the supporting or more compact form of the tissues than to record the tissues at rest. While it is true that this results in better support for the denture, the disadvantage is that the tissues must rebound when the occlusal load is released, at which time the surface of the tissues and the surface of the denture are not the same. The argument for making the complete denture to the resting, or mucostatic, form of the tissues is that this is the constant form of the tissues except when an occlusal load is applied.

The form of the residual ridge recorded under some loading, whether by occlusal loading, finger loading, or the consistency of the recording medium, is called the *functional form*. This is the surface contour of the ridge when supporting a uniformly distributed functional load. How much it will differ from the anatomic form will depend upon the thickness and structural characteristics of the soft tissues overlying the residual bone. It will also differ from the anatomic form in proportion to the total load applied to the denture base. This is the form that is recorded by certain of the mouth-temperature waxes, which are

---

*From Hindels, G. W.: Load Distribution in Extension Saddle Partial Dentures, J. Pros. Den. **2:**92-100, 1952.

capable of displacing those tissues that can be readily displaced without over-loading the firmer areas.

The objective of any functional impression technique is to provide maximum support for the partial denture base, thereby maintaining occlusal contact so as to distribute the occlusal load over both natural and artificial dentition and at the same time minimize movement of the base which would create leverage on the abutment teeth. While some tissueward movement of the free-end base is unavoidable and dependent upon the five factors listed previously, it can be minimized by providing the best possible support for the denture base.

Steffel has classified advocates of the various methods for treating the free-end partial denture as follows:

> 1. Those who believe that ridge and tooth supports can best be equalized by the use of stress-breakers or resilient equilizers.
>
> 2. Those who insist on bringing about the equalization of ridge and tooth support by physiologic basing which is accomplished by a pressure impression or by rebasing the denture under biting stress.
>
> 3. Those who uphold the idea of extensive stress distribution for the purpose of stress reduction at any one point.*

It would seem that there is very little difference in the philosophy behind methods 2 and 3 as given by Steffel, for both the equalization of tooth and tissue support and stress distribution over the greatest area are objectives of the functional type of impression. Many of the requirements and advantages which may be given for the distributed stress denture apply equally well to the functionally or physiologically based denture. Some of these requirements are (1) positive occlusal rests, (2) an all-rigid, nonflexible framework, (3) indirect retainers, whenever practical, to add stability, and (4) well-adapted, broad-coverage bases.

Those who do not accept the theory of functional basing and those who, for one reason or another, do not use some kind of secondary impression technique for partial dentures, should use some form of stress breaker between the abutment and the free-end base. The advantages and disadvantages of doing so have been given in Chapter 11 under stress breakers.

METHODS FOR OBTAINING FUNCTIONAL SUPPORT FOR THE FREE-END BASE

A thorough understanding of the characteristics of each of the impression materials leads to the obvious conclusion that no single material can record both the anatomic form of the teeth and tissues in the dental arch and, at the same time, the functional form of the residual ridge. Therefore, some secondary impression method must be used.

There are several methods by which this may be accomplished. Each of them seems to satisfy the two requirements for providing adequate support to the free-end partial denture base, which are (1) that it records and relates

---

*From Steffel, V. L.: Fundamental Principles Involved in Partial Denture Design, J.A.D.A. **42:**534-544, 1951.

the tissues under some loading, and (2) that it distributes the load over as large an area as possible.

FUNCTIONAL RELINING METHOD

While there are hazards to be overcome in any relining procedure of a free-end base, the *functional relining* method is used satisfactorily in competent hands. The principal hazard is that, unless an open-mouth technique is used whereby the original relationship of the denture framework to the supporting teeth can be positively maintained, indirect retainers may not be seated when the functional impression is made. Since any settling of the denture base will have influenced the occlusion, restoring the denture framework to its original position with indirect retainers seated will result in an elevated occlusion. For this reason, readjustment of the occlusion must be anticipated when an open-mouth relining method is used. In extreme instances, the teeth on the prosthesis will have to be reoccluded to the opposing dentition following relining of the denture base.

On the other hand, if a closed-mouth impression method is used, particularly with a bilateral distal extension, stops of self-curing resin or modeling plastic against resilient tissue may not be adequate to keep the free-end base from settling tissueward under occlusal loading. In such case, the denture inevitably rotates about its fulcrum line and the indirect retainers lift from their terminal position. Although occlusal harmony on the relined prosthesis will have been maintained by this method, the relationship of the denture framework to the supporting teeth will not be the same as it was on the original master cast.

A second hazard of any relining procedure is the possibility of errors occurring during the reprocessing of a resin base. Relining of a resin base frequently results in an increase in vertical dimension. Although this can be minimized by careful laboratory procedures (Chapter 17), by the use of a free-flowing resin, by making sure there is sufficient space inside the original base for the resin to flow, and by the employment of some space in the land area, some increase in dimension is always possible. Any such increase will result in a faulty relationship between the denture framework and the supporting natural teeth, as well as changes in occlusal relationships.

Where a relining method for functional basing is to be used, the original denture base may be processed over a spacer of metal (No. 7 Ash's metal) that has been adapted to the anatomic ridge form. This is the form of the ridge as reproduced on the master cast from a hydrocolloid impression. The relief metal is then stripped away from the resin base, leaving a space on the tissue side for the placement of the impression material and, later, the resin reline.

If this is not done, the underside of the denture base must be relieved by removing sufficient resin to accommodate the impression material. Clearance should also be adequate to assure freedom for the flow of the impression material. It should be remembered that thermoplastic impression materials are sluggish and greater space for their flow is needed than where an impression paste or other fluid material is used. It should also be remembered that impression wax will not overdisplace tissue *only if given sufficient space and time in which to flow.*

Fig. 174. **A,** Modeling composition placed so as to support the distal extensions during the correction of occlusion. **B,** The ridge surfaces of the bases prepared to receive the modeling composition. **C,** The smooth, accurate, muscle-trimmed impression in modeling composition. **D,** Bases prepared for the application of impression wax (Iowa formula). **E,** The finished impression made of modeling composition and wax. Note the escape of wax through holes in the denture bases.

Following is Steffel's procedure for making a functional reline impression:

If the partial denture has only the two clasps with no indirect retainer(s), an effort should be made to refine the occlusion before going forward with the relining impressions, which step-by-step procedure will be carried out in the same manner whether or not an indirect retainer is present. If there is an indirect retainer, or additional points of contact of the framework to make tripoding or stabilization possible, in the technique about to be described, it is preferred to reharmonize the positional relationship of the partial denture to teeth and tissues first, and to correct the occlusion first also, before proceeding with the reline impression. To do this, the technical procedure is as follows: Low-fusing modeling composition is placed in excess on the distal one-third to one-half of the tissue surface of the bases (this amount is sufficient for the purpose intended and in convenient location for subsequent removal). The denture is now mass heated in the 140° F. water, quickly carried to the patient's mouth while the impression material is still readily moldable, and seated with firm pressure against only the framework. The material at the distal ends of the bases (Fig. 174, *A*) will have contacted the tissues and hardened so that the appliance is now reoriented in relation to its own arch, but out of harmony with the opposing arch. With the modeling composition for support distally, and accurate metal-to-tooth support anteriorly, the partial denture is stabilized and positioned, and the occlusion can now be altered and balanced in accordance with our judgment for this specific location.

After the occlusion has been corrected with the denture being supported at its proper relative elevation, the impression substance which has now served its purpose is removed, undercuts are eliminated from the base, and some base material is cut away from the tissue surfaces and from the peripheries of the basal seats (Fig. 174, *B*) to make more room for, and provide better workability of, the impression materials.

An excess amount of low-fusing modeling composition (low-fusing to prevent overdisplacement of tissues) is now applied to the bases. Excess is used so that there will always be some present wherever needed. The appliance is mass heated in the water bath and inserted part way toward the tissues but not seated. The patient is not allowed to close for contact. Seating all the way at the first insertion might result in too-severe pressures against supporting tissues, flowing of the moldable materials into the direct retainers, and the lack of occlusal contacts in the finished denture due to overclosure. Usually about four mass heatings and insertions, progressively, are necessary before allowing the patient to close natural teeth to light centric occlusal contacts. For final closure, the patient should be instructed to proceed just to the point of faint facet-to-facet or interdigitative contact, not asked to close with great force. Doing so might result in an upward mandibular displacement. At this juncture, the bases will be at their correct vertical position, occlusion will be re-established, and because correct occlusal contacts were provided beforehand, the metal work will have accurate adaptation to the natural teeth. Since modeling compositions are always under the operator's control, he can make them do what is required for any specific case; and since they do not soften again at mouth temperatures, there is no danger of his losing subsequently the corrections which he has so painstakingly made.

The border limits are now formed by heating short sections with the torch, then manipulating the cheeks and lips for border outline.

The reline impression (Fig. 174, *C*), at this point, *looks* acceptable, with adequate tissue coverage, rounded smooth borders, smooth impression surfaces, and a stabilized, properly repositioned composite partial denture. However, the borders are really not physiologically trimmed, and as recorded, there will be small inaccuracies in surface detail, excessive stress against the crest of the ridge, and *probably* against the mylohyoid ridge.

Impression substance, and even base material if necessary, is now removed all along the crest of the ridge, and usually along the mylohyoid ridge. Also, if the distal extensions are long, escape holes are bored completely through the base material at these areas requiring relief (Fig. 174, *D*); if they are short, their open ends provide sufficient escape ways. *No* impression bulk is removed along the normal slopes of the ridges.

Impression wax (Iowa) is now painted over the entire impression surface, the partial denture is inserted, and the patient instructed to gradually force it to place, then to continue with the functional movements of chewing. In contrast to modeling composition, the wax must always be well chilled before removal for examination. After a short period in the mouth, five minutes for example, excesses of wax should be removed and the restoration reinserted (with wax additions, if necessary). The patient is again instructed to go through the functional movements of chewing, together with facial and oral gymnastics, for about ten minutes. The wax flows so readily that there is no danger of its remaining on any surface where its contour will not be tolerated later. Limited movement of the base extensions under the functional stresses will mold the soft wax for relief of vulnerable areas. Also, in the completed restoration, the slight movement allowed by the passive retainers will preclude the possibility of tissue strangulation.

This final step in the reline impression (the relieving of areas and the addition of wax) does not change the previously re-established position of the partial denture in the arch, but merely refines the impression, and specializes the fit with reference to the different types of supporting tissues. Obviously, at this point, the impression (Fig. 174, *E*) is ready for accurate conversion into a permanent material as it presents: (1) A surface which is absolutely smooth and tissue adapted. The wax corrects any small surface discrepancies. (2) A surface outline which will place additional stresses on tissues which can tolerate them, giving relief to others. The rationale of this is clearly understood. (3) Borders which have a functional outline molded by physiologic muscular action and not by excessive manual manipulation.°

In the reline impression as advocated by Steffel, the impression wax is used as a final correction material. Iowa formula impression wax is used in much the same manner as for a complete denture impression, except that the impression for a partial denture is coordinated with the terminal position of the cast framework.

FLUID-WAX FUNCTIONAL IMPRESSION METHOD

One must differentiate between the wax "wash," or correction impression, as originally developed by Dr. Earl S. Smith of the University of Iowa, and the full wax impression, as developed by Dr. O. C. Applegate of the University of Michigan and Dr. S. G. Applegate of the University of Detroit. The latter method uses an impression wax (Korecta wax No. 4) that is slightly more fluid than the Iowa wax. Peripheral extention is established by the impression wax and then reinforced by backing it up with a special hard wax (Korecta wax No. 1).

The Applegate method may be used for making a reline impression or for the correction of the original master cast. In either application, the thickness of wax permits a greater flow of material and therefore less muco-compression than the wax "wash." The full wax impression is used with an open-mouth procedure; therefore, there is less danger of overdisplacement of tissues by the application of vertical forces. If adequate space for the flow of the material is provided and sufficient time is allowed for the escape of excess material, the full wax impression will not overdisplace tissues. Only those soft tissues that can readily be displaced or made more compact by the consistency of the wax itself will be recorded in a different form from that recorded by the anatomic impressions.

In addition to less displacement of tissues, the full wax technique records

°From Steffel, V. L.: Relining Removable Partial Dentures for Fit and Function, J. Pros. Den. **4**:496-509, 1954.

the moving border tissues physiologically, resulting in a more accurate denture periphery. The limits of peripheral extension are determined by the wax alone, unencumbered by any influence from the impression tray. Both the length and the width of the periphery are thus established in wax and reproduced in the denture base. The harder wax (Korecta wax No. 1) is used only to back up the impression and should not be allowed to influence the impression record.

O. C. Applegate has named this method the *fluid-wax functional impression.* While it may be used for relining purposes, it is designed primarily for the making of a secondary impression for the correcting of a master cast. The anatomic ridge form, as recorded in hydrocolloid, is thus replaced with the functional form, as recorded in fluid wax, and the denture base processed to the latter form.

Three Objectives in the Making of a Fluid-Wax Impression. There are three objectives to be considered in the making of a fluid-wax impression. First of these is *tissue support,* as evidenced by a glossy appearance of the wax in areas where the tissues have reached their supporting form. No additional wax is needed in these areas, since support without overdisplacement is the primary objective of the fluid-wax impression method. It is necessary, however, that wax be added to dull areas which have not yet recorded the supporting form of the tissues.

The second objective, which is the *extension of the impression to obtain maximum coverage by the partial denture base,* is accomplished by adding wax inside the flanges of the impression until excess wax begins to turn at the periphery of the impression as influenced by the activity of bordering tissues. As the limits of peripheral extension are reached, the soft wax peripheries are then preserved by backing them up with the hard No. 1 wax.

The third objective is the *release of any tissues that may have been overdisplaced.* This is accomplished by allowing sufficient *time* for the excess wax to flow to the peripheries where it can escape as it is turned by the action of moving border tissues. During this period, which should be about eight minutes, functional movements are repeatedly simulated so as to turn the excess wax as it reaches the periphery of the impression.

Methods of Obtaining a Cast of the Functional Ridge Form. The end result of the fluid-wax impression is the making of a cast of the supporting ridge to which the partial denture base can be processed, thereby providing optimal support for that base. While the impression technique does not vary, the manner in which the cast is corrected may be varied in accordance with the preference of the operator and the type of prosthesis, that is, whether it is to have a metal or a resin base. These several methods of correcting the master cast are described as follows:

1. The correction of the master cast subsequent to the making of the denture framework. The cast framework is used as a means of positioning the impression tray in the mouth and, later, back onto the master cast for the purpose of repouring the ridge areas. The components of the cast framework act as a positive guide to the accurate seating of the denture, both in the mouth and on the stone cast. This method is used only where resin bases will be processed to the corrected master cast.

1a. This is identical with *1* except that the stone cast is poured against both the impression and the underside of the denture framework, thereby forming a *processing cast.* Properly done, the cast framework can then be lifted from the processing cast for the purpose of removing the attached impression base and then repositioned on the processing cast with accuracy. The advantages of this method are that the master cast need not be cut, and the possibility of error in reseating the framework on the master cast is eliminated. For the first method to be done with accuracy, the denture framework must bear exactly the same relationship to the master cast as to the mouth when the impression was made. This hazard is avoided by the use of a processing cast. Where only a few natural teeth remain to aid in repositioning the cast framework, as, for example, where only six anterior teeth remain, there may not be enough tooth contact to positively establish the exact position of the framework on the master cast. In such case, the making of a processing cast is perferred over the correction of the original master cast.

1b. Where metal bases are to be cast separately to the functional ridge form and then attached to the original frame by soldering or with resin, the impression may be made as in *1* and the master cast corrected prior to the making of the metal bases. This method is essentially the same as *1* except that separate metal bases will be made rather than resin bases processed directly to the cast.

2. The use of an acrylic tray rather than the denture framework for positioning the impression in the mouth and then back onto the master cast for the correction of the ridges is a method that makes possible the correction of the master cast prior to the making of the denture framework. It was developed primarily to permit the making of a one-piece partial denture with metal bases made to functional ridge form. It may be used also to correct the master cast prior to making the cast framework for a resin-base denture, if the dentist prefers to use this method instead of method 1.

Step-by-Step Procedure for Making a Fluid-Wax Functional Impression. The technique for making a fluid-wax functional impression is the same regardless of the method of application used for making the stone cast. The step-by-step procedure given here is for method 1, using the denture framework as a medium for carrying the impression to the mouth and then back onto the master cast for correction.

1. First outline the limits of the impression tray on the master cast with pencil. A sheet of 26-gauge wax or wet asbestos is adapted to the edentulous areas to be recorded in wax and later to be corrected to their functional form. In this way, the resin impression base may be trimmed to the limits of the spacer before its removal, thereby establishing the peripheral limits as previously outlined.

Provide extra relief in the mandibular arch over the retromolar pad since this is easily deformed by the impression wax. A hole may also be placed in the resin base over the pad to effect the escape of confined wax and to prevent distortion of the glandular portion of the retromolar pad. Should the retromolar pad not be recorded on the master cast, extend the tray onto a molded clay extension of the cast; otherwise that portion of the tray will have to be extended in the mouth with self-curing resin. Since warm wax will be used, it is best not to border mold or extend the impression base in the mouth with modeling plastic. Should extension of the impression base in the mouth be necessary, use a mix of self-curing resin in a soft doughy state; wet the original base with monomer, add the soft resin dough and shape with fingers, muscle-molding it in the mouth. After hardening, trim any excess, and the base is thus extended the desired amount.

2. After painting the spacer and surrounding cast with tin-foil substitute, seat the denture framework to its terminal position on the master cast, making sure that the indirect retainers and occlusal rests are fully seated. If a wax spacer is used, slightly warm the casting to assure its seating into the wax. Then secure it anteriorly with sticky wax. Whether wax or wet asbestos is used, create some clearance around the retentive framework for the attachment of the resin impression base.

3. Sprinkle the resin tray material (Yates Flash Acrylic) onto the retentive framework and beyond the limits of the spacer, sufficiently thick to assure the rigidity of the impression base.

After hardening, remove the cast framework with attached impression base(s) from the cast, trim to the limits of the spacer, and then remove the spacer.

This is all done in the laboratory, preparatory to the appointment for the functional impression. The care with which the impression base is outlined and fabricated will do much to facilitate the impression procedure. This presumes that the dentist or technician will have interpreted the anatomy of the master cast correctly to avoid gross overextension or underextension of the impression base, thereby avoiding the necessity of time-consuming adjustments at the chair. It is entirely possible to complete the functional impression with three insertions in the mouth, as will be seen subsequently.

Equipment and Materials Needed. The following armamentarium should be set up for the making of the functional impression (Fig. 175):

Bunsen burner	One cake Korecta wax No. 4 in a wax cup
Air tip	immersed in an electric compound
Water syringe and chilled water	heater
No. 7 spatula	One cake Korecta wax No. 1
Bard-Parker handle No. 3 with No. 11 blade	A rather stiff bristle brush for applying
attached	the fluid wax

4. After trying in the cast framework and adjusting the impression base for any obvious overextention or impingement, dry the base thoroughly. With broad sweeping strokes, paint the fluid wax onto the impression surface until a uniform thickness in some excess has been applied. (Fig. 176, A-I.)

5. Seat the framework in the mouth and hold for about two minutes, during which time excess fluid wax will flow to the periphery.

It is of utmost importance that the cast framework be seated in its original position each time and that it be held with three fingers of the working hand in the manner of a tripod. The two legs of the tripod are always the two principal occlusal rests. The third is the principal indirect retainer on the anterior portion

Fig. 175. Armamentarium for making a fluid-wax functional impression: wax cup immersed in water bath held at the medium setting, cake of No. 4 Korecta wax which is melted in the wax cup, cake of No. 1 Korecta wax used with a wax spatula to reinforce the impression wax at the peripheries, No. 11 Bard-Parker blade and handle used for bisecting the impression wax at the peripheries prior to adding the No. 1 wax for reinforcement, No. 7 wax spatula, flat bristle brush for applying the No. 4 wax, and Bunsen burner for use when applying the No. 1 wax with the wax spatula at the peripheries.

of the major connector. In this manner, the framework is always seated in its terminal position. At no time should finger pressure be exerted on the impression base for danger of rotating the appliance away from its forward terminal position.

Now remove the impression from the mouth, chill under tap water, dry with air, and inspect. Areas of *support* will appear glossy, and all others will be dull in appearance. Ideally, the entire impression surface should show evidence of supporting tissue contact after the initial insertion.

6. Paint fluid wax onto dull areas only and inside the flanges at the periphery. No wax should be added to the periphery nor on the outside of the impression base.

The framework is reseated in the mouth and held as before, but this time functional border movements are begun for the purpose of effecting *extension of the impression to obtain maximum coverage.* These border movements are done in the following sequence:

(a) Using the opposite hand, pull the mucous membrane reflection area vertically against the borders of the impression, thereby simulating the extreme position of those tissues against the denture. Do this first on one side and then the other, making sure that the denture framework remains seated at all times.

(b) In the mandibular arch, in order to muscle-mold the lingual periphery,

A   B

C   D

Fig. 176. Nine steps in the making of a fluid-wax functional impression. **A,** Korecta wax No. 4 is painted evenly over the impression base. **B,** The denture framework is placed in the mouth and held in its terminal position with three fingers, one on each principal occlusal rest and a third in between, holding the framework forward in its terminal position with any indirect retainers fully seated. The chin is supported with the other hand. **C,** While holding the framework down, the cheek on each side is pulled vertically against the periphery of the impression. This limits the buccal extension to extreme positions of the bordering attachments. **D,** Again keeping the framework fully seated, the patient is asked to place the tongue forcibly into each cheek. This records extreme movement of the sublingual tissues on the opposite side. **E,** Still holding the framework down, the patient is asked to press the tongue forward against the lingual surface of the anterior teeth. This limits the distolingual extension of the impression on both sides. Following this movement, the patient is asked to open wide, to make the pterygomandibular raphe taut and limit the extreme distal portion of the impression. **F,** The impression is removed and examined for a glossy surface which is evidence of tissue contact. Once this is established, the periphery is reinforced by bisecting the impression wax at the periphery with a No. 11 Bard-Parker blade, leaving unsupported the impression wax extending beyond the impression base. **G,** The very hard Korecta wax No. 1 is applied with a hot No. 7 spatula to reinforce the impression wax at the periphery. This must be applied hot enough to effect good attachment to the impression base. Sufficient No. 1 wax is used to act as a reinforcing extension of the impression base and prevent any undesirable shifting of the impression wax at the periphery. **H,** More No. 4 wax is brushed on, just inside the periphery, to provide an excess which will then be turned at the periphery by a repetition of the previous movements. The wax must be hot enough that it can be brushed on with broad sweeping strokes free of brush mark. **I,** The completed functional impression. Note the peripheral extension buccally and lingually and the thickness of the periphery permissible with this particular patient. This varies widely with each patient, but the periphery recorded by this method should always be reproduced in the finished denture.

E   F

G   H

I

Fig. 176 (cont'd). For legend see opposite page.

ask the patient to first place the tongue firmly into the left cheek, then into the right cheek, and then to press firmly against the lower anterior teeth. The first two movements mold the lingual borders and distal lingual borders on the opposite side; the third lifts the floor of the mouth and brings the retromylohyoid curtain of tissue forward against the distolingual borders.

(c) Ask the patient to open his mouth as wide as possible. In the mandibular arch, this tenses the pterygomandibular raphe, identifies the tendon of the temporal muscle, and brings the anterior border of the masseter muscle against the distobuccal portion of the impression. On the finished impression, the pterygo-

Fig. 177. A close view of a completed fluid-wax functional impression.

Fig. 178. A close view of two maxillary fluid-wax functional impressions. **A,** A bilateral free end (Class I). Note the variation in width at the peripheries and note that the impression wax has been trimmed flush with the palatal finishing line of the framework. **B,** A unilateral free end (Class II).

mandibular notch should be evident. Lingual to this is the extension of the impression into the retromylohyoid space. Buccally should be the notch or the 45-degree angle formed by the anterior border of the masseter muscle (and the external oblique ridge) at the distobuccal periphery of the impression.

In the maxillary arch, the pterygomaxillary notch should be evident as a guide to the trimming of the denture base. Also, as a result of opening wide, the distobuccal aspect will frequently show the flattening effect of the coronoid process of the mandible.

These muscle movements are repeated at intervals of one minute or so. In between, time is allowed for excess wax to escape to the periphery where it is turned by the next series of muscle movements.

After approximately five minutes, remove the impression, chill with tap water, then dry with air, and inspect. The length of time the impression is left in the mouth will depend upon the size of impression and how far the excess wax must move to reach the periphery where it may escape and be turned by the activity of bordering tissues.

This time, the entire impression surface should appear glossy and there should be some excess wax at the periphery. Should any dull areas remain or any of the periphery be deficient, brush fluid wax onto these areas in broad, sweeping strokes and return the impression to the mouth, repeating the previous step.

7. Having obtained evidence of support and peripheral extension, the next step is to reinforce the peripheral excess. This is done in the following manner:

Holding the impression tissue side up, use the No. 11 Bard-Parker blade to bisect the peripheral excess back to the resin impression base. Discard that half on the side away from the tissues, as well as remove all wax that has flowed or has been accidentally applied to the outside of the impression base, leaving a wax-free surface for the attachment of the supporting No. 1 wax. The remaining half is unsupported impression wax that has flowed beyond the limits of the impression tray.

With the large end of the No. 7 spatula, apply Korecta wax No. 1 to the outside of the unsupported No. 4 wax. Apply it hot enough to be fluid and to fuse both to the impression wax and to the resin impression base, yet without melting the impression wax. Cool each application of No. 1 wax with compressed air, returning it to its original hard state. Since this wax is unaffected by mouth temperature, it becomes a stable extension of the resin base. Therefore, extend it up onto the tray for some distance. It must have been applied and smoothed with the hot spatula so as to become a reliable backing for the impression wax. Should it be applied in layers, or should it have impression wax incorporated into it, it cannot provide stable support and will tend to move in the mouth under functional movements.

As an alternate method, the impression wax at the periphery may be supported with resin tray material, using a brush technique for applying. The original tray must be exposed, leaving the unsupported impression wax which is then reinforced with the applied resin. Since time must be allowed for polymerization of the resin, this method is generally used only where gross extension of the impression tray is indicated. Minor extension is best accomplished with No. 1 Korecta wax as outlined in the preceding paragraph.

8. Having reinforced the peripheral extensions of the impression wax with the supporting wax, add a final application of fluid impression wax to and over the periphery. Up to this time, impression wax has been added only to the inside of the periphery. This time, not only is the peripheral limits to be recorded under functional movements, but also peripheral thickness. Except for the distolingual borders of the mandibular denture, which are arbitrarily thinned on the finished denture to avoid objectionable thickness in this area, the thickness of the denture periphery should be that recorded in the wax impression. Thus, the functional impression method provides not only support for the free-end base but also a physiologic peripheral thickness as established by functional

Fig. 179. **A,** Following the making of the resin impression base attached to the partial denture framework, the ridge areas recorded in their static or anatomic form are removed from the master cast by sawing with a spiral saw blade in two planes. One cut is made at right angles to the longitudinal axis of the ridge, 1 mm. distal to the abutment tooth. The second cut is made just lingual and parallel to the lingual sulcus as recorded in the original impression. The two are joined anteriorly and the anatomic reproduction of the ridge is removed. At this time, if the saw cuts are not rough enough, the cut surfaces of the cast should be scored with a knife to provide mechanical retention for the attachment of the new stone to the old. **B,** The completed fluid-wax functional impression. **C,** The completed wax functional

Continued on opposite page.

movements. Support for the cheek is thus assured, and food impaction is prevented by properly contoured polished denture surfaces.

Return the functional impression to the mouth for what should be the final insertion. The third objective, that of *effecting a release of any tissue which has been overdisplaced,* is accomplished during this final insertion. For this reason, sufficient time must elapse for the entire impression to return to its fluid state at mouth temperature and for any excess wax to be displaced by rebounding tissues, where it may flow to the periphery and be turned by functional movements. For the average impression, eight minutes is usually sufficient, during which time the same sequence of functional movements is performed at intervals of approximately one minute. For a larger impression, as much as twelve minutes may be necessary since the excess wax will have a greater distance to travel to the periphery as overdisplacement is released. During this period, as before, the denture framework must be held in its terminal position with indirect retainers fully seated.

The finished impression must not be marred during removal from the mouth, since it may not be corrected without reinsertion. For this reason, use chilled water to reduce the temperature of the wax to a more stable form. After emptying one or more syringefuls of chilled water into the mouth, which is then aspirated, remove the denture framework and attached impression. The patient should be cautioned to remain passive and allow the operator to remove the impression unaided. After releasing the clasp retainers, it is sometimes helpful to lift the framework out of the mouth with thumb forceps, although this will depend upon

---

Fig. 179. (cont'd)

impression is seated on the remainder of the master cast after the anatomic ridges have been removed. Note the scored surface for added retention. The cast metal framework is secured to the dry cast with sticky wax after first making sure that no debris interferes with seating and that all occlusal rests and indirect retainers are seated. Utility wax is placed on the original cast just anterior to the saw cut and sealed anteriorly with a hot spatula. Sheet wax of the adhesive type is placed lingually and sealed to the cast and along the side of the impression base. It must be sealed anteriorly, but the hot spatula must not come in contact with the impression. The surface of the cast anteriorly is then painted with sodium silicate or some other separator, such as Microfilm. Just prior to pouring the new ridge areas, the base of the cast is immersed in ½ inch of water for ten minutes to provide saturation of the dry stone. **D,** The wax functional impression attached to the master cast. The anatomic ridge form has been removed and the cut portion of the cast undercut to assure attachment of the new stone to the old. The cast has been saturated by placing it base downward in ½ inch of water for ten minutes prior to pouring. The only vibrating necessary in adding the new mix of stone is to prevent trapping air at the junction of the wax impression with the cut surfaces of the stone cast. **E,** The ridge areas are poured with a stone of a different color, using no more vibration than necessary, and then inverted into additional stone on a glass or ceramic slab. Stone must be brought up well around the distal ends of the impression. After the stone has hardened, the excess is trimmed away until the margins of the impression wax are exposed. The sticky wax is chilled with ice or the cast is chilled and the sticky wax flaked off. The cast is then immersed in water at 110° to 120° F., sufficient to just soften the mouth-temperature wax, and the framework with attached impression base is lifted. Usually, the impression wax remains on the impression base, leaving a clean cast as shown.

its accessibility and the digital dexterity of the operator. The greatest hazard to be avoided is the cusps of the teeth nearest the impression which may touch and mar the periphery during removal.

Now dry the impression with compressed air and inspect. If satisfactory, place the impression tissue side up on two cotton rolls, which preferably have been secured to the bottom of a shallow box. Although the impression need not be poured immediately and may be kept safely at normal room temperature, protect it from damage and heat.

Pouring Up the Functional Impression. This is usually done by removing the anatomic form of the residual ridge from the master cast and repouring it in its functional form as recorded by the wax impression.

1. If the anatomic ridge form on the master cast is to be replaced with the functional, or supporting, form, remove and discard that portion of the master cast. This is done by sawing the cast with a spiral saw blade along lines drawn on the cast. (Fig. 179, A-E.)

Beginning about 1 mm. distal to the abutment tooth, draw a line at right angles to the longitudinal axis of the ridge and down the side of the cast. Then project this line along the bottom of the cast. On the mandibular cast, draw a second line at right angles to the first, beginning just mesial to the lingual sulcus and extending distally along the rim of the sulcus to the dorsal aspect of the cast and down that side. Then project this line anteriorly along the bottom of the cast to join the first line at a right angle. If a Class I cast, do this for both ridges.

With a spiral saw blade, saw the cast along these lines until the cuts meet at the anterior lingual angle. Then remove and discard the anatomic ridge form. If a Class I cast, this leaves the center portion of the cast intact.

On the maxillary cast, make the longitudinal cut on the palatal aspect to

Fig. 180. An occlusal view of the wax blockout before repouring the edentulous area to the form recorded by the fluid-wax functional impression. The framework must be secured in position with sticky wax. Utility wax is used to limit the fresh stone on the buccal surface at the line of junction only. Adhesive sheet wax is used on the lingual surface, which is sealed anteriorly to prevent the new stone from leaking through.

coincide with the edge of the wax impression so that a butt joint is created between the wax and the remaining cast. Otherwise, excess stone will flow beneath the denture framework. This is facilitated by scoring the cast along the wax relief at the time of blockout. Trim the palatal aspect of the relief abruptly so that a raised platform will be evident on the investment cast and a step will exist on the denture casting. This serves as a finishing line on the tissue side, first to limit the wax impression and later to establish the finishing line for the resin base. Having scored the cast previously, cut the cast longitudinally along this line. A precise junction between the impression wax and the remaining portion of the cast will thus be possible to assure a smooth junction between the new functional ridge form and the anatomic form of the palate. (If a slight step results from tissue displacement, it may then be removed by scraping the cast along the line of junction.)

After removing the anatomic ridge, roughen or undercut the fresh edges of the cast to create some mechanical retention between the new and the old stone.

2. Being sure that the denture framework and the master cast are free of any debris, seat the framework in the same terminal position as it was when in the mouth. Secure it anteriorly with sticky wax. Some wax blockout is necessary to confine the new stone, but complete boxing is neither necessary nor advisable.

Beginning at the base of the abutment tooth, adapt a stick of utility wax on the buccal surface down to the bottom of the cast. Seal this along its anterior border without covering the freshly cut surface to which new stone must attach. This is the only blockout on the buccal surface, and on the maxillary cast, the only blockout that is needed.

On the mandibular cast, adopt a sheet of soft wax, such as utility wax or adhesive wax, along the lingual sulcus. Seal this anteriorly around the lingual bar and the minor connector, all along its junction with the cast, and to the impression base some distance above the periphery of the impression. It is important that the hot spatula not approach the impression periphery as the mouth-temperature wax is easily melted.

The exposed remainder of the original cast should now be painted with a separating film, such as tin-foil substitute, to prevent new stone from attaching to critical areas of the cast.

Place the base of the cast in a pan of water no more than one-half inch deep, so that it may become saturated without immersing the impression itself. Five to ten minutes' soaking is sufficient.

3. Pour the impression with the same type of stone as the original cast or with stone of a different color for contrast. For example, if the master cast was poured in Duroc or Vel-Mix, the wax impression may be poured in Castone. Any excess is more easily identified by using stone of contrasting colors. The object in using a separator on all but the cut surfaces is, of course, to facilitate the removal of any unwanted stone. Such excess can be prevented, however, by carefully sealing the blockout wax and by avoiding excessive vibration when filling the impression. The only reason for vibrating the impression is to avoid trapping air at acute angles where the impression joins the cast. After this area has been filled, the

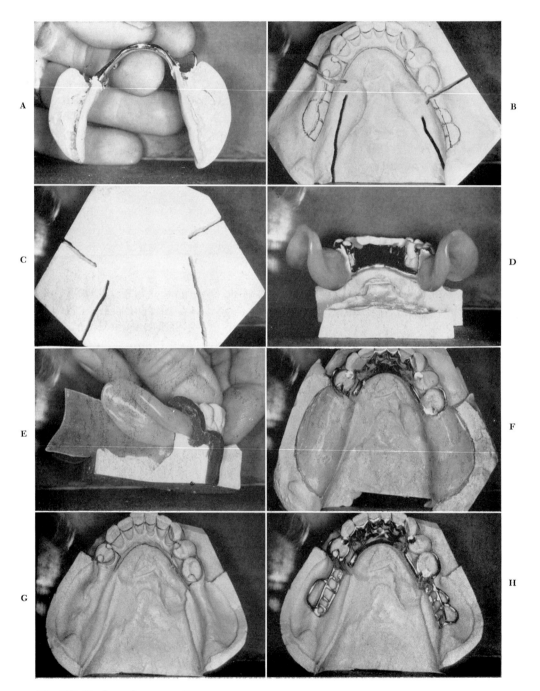

Fig. 181. For legend see opposite page.

remainder may be filled without vibrating. Add stone in excess, piling still more stone onto a glass slab; then invert the impression carefully onto the glass slab. Then smooth the sides of the cast with the spatula, and, as the stone stiffens, trim away the gross excess. It is not necessary to immerse the impression, for by the time the stone gives off exothermic heat, the initial set has occurred. At this point, immersing the cast for the purpose of supplying additional water for crystallization may be advisable.

4. To separate the impression from the cast first chill the sticky wax and blockout wax to aid in its removal, trimming away any interfering stone around the peripheries and finally immersing the wax impression in water just above mouth temperature (approximately 110° F.). This latter precaution is to avoid melting the wax which would cause wax impregnation of the cast surface and later interfere with the action of the tin-foil substitute. Failure of the tin-foil substitute to adequately act as a separating film between the cast and the denture base resin is usually due to wax contamination of the stone cast. This is particularly true where molten wax has impregnated the cast to some depth. Not only for this reason should melting of the impression wax be avoided but also because of the orange-colored pigment in the wax which, if allowed to impregnate the stone, may cause discoloration of the resin base.

After separation of the cast from the impression, trim the corrected cast, remove any excess, and prepare for the making of a denture base upon which jaw relations may be established. Since any previous base will not now fit the functional ridge form it is necessary that new bases be made, or the original impression base corrected, before final jaw relations can be recorded.

Fig. 181. Eight steps in the correction of a master cast to functional ridge form. **A,** The resin impression base is made with sufficient relief to accommodate the impression wax. This may be either sheet wax or over a sheet of asbestos as shown. If a separating film is not used, the fibers remaining after stripping out the asbestos aid in the retention of the wax to the resin base. **B,** Upon this master cast the denture framework and, subsequently, the attached impression base are made. After the impression base has been made, the cast may be partially sectioned with a spiral saw blade as shown. **C,** The underside of the cast shows the relationship of the two saw cuts. Some irregularity is desirable to provide mechanical attachment of the new and old stone. **D,** The completed functional impression is returned to the master cast. The metal framework must be completely seated and secured with sticky wax. The anatomic ridges have now been removed. **E,** Utility wax is placed and seated just anterior to the wax cut on the buccal surface. Adhesive sheet wax is placed on the lingual surface and sealed to prevent leakage. The remainder of the cast other than the portion to be repoured is painted with tin-foil substitute, Microfilm or sodium silicate, as a protective film. The base of the cast is then immersed for ten minutes in ½ inch of water. **F,** After repouring the ridge areas, the cast is inverted on a glass slab and the fresh stone brought up around the heels. After setting, excess stone is cut away until the impression wax is visible. **G,** The sticky wax is chilled and flaked off. Then the impression wax is softened in warm water and the impression base with wax still attached is lifted from the cast. The corrected cast is then trimmed as shown. Compare the new functional ridge form with the anatomic ridge form shown in **B. H,** The resin impression base is removed from the framework and the framework is cleaned free of any debris and returned to the corrected cast for the purpose of making a new resin jaw relation record base which will be essentially identical to that of the finished denture.

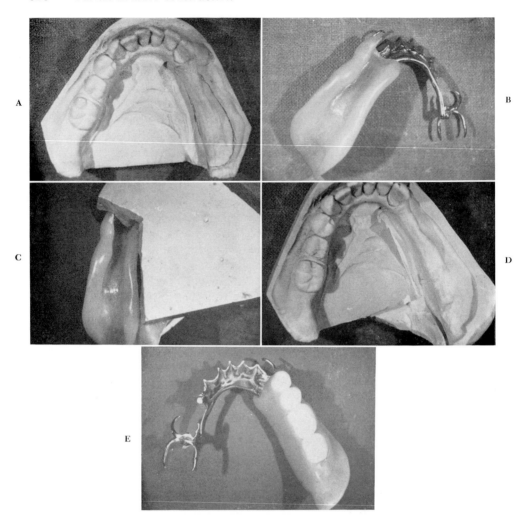

Fig. 182. A sequence in the correction of a lower Class II cast to functional ridge form. **A,** The master cast with anatomic ridge form as recorded from a hydrocolloid impression. The outline of the proposed impression base is drawn in pencil. **B,** The completed functional impression. **C,** The impression seated on the cut-away cast, boxed anteriorly with sticky wax and lingually with adhesive sheet wax. **D,** The corrected master cast. Compare this with **A.** **E,** An occlusal view of the completed denture showing the broad coverage made possible by this impression method. This denture base, although much larger than the denture worn previously, was accepted by the patient with no adjustment whatsoever.

Pouring a Processing Cast. Occasionally a processing cast may be preferable to a corrected master cast. This cast will then be used instead of the master cast for completion of the denture, the master cast having served its purpose for the making of the denture framework and the impression base. (Fig. 184.)

The sole advantage in using a processing cast is that possible errors in returning the impression to the master cast are thus avoided. It must be created

Fig. 183. The correction of a lower Class I master cast with only six anterior teeth remaining. **A,** The original master cast with edentulous areas reproduced in their anatomic form. The penciled design of the denture framework is evident. **B,** The same cast with edentulous areas corrected to their functional form. Compare with **A. C,** The framework returned to the corrected cast for the purpose of making jaw relation record bases.

Fig. 184. Two steps in the making of a processing cast instead of correcting the master cast. **A,** The functional impression. This is poured completely in new stone, which is brought up anteriorly to provide a surface for reseating the denture framework. Any stone that might interfere with removal must then be trimmed away before attempting separation of the framework from the cast. **B,** The completed processing cast. Note the functional form of the edentulous areas and the index areas remaining to assure accurate repositioning of the denture framework. This method is not used where anterior tooth replacements are involved.

with care, however, so that the denture framework may be removed and reseated with accuracy during subsequent steps in finishing the denture. In pouring the cast, the stone must be brought up around the underside of all of the components of the denture framework to positively establish its future relation to the cast, and yet any excess which would interfere with its removal must be eliminated. For this reason, the individual pouring the impression must give it his undivided attention and trim away excess as soon as the consistency of the stone permits. If this is done, the denture framework and impression may be separated from the cast without interference, leaving an accurate imprint of the underside of the denture framework for later repositioning. Those portions of the cast lying within denture clasps should be trimmed flush with the occlusal border of the clasp arms and the occlusal rests, thereby simulating occlusal surfaces which may later be used as vertical stops on the articulator. Those portions lying beneath major connectors and indirect retainers must remain intact to assure accurate repositioning of the framework.

Using a Resin Tray for the Functional Impression. Although the majority of free-end partial dentures are made with resin bases which can later be relined, there are occasions when the use of metal bases is desirable. There is good reason to believe that ridge tissues remain healthier and ridge resorption is minimized by the stimulating effect of metal bases. (See advantages of metal bases, Chapter 11.)

Since metal bases may not be satisfactorily relined, they are used only where resorption of the edentulous ridge is not anticipated. It is generally considered that where sufficient time has elapsed since extractions for a firm ridge to be established, there will be less resorption beneath the denture base. It should be remembered that the age and health of the patient and the response of the ridge to occlusal loading will influence the rapidity of tissue change beneath a denture base. It is impossible to predict with any accuracy the response of any given ridge to loading. Still, the beneficial effects of using a metal base with harmonious and moderate occlusion may prevent changes which would ordinarily occur beneath resin bases or under traumatic occlusion. In such cases, the calculated risk of using a metal base, even though it cannot be relined, may be justified.

On the other hand, a ridge that has been satisfactorily supporting a previous denture may be expected to remain constant beneath a new metal base if not subjected to excessive occlusal loading or trauma. While disuse atrophy of an unused ridge may lead to immediate changes under loading, the fact that a ridge has been supporting a denture previously without unfavorable response leads to the obvious, and valid, assumption that it may do so in the foreseeable future. In such case, metal bases may be used satisfactorily and to advantage.

A metal-based free-end denture is no different than a resin-based denture insofar as support is concerned, for any free-end denture should have the best possible tissue support. But for the metal bases to be cast to the supporting or functional form of the ridge, the master cast must be corrected prior to the blockout and duplication of the master cast. Otherwise, the metal bases must be cast separately and attached to the supporting framework by soldering or other means. A technique for doing the latter will be given later in this chapter.

Several years ago, Applegate and Hall worked out a technique for using a resin tray instead of the denture framework as a means of positioning the impression tray in the mouth and then back onto the master cast for correction. In this method, three or more occlusal surfaces on natural teeth are used for tripoding the resin tray.

Originally, the tray was waxed on a duplicate master cast, reinforced with piano wire, and invested and processed in acrylic resin. Later a technique was developed for blocking out the cast with modeling clay and forming the tray by sprinkling with self-curing acrylic resin. The sprinkled resin tray was found to be just as accurate as the processed tray, and the technique was thereby simplified.

A resin tray may be made on an accurate study cast or a duplicate thereof. The ridge areas to be corrected are covered with one thickness of 28-gauge wax to provide space for the impression material. The remainder of the cast, with the exception of three widely spaced occlusal seating areas, is blocked out with modeling clay. A trough of baseplate wax may be added anteriorly to provide a form for the molding of the tray handle, or a resin or wire handle may be added later. (Fig. 185.)

The three occlusal stops are painted lightly with a tin-foil substitute which is then permitted to dry. A separating medium such as Microfilm should never be used, as it may have a retarding effect on the self-curing resin tray material.

A self-curing acrylic resin (Yates Flash Acrylic) is used with a sprinkling technique to form the tray. The area to be covered is first wet with monomer and then sprinkled with polymer, which is again wetted with monomer. This process is repeated until a tray of adequate thickness has been formed. (Fig. 186.) An

Fig. 185. Clay matrix for making a sprinkled acrylic resin impression tray. The ridge areas are first relieved with 28-gauge sheet wax. Three or four occlusal surfaces are left exposed for index areas for positioning the impression tray in the mouth and back onto the master cast for repouring the ridge areas. The clay is grooved from one side to the other to provide a reinforcing rib on the underside of the impression tray.

Fig. 186. Six steps in the correction of a master cast to functional form, using the resin tray method. **A,** The clay matrix has been formed, with the edentulous area relieved with 28-gauge sheet wax and three occlusal surfaces left exposed to form the legs of a tripod. Note the wax form for the handle extending anteriorly. **B,** Acrylic resin has been sprinkled into the clay matrix. **C,** The resin tray has been trimmed and tried in the mouth. The three bearing areas of contact are then perfected with a fresh application of self-curing resin (visible at the incisal edge of the canine teeth). Note that there is no other contact either with teeth or in the edentulous area where the impression wax will be placed. **D,** The fluid-wax impression is shown, completed. In this method, the amount of palatal area included is arbitrary, but whatever is included in the impression must be cut away from the master cast before the tray is seated upon it. Note the three bearing areas which determine accurately the position of the tray in the mouth and when returned to the master cast. **E,** That portion of the master cast to be corrected has been cut away and undercut. The resin tray is seated accurately upon it, secured with sticky wax, and blockout placed anteriorly and palatally. The cast, only, is then soaked before repouring the edentulous portion of the cast. **F,** The corrected master cast shows the line of junction which must now be trimmed until flush.

Fig. 187. The completed functional impression, whether with resin tray or denture frame-work, should be supported by cotton rolls until poured. If it must be transported to the laboratory, it may be secured to the bottom of a shallow box with sticky wax.

upper cast is treated the same as a lower, without covering the palate. The tray is then covered so as to prevent too rapid evaporation of the monomer and is set aside for one hour or more. Following the polymerization period, the tray is lifted and trimmed and is ready to be taken to the mouth where it should seat accurately on three occlusal legs in the manner of a tripod. The tray, when finished, should be of uniform thickness, with a handle that projects over and beyond the incisal edges of the anterior teeth. It should not contact the teeth at any points other than at the three occlusal stops. Using this tray as the impression base, a fluid-wax functional impression is then made of the edentulous areas, the same as when a cast framework is used. The completed impression is then positioned on the cut-away master cast for the repouring of the edentulous areas.

It was mentioned previously that the tray may be formed upon an accurate study cast. This can only be done if the study cast is made with the same care as is used in making a master cast. (Any study cast should be an accurate reproduction of the conditions present, so that diagnosis and treatment planning may be effectively accomplished.) However, whether the impression tray is made on the study cast or the master cast, the three occlusal areas should be corrected in the mouth with a thin mix of self-curing acrylic resin just prior to making the fluid-wax impression of the edentulous areas. Any change in tooth form, such as the preparation of guiding planes and occlusal rest seats, will be subtractions rather than additions to the teeth and therefore will not interfere with the seating of the impression tray. The three seating areas should be selected with the design of the partial denture framework in mind.

To conserve chair time, the appointment for the making of the wax functional impression in the previously prepared tray may be made to coincide with the making of the final hydrocolloid impression for the master cast. The wax functional impression is made first, and then the hydrocolloid impression of the anatomic form of the teeth and adjoining structures is made. In this case, the edentulous areas to be recorded in their functional form are blocked out on the hydrocolloid impression with stainless steel strips and left unpoured. After the separation of the master cast from its impression, the resin tray, with its functional wax impression, is seated onto the cast and attached to it securely with sticky wax. The edentulous areas are then poured. The resulting master cast, complete with corrected saddle areas, is then ready for the construction of either a resin or a metal partial denture base without further need for seeing the patient until the denture is ready for the recording of occlusal relationships.

Although the resin tray method was developed with metal bases in mind, it may be used regardless of the type of denture bases to be used. If the dentist prefers, he may thus send a corrected master cast to the technician rather than have the cast framework returned for the purpose of making the fluid-wax impression.

While it is basically just as accurate a method, the resin tray will not give results equal to those obtained with the denture framework unless the tray is used with considerable care to assure accurate positioning both in the mouth and upon return to the master cast. Some of the precautions to be taken when the resin tray method is used are as follows:

1. The resin tray must be made rigid and should be braced by a reinforcing cross-arch strut. It should have sufficient bulk to assure rigidity without interference to insertion, removal, or functional movements.

2. The resin tray must seat in the mouth and on the master cast identically. This is facilitated by correcting the seating areas in the mouth just prior to making the impression and rechecking the accuracy of its position on the master cast. There must be no interference or resistance to seating, nor should any instability be present. The corrected areas should extend onto suprabulge buccal or labial surfaces of the supporting teeth for added stability. Foreign particles or folded-under pieces of resin material must be eliminated beneath all seating areas to assure accurate repositioning of the tray.

3. The tray must have three or more widely spaced seating areas. Ideally, this would be three legs of a tripod, resting on the occlusal surface of two posterior teeth and one anterior tooth. For a Class I arch, two second premolars and one or both canines are best suited for stable support. For a Class II arch, the free-end abutment on one side, the most posterior tooth on the opposite side, and the canine farthest from the free end are preferred for optimal support of the tray.

The mandibular incisors should seldom be used for support of the resin tray, but when they are, the incisal edges of two or more adjacent teeth are considered one area. The anterior support should not be located beneath the handle but should be freely visible, both in the mouth and on the master cast.

4. The resin tray must be held in the mouth during the entire impression sequence by direct finger pressure over the seating areas *only*. Since there are no clasps, minor connectors, and bracing components to help stabilize the position of the impression tray, only vertical forces may be used to stabilize the tray on the supporting teeth.

5. The master cast and the seating areas of the tray must be free of any debris when it is reseated onto the master cast. The cast must be dry so that

sticky wax will adhere to it. The tray should be attached to the cast with sticky wax at places other than the seating areas. These should remain uncovered at all times so that any change in position or inaccuracy in seating may be detected.

6. Blocking out the master cast prior to pouring up the wax impression must be done with extreme caution to prevent dislodgment of the tray. The application of a separating medium, such as a tin-foil substitute, to exposed cast surfaces is very important since the tray may interfere with a complete blockout of areas not to be corrected.

7. The sticky wax should be chilled with cold water and removed before removal of the tray so as to prevent damage to the surfaces of the cast to which it was attached. The impression wax is then warmed in water just above mouth temperature and lifted off.

8. Any excess stone must be carefully removed and the junction between anatomic and functional cast surfaces smoothed by light scraping. The resulting master cast, with ridges corrected to functional form, can be entirely accurate

Fig. 188. Four steps in the making of a replaceable metal base for a unilateral free-end partial denture. **A,** The master cast is corrected to reproduce the supporting form of the residual ridge beneath the distal extension. The cast metal framework was used in the conventional manner to carry an impression base to the mouth and then back on the master cast for correction. **B,** The wax pattern is formed on an investment cast duplicate of the corrected cast and the original framework seated upon it to properly relate one to the other. **C,** The metal base is cast and fitted to the master cast. **D,** The original framework and separate metal base are now on the master cast. These are next united by self-curing acrylic resin, using a brush or sprinkling method of applying the resin,

if the preceding precautions are taken. The master cast is now ready for final surveying, blocking out, duplication, and the making of either a metal-base denture or a casting with retention lugs for the attachment of a resin base.

Assembled Metal Bases. The preceding technique permits correction of the master cast for the purpose of making a one-piece casting with metal bases made to the functional, or supporting, form of the edentulous ridge. This type of free-end partial denture is not designed to be rebased; therefore, it is only used in selected cases. There has been some demand for partial dentures that combine the advantages of metal bases with the opportunity of replacing those bases in the event of changes in tissue support. The solution lies in replaceable metal bases attached to the denture framework with resin rather than by soldering. (Fig. 188, *A-D*, and Fig. 189, *A-E*.)

In this method, the denture framework is designed and cast as for a resin-base denture, except that an open retentive framework is made which will fit inside the finishing line of the future metal base. If, because of recent extractions or the possibility of changes due to disuse atrophy, any change in the supporting ridge is anticipated, the denture may be made first with a resin base. Such a base is preferably made to functional form, even though it is to be replaced later with a metal base. Better support and better stimulation of the residual ridge will result if the functional form is used to support reasonable occlusion. Under such conditions, the amount of change in ridge form will be held to a minimum.

Although occlusion is usually added, the resin base alone may be used, permitting stimulation as an exercise prosthesis as advocated by Applegate, who has this to say about the reconditioning of alveolar bone:

> One of the most difficult situations with which the prosthodontist must deal is that existing when disuse atrophy (osteoporosis) has occurred in the edentulous area. Frequently, the missing teeth may have been extracted many years before their prosthetic replacement is accomplished. Bone is maintained only in response to the stimulation associated with its functional use. Of this, Weinmann and Sicher say, "If the loss of teeth is extensive or if the teeth bordering the edentulous area have lost their function, for instance, through the elimination of their antagonists, the osteoporosis is much more severe and the loss of bone substance at the alveolar ridge is much greater." One of the most common errors in prosthodontics is to assume that, because the bone is being maintained normally in the area of remaining teeth which have received greater than normal function the edentulous ridge in the same mouth also will furnish stable support immediately.
>
> Frequently, the replacement of teeth is done in a manner to restore a nearly normal functional load to such edentulous areas, only to have a rapid resorptive change occur beneath the denture base. I make a plea for the preconditioning of the residual alveolar ridge, where there has been long disuse, before the normal stress load is restored. This can be done by one of the following procedures:
>
> 1. Supply a temporary exercise prosthesis for use over a period of a few months.
> 2. Construct the appliance with the base adapted to functional form and extended to maximum area, but do not replace the teeth until later.
>
> In addition, have the patient exercise the ridge area with finger massage prior to the prosthetic service, while restorative and other mouth preparation is being done. Be certain, also, that the diet and vitamin intake is proper and that the physical condition of the patient is such as to assure the best possible metabolic function. . . .

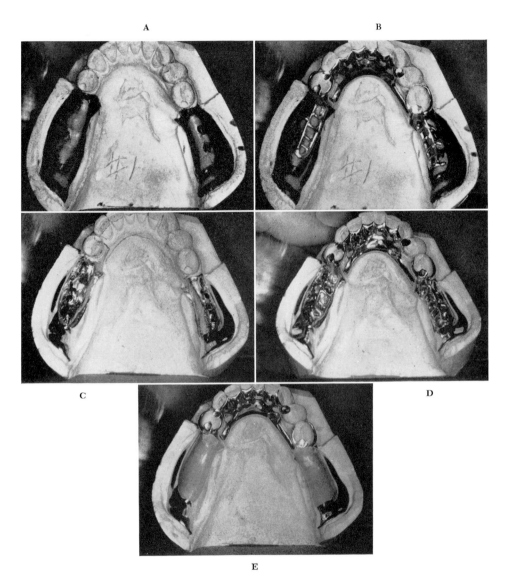

Fig. 189. Five steps in the making of replaceable metal bases for a bilateral free-end partial denture. **A,** The wax patterns for the metal bases are formed on an investment cast duplicate of the corrected master cast. **B,** The original metal framework is placed over the wax pattern and the two are relieved or re-formed as needed to eliminate interference and provide retention and finishing lines for the resin attachment. **C,** The cast bases are returned to the master cast. **D,** The three pieces are assembled on the master cast. This should be done by the laboratory, at which time any remaining interference is eliminated. **E,** The pieces have been assembled with self-curing acrylic resin. Final jaw relations may now be established on this assembled denture, or this may be deferred until the patient and the tissues have become accustomed to the wearing of the prosthesis for a period of time before adding occlusion.

To be of value, the ridge surfaces of the exercise bases should not only be maximum in area, but they should be related to the basal structures exactly as the bases of the finished partial denture will be. The daily two or three exercise periods of intermittent biting pressure will then direct stimuli through the base into the substructures in the same manner that work stimuli will later be induced by tooth surface contacts. Under this method of bone reconditioning, the edentulous ridge may be expected to undergo a process of reorganization which will prepare it to accept a reasonable occlusal load, at a later time, with much less resorptive change.*

Adding Metal Bases to the Partial Denture. When it may be presumed that the residual ridge has undergone its initial changes under the load of supporting a denture, the metal bases may be added in the following manner:

The original resin base may be relieved and used as an impression base or it may be removed entirely and replaced with a resin impression base as outlined previously in this chapter. A new fluid-wax functional impression is made and the original master cast or a new master cast is corrected to the existing functional ridge form as though for a resin base. The corrected master cast is then duplicated and an investment cast made.

Upon the investment cast, a metal base or bases is waxed, using 26-gauge wax over the ridge. The peripheries are reinforced using 14- or 16-gauge round wax and free-hand waxing. Prior to locating the finishing line for the resin attachment, the cast framework must be tried on the investment cast to see if the retentive frame will interfere. Any extension loops that were added for the purpose of supporting resin bases are removed, leaving only the ladderlike retentive frame. The cross pieces should have been made originally far enough apart to accommodate nailhead retentions on the metal base.

An undercut finishing line is added, forming a recess for the resin attachment beyond the limits of the retentive frame. The original cast framework may have to be warmed slightly to assure its seating into the wax pattern for the metal base. Within the boundaries of the retentive frame, two or more nailhead retentions are added for the purpose of securing the metal base to the resin attachment which will be, in turn, attached to the retentive frame. Some care must be taken in waxing around the major connector to form a neat junction without interfering with separation of the cast framework from the wax pattern.

The cast framework may now be lifted and the metal base or bases sent to the laboratory for casting and polishing. The original framework and the master cast must also be sent to the laboratory so that the separate pieces may be fitted together on the master cast. On return from the laboratory, there must be no definite contact between the separate pieces. Rather, the metal base or bases must seat easily and the original framework go to its terminal position with clearance to spare. Since the attachment between the pieces will be with a self-curing acrylic resin, there is no need for their making contact which could lead to errors in positioning.

Each piece should be tacked separately to the master cast with sticky wax.

*From Applegate, O. C.: The Removable Partial Denture in the General Practice of Tomorrow, J. Pros. Den. **8:**609-622, 1958.

With the use of a brush technique first and then sprinkling, the pieces are secured to each other with sufficient acrylic resin to assure stability. Occlusal relations may then be established on this assembled denture.

Since the teeth will be attached to the metal base with resin, it is preferable that there be no line of junction between the acrylic resin attaching the separate pieces and the resin supporting the teeth. For this reason, before setting teeth in wax the original resin should be cut back short of the finishing line. In this way, the only resin visible will be that supporting the denture teeth.

The principal advantage of this method is that the metal base or bases may be easily removed at some future date by point flaming the underside of the metal base enough to soften the resin attachment. The original metal base may then be separated from the original framework and discarded, leaving the denture framework intact to support a new metal base and new occlusion.

By this method it is possible to replace metal bases when it becomes necessary due to changes in support, accomplishing much the same thing as with the relining of resin bases but with all of the desirable advantages of using metal bases.

Chapter 16

Occlusal relationships for
partial dentures

The third phase* in the construction of a partial denture is the establishment of a functional and harmonious occlusal relationship between opposing dentition. This has long been one of the most neglected aspects of partial denture construction.

Failure to provide and maintain adequate occlusion on the partial denture is primarily due to (1) lack of support for the denture base and (2) the fallacy of establishing occlusion to a static jaw relation record only. Support for the jaw relation record base must be the same as for the finished prothesis, either through occlusal rests or through a combination of occlusal and tissue support. The establishment of functional occlusal records will be covered later in this chapter.

Balanced occlusion is desirable on complete dentures because occlusal stresses may cause instability of the dentures and/or trauma to the supporting structures. And yet, these stresses can reach a point beyond which movement of the dentures takes place. The stresses therefore are eliminated at the expense of denture stability and retention.

In partial dentures, however, because of the fixation to abutments, occlusal stresses are transmitted directly to the abutment teeth and other supporting structures, resulting in sustained stresses which are far more damaging than those transient stresses found in complete dentures. Therefore, occlusal harmony between a partial denture and the remaining natural teeth is a major factor in the preservation of the health of their surrounding structures.

In the fabrication of complete dentures, only one factor, which is the inclination of the condyle path, is not within the control of the dentist. All other factors may be altered to obtain occlusal balance and harmony in eccentric positions to conform to the dentist's particular concept and philosophy of denture occlusion.

In establishing occlusion on a partial denture, the influence of the remaining

---

*See Chapter 2, under Three Phases of Partial Denture Service.

natural teeth is usually such that the occlusal forms of the teeth on the denture must conform to an already established occlusal pattern. This pattern may have been improved upon by occlusal equilibration or rehabilitation, but the pattern present at the time the partial denture is made dictates the occlusion on the partial denture. The only exceptions are those where an opposing complete denture can be made to harmonize occlusally with the partial denture or where only anterior teeth remain in both arches and the incisal relationship can be made noninterfering. In these situations, the recording of jaw relations and the arrangement of the teeth may proceed in the same manner as with complete dentures, and the same general principles apply.

With all other types of partial dentures, the remaining teeth must dictate the occlusion, unless the dentist is willing to accept nothing more than centric occlusal contacts and ignore interference in lateral movement or has reason to believe that he can achieve occlusal harmony on the partial denture by adjusting the occlusion in the mouth. While some claim that a functional relationship of the partial denture to the natural dentition may be adjusted satisfactorily in the mouth, it is doubtful that this is or ever can be done adequately. Partial denture occlusion thus established can at best only perpetuate malocclusions that existed previously and help to maintain the existing vertical relationship, however inadequate it may be.

The establishment of a satisfactory occlusion for the partial denture patient should include the following: (1) an analysis of the existing occlusion, (2) the correction of existing occlusal disharmony as a necessary step in preparing the mouth for the partial denture, (3) the recording of an adjusted centric occlusion, and (4) the recording of functional eccentric occlusion. An adjusted and corrected occlusion on the natural teeth is the occlusion which the dentist attempts to transfer to an instrument in such a manner that occlusal harmony on the partial denture is made possible.

Wilson and also Osborne and Lammie have described four ways of establishing interocclusal relations for partial dentures. Five methods instead of four will be given in this chapter.

Before describing any of these, it is necessary that the use of a face-bow mounting and the pertinent factors in partial denture occlusion be considered. A description of the face-bow is found in most prosthetic textbooks and will not be repeated here. The technique for applying the face-bow has been described briefly in Chapter 3, Diagnosis and Treatment Planning.

While a hinge axis mounting may be desirable for complete oral rehabilitation procedures, the common face-bow will facilitate the mounting of the upper cast in relation to the condylar axis of the articulating instrument with reasonable accuracy. As suggested in Chapter 3, it is still better that, in addition to mounting the casts at a comparable radius, the plane of occlusion be related to the orbital-axis plane. Since the dominant factor in partial denture occlusion is the remaining natural teeth and their proprioceptor influence on occlusion, a comparable radius at the oriented plane of occlusion on an acceptable instrument will allow reasonably valid mandibular movements to be reproduced. Such instruments are the Hanau models S-M and H-2 and the Dentatus model ARH.

METHODS FOR ESTABLISHING
OCCLUSAL RELATIONSHIPS

The recording of occlusion for the partially edentulous arch may vary from the simple apposition of opposing casts by occluding sufficient remaining natural teeth to the recording of jaw relations in much the same manner as for a completely edentulous patient. As long as there are natural teeth remaining in contact, however, some consideration must be given the cuspal influence that those teeth will have on functional jaw movements.

Direct Apposition of Casts. The *first method* is used where there are sufficient opposing teeth remaining in contact to make the existing jaw relationship obvious and where only a few teeth are to be replaced on short denture bases. In this method, opposing casts may be occluded by hand and the relationship recorded by projecting several pencil lines from one arch to the other to guide the technician in reoccluding the casts. The occluded casts should be held in apposition with wooden sticks or wire nails attached with sticky wax to the bases of the casts until they are securely mounted on the articulator.

At best, this method can only perpetuate the existing vertical dimension and any existing occlusal disharmony present between the natural dentition. Occlusal analysis and the correction of any existing occlusal disharmony should precede the making of such a jaw relation record. The limitations of such a method are obvious. Yet, such a jaw relation record is better than an inaccurate interocclusal wax record between the remaining natural teeth. Unless a record is made which does not influence the closing path by reason of its bulk and the consistency of the recording medium, direct apposition of opposing casts at least eliminates the possibility of the patient giving the dentist a faulty or strained jaw relationship.

Interocclusal Records With Posterior Teeth Remaining. A *second method*, which is a modification of the first, is used when sufficient teeth remain to support the partial denture (Kennedy Class III) but the relation of opposing teeth does not permit the occluding of casts by hand. In such cases, jaw relations must be established as for fixed bridge restorations, using some kind of interocclusal record.

The least accurate of these is the interocclusal wax record. The successful recording of centric relation with an interocclusal wax record will be influenced by the bulk and the consistency of the wax and the accuracy of the wax after chilling. Excess wax contacting mucosal surfaces may distort soft tissues, thereby preventing accurate seating of the wax record onto the stone casts. Distortion of wax during or following removal from the mouth may also interfere with accurate seating. Therefore, a definite procedure for making interocclusal wax records is given as follows:

A uniformly softened roll of baseplate wax is inserted between the teeth and the patient is asked to close in centric relation. Correct closure should have been rehearsed prior to inserting the wax so that there will be no hesitancy or deviation on the part of the patient. The wax is then removed and immediately chilled thoroughly with ice water. After inspecting the wax record to make sure that opposing teeth were in centric contact, it should be reinserted a second time to correct the distortion resulting from chilling and again chilled after removal.

With a sharp knife, all excess wax should now be removed. It is most important at this time that all wax contacting mucosal surfaces be trimmed free of contact. The chilled wax record should again be reinserted to make sure there is no contact with soft tissue.

A wax record may be further corrected with an impression paste which is used as the final recording medium. Some impression pastes are more suitable than others for this purpose. Generally, a material that sets quite hard is preferred.

In making such a corrected wax record, the opposing teeth (and also the patient's face and the dentist's fingers) should first be coated with petroleum jelly on a silicone preparation. The impression paste is then mixed and applied to both sides of the wax record. It is quickly inserted and the patient asked to close in the rehearsed path, which will this time be guided by the previous wax record. After the paste has set, the corrected wax record is removed and inspected for accuracy. Any excess projecting beyond the wax matrix should then be removed with a sharp knife.

Such a record should seat on accurate casts without discrepancy or interference and will provide an accurate interocclusal record. When an intact opposing arch is present, use of an opposing cast may be dispensed with and a hard stone poured directly into the impression paste record to serve as an opposing cast. However, although this may be an acceptable procedure in the construction of a unilateral fixed bridge, the advantages of having casts properly oriented on a suitable articulator contraindicates the practice. The only exception to this is where the upper cast upon which the partial denture is to be fabricated has already been mounted previously with the aid of a face-bow. In such case, an intact lower arch may be reproduced in stone by pouring a cast directly into the interocclusal record.

An interocclusal record may also be made using an adjustable bite frame (Fig. 16). Reference to this method has previously been made in Chapter 3, Diagnosis and Treatment Planning. The adjustable bite frame was devised for use with materials that offer no resistance to closure, such as zinc oxide and eugenol impression pastes.

Some of the advantages of using a metallic oxide paste over wax as a recording medium for occlusal records are as follows: (1) uniformity of consistency, (2) ease of displacement on closure, (3) accuracy of occlusal surface reproduction, and (4) dimensional stability; also (5) some modification in occlusal relationship is possible after closure, if made before the material sets, and (6) distortion is unlikely during mounting procedures.

The technique for using the adjustable bite frame is as follows:

1. Adjust the bite frame to the mouth so that the patient can close into the desired relation without interference.

2. Trim the gauze bibs to correspond to the size of the arch being recorded.

3. Mix the impression paste and apply it to both sides of the gauze.

4. Carefully insert the frame into the mouth and have the patient close into

centric occlusion (or to the desired position). Lateral and protrusive records may also be recorded if desired, by making separate records for each. Slight changes in jaw position may be effected after closure before the material has set.

5. Upon completion of the set, have the patient open the mouth, and remove the frame from the mouth. The individual records are then removed from the frame before transferring them to the casts for mounting.

Three important details to be observed when using this method are as follows:

1. Make sure that the occlusion is satisfactory before making the interocclusal record.

2. Be sure that the casts are accurate reproductions of the teeth being recorded.

3. Trim the record with a sharp knife whenever it engages undercuts, soft tissues, or deep grooves.

Occlusal Relations Using Occlusion Rims on Jaw Relation Record Bases. A *third method* is used where one or more distal extension areas are present, where a tooth-bounded edentulous space is very large, or where opposing teeth do not meet. In these instances, occlusion rims on accurate jaw relation record bases must be used. It should not be necessary to add that simple wax records of edentulous areas are never acceptable, despite the unfortunate continuation of this practice. Any wax, however soft, will displace soft tissues. It is totally impossible to seat such a wax record on a stone cast of the arch with any degree of accuracy. Commercial dental laboratories would do prosthetic dentistry a great service if they would refuse to accept wax records of edentulous spaces.

In this method, the recording proceeds much the same as in the second method, except that occlusion rims are substituted for remaining teeth. It is essential that accurate bases be used to help support the occlusal relationship. Shellac bases may be adapted to the casts and then corrected with some kind of impression paste. This is best done by first burnishing tin foil onto the lubricated cast, mixing a suitable zinc oxide and eugenol impression paste and applying it to the shellac base, and then seating the shellac base onto the cast until the paste has set. The tin foil adheres to the impression paste, giving a tin-foil-lined correction of the original base. Such a corrected base is entirely acceptable for jaw relation records. Shellac bases may also be lined with some self-curing resin to accomplish the same purpose. In either case, undercuts on the cast must first be blocked out, and tin foil or, where resin is used, a tin-foil substitute, must be used.

Record bases may also be made entirely of self-curing resin. Those materials used in dough form lack sufficient accuracy for this purpose unless they are corrected by relining. A resin base may be formed by sprinkling monomer and polymer into a shallow matrix of wax or clay, after blocking out any undercuts. If the matrix and blockout have been formed with care, interference to removal will not occur, and little trimming will be necessary. When the sprinkling method is used and sufficient time is allowed for progressive polymerization to occur, such bases are the most stable and accurate obtainable short of using cast metal, vulcanite, or pressure-molded resin bases for jaw relation records.

Occlusal rest lugs may be formed of stiff wire and located where they will not interfere with the occlusion. These are first attached to the occlusal surfaces with sticky wax, with a retention loop or hook extending into the area to be filled by the sprinkled acrylic resin. The rest lug is thus attached to the record base in much the same manner as a wrought-wire clasp is attached to a temporary appliance or an orthodontic retainer.

Jaw relation records made by this method accomplish essentially the same purpose as the two previous methods, which is to record centric occlusion of the remaining natural teeth. The fact that record bases are used to support edentulous areas does not alter the effect. Articulatory movements will still be governed by the cuspal guidance of the remaining teeth, and occlusion will still have to be perfected in the mouth. Therefore, in any of these three methods, the skill and care used by the dentist in making intraoral adjustments on the finished prosthesis will govern the accuracy of the resulting occlusion.

Methods for Recording Centric Occlusion on Record Bases. There are many ways by which centric occlusion may be recorded where record bases are used. The least accurate is the use of softened wax occlusion rims. Modeling plastic occlusion rims, on the other hand, may be uniformly softened by flaming and tempering, resulting in a generally acceptable occlusal record. This method is time proved, and when competently done it is equal in accuracy to any other method.

Where wax occlusion rims are used they should be reduced in height until just out of occlusal contact. A single stop is then added to maintain its terminal position while a jaw relation record is made in some uniformly soft material which sets to a hard state. Quick-setting plaster of Paris, impression paste, or self-curing resin may be used. With any of these materials, opposing teeth must be lubricated to facilitate easy separation. Whatever the recording medium, it must permit normal closure into centric occlusion without resistance and must be transferable with accuracy to the casts for mounting purposes.

Relative to the third method, some mention must be made of the ridge upon which the record bases are formed. If the prosthesis is to be tooth supported or a free-end base is to be made upon the anatomic ridge form, the bases will be made to fit that form of the residual ridge. But, if a free-end base is to be supported by the functional form of the residual ridge, it is necessary that the recording of jaw relations be deferred until the master cast has been corrected to that functional form. Record bases must be as identical as possible to those of the finished prosthesis. Jaw relation record bases are useless unless they are made upon the same cast to which the denture will be processed, or a duplicate thereof, or are themselves the final denture bases. The latter may be either of cast alloy or a processed resin base. Therefore, for free-end dentures that are to be made to conform to the functional form of the edentulous ridge, the making of final jaw relation records must be deferred until the functional impression has been made, the functional ridge form has been reproduced on the stone cast, and accurate record bases have been made to fit that functional form.

Jaw Relation Records Made Entirely on Occlusion Rims. The *fourth method* is used when no occlusal contact exists between the remaining natural teeth, such as when an opposing maxillary complete denture is to be made concurrently with a lower partial denture. It may also be used in those rare cases where the few remaining teeth do not occlude and will not influence eccentric jaw movements.

In either case, jaw relation records are made entirely upon occlusion rims. The occlusion rims must be built upon accurate jaw relation record bases. Although baseplate wax rims may be used, modeling plastic is preferable because it may be uniformly softened to the desired depth by flaming and is dimensionally stable when chilled.

Here the choice of method for recording jaw relations is much the same as that for complete dentures. Either some direct checkbite method or a stylus tracing may be used. As with complete denture construction, the use of a facebow, the choice of articulator used, the choice of method for recording jaw relations, and the use of eccentric positional records are optional according to the training, ability, and desires of the individual dentist.

The same principles of occlusion apply to such a partial denture as to a complete denture. If the dentist believes that he can adjust occlusion adequately in the mouth, a simple hinge mounting is all that is needed. On the other hand, if he believes in the use of a fully adjustable instrument with the casts mounted to the hinge axis, then he should do so with a partial denture. In between these two extremes we find the majority of dentists who are trained in prosthodontics using a simple face-bow mounting on a semiadjustable articulator (Hanau, Dentatus, etc.) and recording jaw relations by means of either a static record or a stylus tracing.

Establishing Occlusion by the Recording of Occlusal Pathways. The *fifth method* of establishing occlusion on the partial denture is the registration of occlusal pathways and the use of an occluding template rather than a cast of the opposing arch. When a static jaw relation record is used, with or without eccentric articulatory movements, the denture teeth are set to occlude according to a specific concept of occlusion. On the other hand, when a functional occlusal record is used, the teeth are modified to accept every possible eccentric jaw movement.

These movements are made more complicated by the influence of the remaining natural teeth. Occlusal harmony on complete dentures and in complete mouth rehabilitation may be obtained by the use of modern instruments and techniques. Schuyler has emphasized the importance of establishing first the anterior tooth relation and incisal guidance before proceeding with any complete oral rehabilitation. Others have shown the advantages of establishing canine guidance as a key to functional occlusion before proceeding with any functional bite registration against an opposing prosthetically restored arch. This is done on the theory that the canine teeth serve to guide the mandible during eccentric movements when the opposing teeth come into functional contact. It has also been pointed out that the canine teeth transmit periodontal proprioceptor impulses to the muscles of mastication and thus have an influence on mandibular movement even without actual contact guidance. But as long as the occlusal surfaces of unrestored natural teeth remain in contact, as in many a partially dentulous mouth, these will always be the primary influence on mandibular movement, and the degree of occlusal harmony obtainable on a fixed or removable restoration will depend upon the occlusal harmony existing between those teeth.

Regarding occlusion, Thompson has said:

> Observing the occlusion with the teeth in static relations and then moving the mandible into various eccentric positions is not sufficient. A dynamic concept is necessary in order to produce an occlusion that is in functional harmony with the facial skeleton, the musculature, and the temporomandibular joints.*

To this needs only be added "and with the remaining natural teeth," and we have defined the requirements for partial denture occlusion.

In the registration of occlusal pathways, an occlusion rim of a suitable hard wax, such as Peck's purple hard inlay wax, is attached to an accurate jaw relation record base. This base must be securely attached to the partial denture framework. It may be the final denture base of processed resin or metal. The occlusion rim is worn by the patient for a period of time, preferably for twenty-four hours or more and preferably during sleep. It is removed by the patient only while eating.

While some of the methods described previously may be applied to the construction of partial dentures in both arches simultaneously, this method requires that an opposing arch be intact or restored to the extent of planned treatment. Should partial dentures be planned for both arches, a choice must be made as to which denture is to be made first and which is to bear a functional occlusal relation to the opposing arch. Generally, the maxillary arch is restored first and the mandibular partial denture occluded to that restored arch. Similarly, if the maxillary arch is to be restored with a complete denture or fixed bridgework and/or crowns, this is done before establishing the occlusion on the opposing partial denture.

Regardless of the method used for recording jaw relations, when one arch is completely restored first, that arch is treated as an intact arch even though it is wholly or partially restored by prosthetic means. It is well to consider at the time of treatment planning the possible advantages of establishing the final occlusion to an intact arch.

By wearing and biting into a wax occlusion rim, a record is made of all extremes of jaw movement. The wax occlusion rim must maintain positive contact with the opposing dentition in all excursions and must be left high enough to assure that a record of the functional path of each cusp will be carved in wax. This record should include not only voluntary excursive movements but also involuntary movements and changes in jaw movement caused by changes in posture. Extreme jaw positions and habitual movements during sleep should also be recorded.

The occlusal paths, thus recorded, will represent each tooth in its three-dimen-

---

*From Thompson, J. R.: In Sarnat, B. S. (editor): Temporomandibular Disorders: Diagnosis and Dental Treatment in the Temporomandibular Joint, Springfield, Ill., 1951, Charles C Thomas, Publisher.

sional aspect. Although the cast poured against this will resemble the opposing teeth, it will be wider than the teeth which carved it because it represents those teeth in all extremes of movement. The recording of occlusal paths in this manner eliminates entirely the need for attempting to reproduce mandibular movement on an instrument.

Occlusion thus established on the partial denture will have more complete harmony with the opposing natural or artificial teeth than can be obtained by adjustments in the mouth alone, because occlusal adjustment to accommodate voluntary movement does not necessarily prevent occlusal disharmony in all postural positions or during periods of stress. Furthermore, occlusal adjustment in the mouth without occlusal analysis is limited by the dentist's ability to interpret correctly occlusal markings made intraorally, whether by articulation ribbon or by other means.

The registration of occlusal pathways has still further advantages. It makes possible the obtaining of jaw relations under actual working conditions, with the denture framework in its terminal position, the opposing teeth in function, and an opposing denture, if present, fully seated. In some instances, it also makes possible the recovery of lost vertical dimension, either unilaterally or bilaterally, where overclosure or mandibular rotation has occurred, instead of perpetuating an abnormal mandibular relationship.

Step-by-Step Procedure for Registering Occlusal Pathways. The technique for the registration of occlusal pathways is as follows:

1. Support the wax occlusion rim by a denture base having the same degree of accuracy and stability as the finished denture base. Ideally, this would be the final denture base, which is one of the advantages of making the denture with a metal base. Otherwise, make a temporary base of sprinkled self-curing acrylic resin which is essentially identical to the final resin base. In any free-end partial

Fig. 190. A, Following the correction of the edentulous area to functional form, the framework is reseated accurately on the corrected master cast, any undercuts are blocked out with clay, and a tin-foil substitute is applied to the surface of the cast. **B,** A new resin base is made with self-curing acrylic resin by sprinkling to form a record base that is as nearly as possible identical to the form of the finished denture base. After curing, the framework is lifted and any flash or excess is trimmed away. This base is then used to establish occlusal relations by whatever method is indicated, depending upon the opposing dentition and the operator's preference.

denture make this base on a cast that has been corrected to the functional, or supporting, form of the edentulous ridge (Fig. 190, *A* and *B*.)

Place a film of sticky wax upon the base before the wax occlusion rim is secured to it. The wax used for the occlusion rim should be hard enough to support biting stress and should be tough enough to resist fracture. Peck's purple hard inlay wax has proved to be suitable for the majority of cases. However, some individuals with weak musculature or tender mouths may have difficulty in reducing this wax. In such cases, use a slightly less hard wax. Make the occlusion rim wide enough to record all extremes of mandibular movement.

2. Have the patient wear the occlusion rim for a period of twenty-four hours or longer. It should be worn constantly, including nighttime, except for removal during meals. Instruct the patient in the removal and insertion of the partial denture supporting the occlusion rim and advise him that by chewing and gliding, the wax will be carved by the opposing teeth. Therefore, the opposing teeth must be cleaned occasionally of accumulated wax particles. It is necessary that the patient comprehend what is being accomplished and that he understand that both voluntary and involuntary movements must be recorded.

Before dismissing the patient, add or remove wax where indicated, to provide continuous contact throughout the chewing range. To accomplish this, repeatedly warm the wax with a hot spatula and have the patient carve the warmed wax rim with the opposing dentition, each time adding to any areas that are deficient. Support with additional wax any wax left unsupported by its flow under occlusal forces. It is important that the wax rim be absolutely dry and free of saliva moisture before additional wax is applied. Each addition of wax must be made homogenous with the larger mass to avoid separation or fracture of the occlusion rim during the time it is being worn. Leave the wax occlusion rim from 1 to 3 mm. high, depending on whether or not vertical dimension is to be increased.

3. After twenty-four hours, the occlusal surface of the wax rim should show

Fig. 191. Two examples of a completed occlusal registration in a hard inlay wax supported by accurate record bases. Note that the width of each cusp in all extremes of mandibular movement is recorded as a continuous glossy surface. Yet the anatomy of each opposing tooth is well defined. The completed registration must be placed back onto the master cast without intervening debris or discrepancy and secured there with sticky wax so that the accuracy of the occlusal registration will be maintained.

Fig. 192. Four views of an occlusal registration for a lower Class II partial denture. **A,** The occlusal registration in wax returned to the master cast. Note the extreme horizontal movement recorded. **B,** The same cast boxed with clay, leaving multiple occlusal surfaces exposed as vertical stops. **C,** The effect of the occlusal stops, eliminating any possible changes in vertical dimension on the articulator. **D,** The processed denture remounted for occlusal readjustment. Note the modification in the occlusal anatomy of the stock denture teeth and the slight increase in the height of the occlusal plane. This is in harmony with natural tooth contact elsewhere in the arch.

a continuous gloss, indicating functional contact with the opposing teeth in all extremes of movement (Fig. 191). Any areas deficient in contact should be added to at this time. The reasons for maintaining positive occlusal contact throughout the time the occlusion rim is being worn are (a) all of the opposing teeth may be placed in function; (b) an opposing denture, if present, will become fully seated; and (c) vertical dimension in the molar region will be increased, thus repositioning the head of the mandibular condyle and allowing temporomandibular tissues to return to a normal relationship.

On the other hand, if during this period the wax occlusion rim has not been reduced to natural tooth contact, warm it by directing air from the air syringe through a flame onto the surface of the wax. By holding the wax rim with the fingers while warming, a gradual softening process will result, rather than a melting of the surfaces already established. Repeatedly warm the occlusion rim and reinsert in the mouth until the occlusal height has been reduced and lateral excursions have been recorded. At this time, support with additional

Fig. 193. Five views of an occlusal registration for an upper Class II partial denture. **A,** A partial view of the occlusal registration returned to the master cast. Again, note the extreme horizontal movement recorded. **B,** The same cast boxed with clay, leaving multiple occlusal surfaces exposed as vertical stops. **C,** The occlusal view of the occluding template. **D,** The processed denture remounted for occlusal readjustment. Note the modification of the teeth, even to the point of disregarding interdigitation, to effect good occlusion with the template. The anterior teeth must be tried in the mouth and positioned for esthetics before setting the posterior teeth. **E,** The occlusal stops in full contact after processing and occlusal readjustment following remounting.

wax those areas left unsupported by the flow of the wax to the buccal or lingual surfaces. At the same time, trim the areas obviously not involved, thus narrowing the occlusion rim as much as possible. Remove also those areas projecting above the occlusal surface which, by their presence, might limit functional movement.

Having accomplished seating of the denture and changes in mandibular position by the previous period of wear, it is possible to complete the occlusal registration at the chair. However, if all involuntary movements and those caused by changes in posture are to be recorded, the patient should again wear the occlusion rim for a period of time.

4. After a second twenty-four to forty-eight hour period of wear, the registration should be complete and acceptable. The remaining teeth serving as vertical stops should be in contact and the occlusion rim should show an intact glossy surface representing each cusp in all extremes of movement.

Not all natural teeth formerly in contact will necessarily be in contact upon completion of the occlusal registration. Those teeth that have been depressed over a period of years and those that have been moved to accommodate over-closure or mandibular rotation may not be in contact when mandibular equilibrum has been re-established. Such teeth may possibly return to occlusal contact in the future or may have to be restored to occlusal contact after delivery of the denture. Since the mandibular position may have been changed during the process of occlusal registration, the cuspal relation of some of the natural teeth

Fig. 194. The completed occlusal registration boxed with clay prior to pouring the template in a hard die stone. The occlusal surfaces of adjacent abutment teeth are left exposed to serve as stone-to-stone vertical stops. The clay is trimmed just to the margins of the registration and raised in the center to provide an arch for lingual access while setting teeth to occlude with the template.

Fig. 195. Rather than use clay sufficient to arch across from one side to another, the same may be done with wax with less time and material. It is better that the clay form a more acute angle with the occlusal wax registration and exposed occlusal surfaces than illustrated here.

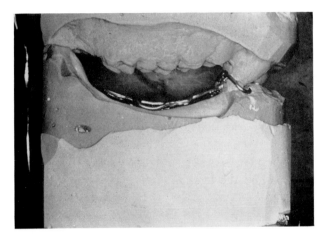

Fig. 196. A profile view of an occlusal template and one of its vertical stops. Despite the fact that this is a record of all extremes of mandibular movement for this patient, the anatomy of the occluding teeth can easily be identified.

may be different than before. This fact must be recognized in determining the correct restored vertical dimension.

The completed registration is now ready for conversion to an occluding template. This is usually done by boxing the occlusal registration with modeling clay after it has been reseated and secured onto the master or processing cast (Fig. 194). Only the wax registration and areas for vertical stops are left exposed. It is then filled with a hard stone to form an occluding template. (See Chapter 17, Laboratory Procedures.)

It is necessary that stone stops be used to maintain the vertical relation rather than relying on some adjustable part of the articulating instrument which might be changed accidentally. Also, by using stone stops and by mounting

Fig. 197. A completed upper partial denture with teeth set and modified to occlude with a template made from a wax occlusal registration. The Hagman Junior Balancer is used as a hinge alone, with all adjustable elements securely locked before mounting the cast and template. Stone stops are used to preserve the vertical relation. Note the notch in the upper cast for keying the cast to the articulator to facilitate accurate remounting following processing.

both the denture cast and the template before separating them, a simple hinge instrument may be used.

Because of its simplicity and the accessibility it affords in setting teeth, the Hagman Junior Balancer is preferred as an articulating instrument for use with an occluding template (Fig. 197). In this application, the instrument is used as a hinge only, with all other moving elements securely locked in a fixed position. However, any hinged articulator may be similarly used.

Setting Teeth to an Occluding Template. The occlusal surface of the denture teeth, porcelain or resin, must be modified to occlude with the template. In this method, they are actually only raw materials from which an occlusal surface is developed which is in harmony with an existing occlusal pattern. Therefore, the teeth must be occluded too high and then ground to fit the template at the established vertical dimension.

Modern resin teeth are preferred over porcelain teeth because they are more readily modified and more nearly resemble enamel in their action against opposing teeth. Resin teeth are usually used in opposition to enamel and gold occlusal surfaces, whereas porcelain teeth are usually used in opposition to other porcelain teeth.

Some changes in this concept have occurred in recent years. Sears and, later, Myerson have shown the feasibility of using porcelain and resin teeth in opposition and the advantage of reduced frictional resistance by doing so. Myerson has compared the effect of porcelain teeth against resin teeth to that of a diamond stylus against a vinyl phonograph record which results in less wear by friction than the less hard sapphire stylus. For this to be truly comparable, the porcelain tooth should possess a glazed surface, but experience has shown that even a polished vacuum-fired porcelain surface causes relatively little wear and greatly reduced frictional resistance when in opposition to a modern resin denture tooth.

A second fact has also been recognized, which is that resin tooth surfaces may in time become impregnated with abrasive particles, thereby becoming an abrasive substance themselves. This may explain why resin teeth are sometimes capable of wearing away opposing gold surfaces. With these facts in mind, the use of resin teeth need not be avoided for fear they will wear away too rapidly.

While there may still be some controversy in regard to the use of porcelain or resin denture teeth, there is broad agreement that narrow occlusal surfaces are desirable. Posterior teeth should be selected which will satisfy this requirement, and the use of tooth forms having excessive buccolingual dimension should be avoided.

Teeth set to an occluding template should ordinarily be placed in the center of the functional range. Wherever possible, the teeth should be set buccolingually in the center of the template. Where natural teeth have registered the functional occlusion, this may be considered the normal physiologic position of the artificial dentition regardless of its relation to the residual ridge. On the other hand, if some man-made occlusion in the opposing arch has been recorded, such as that of an opposing denture, the teeth should be set in a favorable relation to their

A   B

Fig. 198. A, A view of the interdigitation sometimes possible when teeth are set to an occlusal template. This is possible only where gross migration of the opposing teeth has not occurred. **B,** A view of the modification to occlusal surfaces necessary where interdigitation is not possible without leaving objectionable spaces. Note that the original cusp-to-cusp relation of the denture teeth has been altered until marginal ridges have actually become the interdigitation cusps. Such an occlusal relationship is entirely permissible and effective.

Fig. 199. Occlusal surfaces after remounting and final occlusal readjustment to the template. Note the functional occlusal anatomy resulting. This is an entirely different occlusal surface than was present on the stock denture teeth as manufactured.

foundation, even if this means setting them slightly buccally or lingually from the center of the template.

The teeth are usually set so as to interdigitate with the opposing teeth in a normal cuspal relationship. As is customary, whenever possible the mesiobuccal cusps of the maxillary first molar is set in relation to the buccal groove of the mandibular first molar and all other teeth set accordingly. With functional occlusion, however, it is not absolutely necessary that a normal anteroposterior relation be re-established. (Fig. 198, *A* and *B*.) In the first place, the opposing teeth in a broken dental arch may not be in normal alignment and interdigitation may be difficult to accomplish. In the second place, the occlusal surfaces will be so modified that they will function favorably regardless of their anteroposterior position. Since cusps modified to fit an occlusal template will always be in harmony with the opposing dentition, it is not necessary that the teeth themselves be set to conform to the usual concept of what constitutes a normal anteroposterior relationship.

Making the Occluding Template of Metal. Some indicator must be used to guide the machining of occlusal surfaces to fit the template. Articulating paper has several disadvantages when used for this purpose. One is that it does not conform readily to irregular surfaces and quickly becomes perforated, giving irregular markings. Another is that the waxlike substance with which the paper is impregnated tends to accumulate on the surface of the template, changing the vertical relation somewhat and giving false marks on the teeth. An inked marking tape (silk ribbon, dental tape, or typewritter ribbon) is superior to articulating paper because it will not tear and yet will conform better to irregular surfaces (Fig. 200). In this regard it also permits more accurate marking of proximal surfaces as they are being ground to fit the denture framework. An ink mark may be more reliably interpreted than a crayon mark made with articulating paper.

Fig. 200. When setting teeth to an occluding template, marking tape should be used in positioning and modifying each tooth to fit the template. Note that at this early stage the articulator has been opened approximately 0.5 mm., as evidenced by the slight space at the vertical stop.

Fig. 201. Drawing of a wire holder for marking tape or typewriter ribbon. The wire used is .036 orthodontic wire. The ribbon is held taut at either end after passing over the inner arch (over, under, and then over).

Fig. 202. A stone occlusal template before and after use. **A,** The occlusal surfaces are unmarred by abrasion. **B,** Evidence of abrasion through the articulating marks shows the damage and therefore the inaccuracy resulting from abrasion and crushing forces as the template is tapped against the opposing teeth. If the occlusal surfaces during remounting are readjusted to fit this altered surface, some occlusal inaccuracies are inevitable, which must then be compensated for by intraoral adjustment of the completed denture.

The inked ribbon may be held with forceps, such as the Miller articulating paper forceps, or in a wire frame (Fig. 201). The latter is easily made of orthodontic wire and holds the ribbon taut at all times, whereas the forceps are designed primarily for use with articulating paper.

One of the hazards of setting teeth to a stone template is that the template becomes abraded by continuous closure against the denture teeth as they are being adjusted to occlude with the template. It is inevitable that during the process of alternately marking and grinding occlusal surfaces the stone template is subjected to considerable abuse and wear (Fig. 202, *A* and *B*). This abrasion can be minimized by using the hardest dental stone available for the template and by avoiding forceful contact of the template with the occlusal surfaces of the teeth. It can also be avoided by electroplating the wax occlusal registration, thus forming a relatively indestructible occlusal template. (Figs. 203 to 208.) The technique is as follows:

Low-fusing metal has been preferred to stone as an occluding cast material, but molten metal cannot be poured into a wax mold. Electroplating permits a metallic surface to be formed on the wax record with accuracy and with greater hardness than low-fusing metals. Electroforming with silver has proved to be the simplest and most satisfactory method.

Interest in electroplating has been revised since the advent of the Thiokol and Silicone impression materials. The change from time-honored copper dies to silver dies was made necessary by the introduction of these new impression materials when electroformed dies were preferred to stone dies.

The technique for electroplating the occlusal template is basically identical with electroplating of Thiokol and Silicone impressions. The main differences are that the vessel containing the electrolyte must be larger, the leads must be attached bilaterally in a manner that will allow the denture to be suspended in the solution, and the denture framework must be protected from the electrolytic current.

Ten milliamperes of current per tooth, plus 10 for the leads, is sufficient. Greater amperage would cause the electroplating to be too soft. The total area of the anode immersed in the solution should not be more than twice the area to be plated. The distance from the anode to the surface to be plated should be about 4 inches.

Since the number of teeth involved will vary, the plating machine must have a widely variable output. The machine being used is a self-made device with a variable output of from 35 to 200 Ma., although suitable machines ready for use may be purchased.

The wax occlusal registration is metallized with Staco silver lacquer, and the leads are painted down the lingual side to join with a T-shaped wire lead. This lead is attached to the wax rims with sticky wax. It is very important that all parts of the denture framework be painted with a protective lacquer, such as Kerr's Plate Mask, to prevent the casting itself from being plated.

At 10 Ma. per tooth, the occlusal registration to be plated should be left in the solution approximately 5 hours. A uniform plate of sufficient thickness will result. A heavier plate seems to cause some curling at the edges and pulling away from the wax surface. This leads to inaccuracies and must be avoided. Since the plated surface will be backed up with stone, a thin plate is all that is needed.

The attachment of the stone backing to the silver plate was a problem at first. In some cases, the metal separated from the stone backing due to the absence of mechanical attachment. The problem has been solved by imbedding two or more wire

Fig. 203. Homemade equipment for electroplating the wax occlusal registration. Milliamperage can be varied from 35 to 200 Ma. The electrolyte in the glass container is silver potassium cyanide; the anode is pure silver. Commercial electroplating equipment may be purchased, or the equipment may be assembled as shown by the diagram in Fig. 204. The work is suspended in the solution from an alligator clip superstructure attached to one side of the electric circuit. The anode may be suspended or placed in a refrigerator dish as illustrated. The variable factor of the distance from anode to work may be eliminated by agitating the solution with an aquarium aerator pump, the open end of the plastic tubing being held in the solution by passing it through an egg-shaped fishing sinker.

staples into the wax surface of the occlusal registration before plating. These staples become part of the plated surface and aid in securing the metal to the stone. The small tip end of each staple projecting through the metal template can easily be ground away without marring the surfaces of the template.

The plated surface is boxed with clay, and stone is poured against it in the same manner as an unplated wax record. The articulator mounting and occluding the teeth to the template is the same, except for the advantages of the metal surface over a stone surface.

It is not expected that the silver plating of a wax occlusal record will receive wide acceptance because of the added step of electroplating. But just as there are those who prefer to work with electroformed dies, so there may be some who would prefer to set teeth to a metal template.*

---

*From McCracken, W. L.: Functional Occlusion in Removal Partial Denture Construction. J. Pros. Den. **8**:955-963, 1958.

Fig. 204. Diagram and parts needed for making electroplating device for silver plating Thiokol and silicone impressions and wax occlusal registrations. **S.W.**, Toggle switch; **T**, small filament transformer; **P.L.**, pilot light; **B.R.**, full-wave bridge rectifier; **V.R.**, variable rheostat; **M.A.**, milliammeter; **F.R.**, fixed resistor. Parts required include 6.3-volt filament transformer, milliammeter, 1.5 Å full-wave bridge rectifier, 50-ohm, 4-watt variable rheostat, pilot light, 2 SPST switches, 10-watt, 50-ohm wire-wound resistor, and utility cabinet. (Diagram courtesy Dr. Paul E. Hammons.)

Fig. 205. Leads are attached below the wax occlusal registration with sticky wax, and the denture framework is coated with a protective lacquer (Kerr plate mask). The occlusal registration is then metalized with a silver lacquer, which is carried down the lingual surface to join the wire leads. (From McCracken, W. L.: Functional Occlusion in Removable Partial Denture Construction, J. Pros. Den. 8:955-963, 1958.)

Fig. 206. A wax occlusal registration after electroplating. Note the wire staples added to the wax to provide retention to the stone which will be poured against the silver surface. The leads and the protective lacquer over the metal framework are now removed prior to reseating the occlusal registration onto the master cast.

Fig. 207. After accurately reseating the denture framework onto the master cast and securing it there with sticky wax, a clay matrix is formed, leaving one or more occlusal surfaces on each side exposed to serve as vertical stops. The clay is made to rise from the borders of the registration at a 45-degree angle and is arched across the midline to provide lingual access when setting teeth to the template. The exposed occlusal surfaces are painted with a separator and stone vibrated into the clay matrix to form the remainder of the occluding template.

Fig. 208. **A,** An electroformed silver occluding template with stone stops anteriorly to preserve the vertical dimension. **B,** Another electroformed occluding template involving six opposing teeth (the functional width of each cusp is readily discernible). (**A,** from McCracken, W. L.: Functional Occlusion in Removable Partial Denture Construction, J. Pros. Den. **8:**955-963, 1958.)

Functional Registration of Occlusal Surfaces for Fixed Bridges and Single Crowns. Many of the advantages to be found in the registration of occlusal pathways for removable partial dentures may be applied also to the construction of fixed bridges and individual crowns. A more harmonious occlusion results from establishing a functional relationship than when only a centric occlusal relation is recorded.

Since fixed bridges and individual crowns are often essential to adequate mouth preparations for partial dentures, it is necessary that methods for obtaining occlusal harmony on those restorations be considered in this chapter. It has been stated previously that analysis and adjustment of the natural occlusion is an essential part of mouth preparations. It is equally essential that any occlusal reconstruction be done in harmony with the accepted or corrected natural occlusion. It is doubtful that this is possible without having some record of the existing occlusal pattern.

Functional occlusion for bridges and crowns must be established entirely at the chair, because the patient cannot be given an appliance that they can remove at mealtime. While such a jaw relation record does not possess all of the advantages of an occlusal registration made during a twenty-four-hour period, it does create an occlusion that is in harmony with the majority of jaw movements. Occlusal discrepancies on the finished restoration caused by changes in posture can only be recorded and eliminated by having the patient wear an unpolished gold restoration or one made dull by sandblasting for a period long enough to register any remaining interference. This limitation of a functional registration done at the chair should be recognized and then corrected for on the finished restoration.

Establishing Functional Occlusion on a Single Crown. The method of registering functional occlusion on a single crown was mentioned previously in conjunction with the making of a crown pattern to fit a denture clasp (see Chapter 13, Preparation of Abutment Teeth). In this technique, a thin coping of self-curing resin is made to support the wax pattern. An occlusal pattern is then established directly in the mouth with little danger of fracture or distortion. Any hard inlay wax may be used for this purpose.

Either removable dies or individual dies in conjunction with a solid cast may be used to establish vertical surfaces on the wax pattern which will satisfy requirements for marginal contact, guiding planes, and contours for clasp retention and reciprocation. This may be done prior to establishing occlusal relations, or the occlusal aspect of the pattern may be completed first and the pattern then returned to the cast for the shaping of vertical surfaces.

Where individual dies are used, occlusion is usually established first and then the pattern is placed on a solid cast of the arch for the purpose of contouring the crown in relation to the path of insertion. This is done with the aid of a surveyor. Finally, the pattern is returned to the individual die for the purpose of refining the margins. Where removable dies are used, the contouring of vertical surfaces may be done first, then the occlusal relationship may be established in the mouth, and finally the pattern is returned to the die for the refinement of the margins.

Where several such restorations are to be made for the same arch, it is best that as many wax patterns be made concurrently as possible. On the other hand, it may be necessary to restore only one or two teeth at a time in order to preserve vertical and horizontal relations. This may sometimes be facilitated by making plastic temporary crowns for all prepared teeth in harmony with the existing occlusion, and then using these temporary crowns alternately as guides while establishing a functional occlusion on the wax patterns.

As with an occlusal registration for a partial denture, the completed occlusal registration should have a glossy surface and should make contact with the opposing teeth throughout the functional range. Sufficient chewing time must be allowed for any excess wax to be eliminated, with the teeth elsewhere in the arch again in contact.

The occlusal surface thus established will be broader than a natural tooth. In the registration for a partial denture or a bridge this is converted to a template and an occlusal surface of acceptable width formed to occlude with only a part of the template. The occlusal registration for a crown pattern, on the other hand, is the wax pattern which becomes the finished casting. This occlusal surface is much too wide and has too much occlusal contact to be within the toleration limits of periodontal support. The wax pattern must therefore be narrowed to reduce the width of the occlusal table. Spillways should be added to further reduce the occlusal area and to increase masticating efficiency. This is generally done so as to conform to concepts of normal occlusal anatomy, the objective being to further reduce the area of occlusal contact and to assure maximum efficiency. A crown restoration thus formed will possess maximum efficiency without interference, in harmony with all eccentric movements and with the other teeth in the arch.

Step-by-Step Procedure for Recording Occlusal Pathways for a Fixed Bridge. The objectives in establishing functional occlusion on a fixed bridge are the same as for a single crown. The method, however, is somewhat different.

Occluding template poured against wax registration with stone stops anterior and posterior.

Functional registration and frame removed to reveal occluding template

B

C

Hard inlay wax

Acrylic resin frame

A

Fig. 209. Establishing functional occlusion for a fixed bridge by means of an occlusal registration of the opposing teeth. **A,** The acrylic resin frame with hard inlay wax occlusal surface. **B,** The occluding template poured against the wax registration with stone stops anterior and posterior. **C,** The resulting template to which the occlusal surfaces of the bridge will be formed.

Functional occlusion for a fixed bridge is established by means of an occlusal registration on an acrylic resin or cast metal frame or platform. The technique of occlusal registration is much the same as for partial denture occlusion except that the frame is not removable by the patient, and therefore occlusal registration must be done entirely at the chair. (Fig. 209, *A-C.*)

The technique for establishing functional bridge occlusion is as follows:

1. Although a cast metal frame may be used, one made of acrylic resin is adequate for the purpose. The frame may be made on a cast from a separate alginate hydrocolloid impression of the prepared teeth or from a second pour of a rubber-base impression. The cast containing trimmed dies is not used for the purpose, for fear of marring its surface.

Clay or utility wax is added to block out the gingival one-fourth of the prepared teeth and the adjacent soft tissues and edentulous areas. This is for the purpose of eliminating any interference to the seating of the frame onto the working cast. Any irregularities in the preparations are also blocked out. Then a wax or clay matrix is formed to confine the self-curing acrylic resin within the desired limits.

The cast is painted with tin-foil substitute, which is allowed to dry. Self-curing acrylic resin is then applied, using the sprinkling method, until a resin platform of the desired thickness has been obtained. The occlusal portion is left wide but thin.

After polymerizing at least an hour, but preferably overnight, the frame is lifted from the cast and trimmed of excess. It should be no bulkier than necessary for strength. The only adjustment that should be necessary in the mouth is the reduction of the occlusal plane to provide space for the registration wax.

2. The resin frame must seat accurately on the abutment teeth, and there must be no contact with soft tissues. The occlusal surface should be reduced sufficiently to provide ample clearance for the registration wax. Apply a film of sticky wax to the dried frame and then add a hard inlay wax to the occlusal surface.*

While the wax is still soft, place the resin frame in the mouth and ask the patient to make centric contact and excursive movements. Add wax where deficient and support the width buccally and lingually with additional wax. Reduce excess width as well as excess height at the limits of excursive movements. Do not add to glossy areas, but only those areas where contact is deficient. This registration differs from the partial denture registration, where the occlusion rim is left 1 to 3 mm. high for the patient to reduce during a twenty-four-hour period. The bridge registration is done entirely at the chair and can only record voluntary movements at the vertical level determined by the other teeth in the arch. As mentioned repeatedly in preceding paragraphs, this should be an occlusion that is acceptable or made so by previous occlusal adjustments and/or reconstruction.

The completed registration should make contact with the opposing teeth throughout the functional range, with the remaining teeth in contact in centric and eccentric positions. The registration should have an intact glossy surface and will be much wider than the occlusion on the finished restoration.

3. The completed occlusal registration is treated much the same as a registration for a partial denture. A hard die stone is poured against it, or it may be metallized and electroplated. In either case, seat it accurately on the working cast and secure it there with sticky wax.

Form a clay matrix at a 45-degree angle from the margins of the registration, leaving the cast exposed anterior and posterior to provide vertical stops. Pour stone directly against the wax registration or the electroplated surface. After this has set, mount the cast and opposing template on some kind of bridge articulator before the two are separated. The resulting mounting will not be dependent upon the articulator for maintaining the vertical relation because stone-to-stone stops will have been provided for this purpose.

---

*For an occlusal registration done entirely at the chair, any inlay wax may be used rather than the harder Peck's purple inlay wax that is used for recording occlusal pathways on a partial denture.

In recent years interest in the functionally generated path has led to the development of special waxes for this purpose, such as the Jelenko "Hi-Fi" wax. These waxes are suitable only for direct registration at the chair and cannot be worn by the patient away from the operatory; but then neither can a bite registration frame be worn outside the dental office because it must be removed by the patient during mealtime, which would leave prepared abutment teeth exposed. When this softer type of wax is used at the chair, it is best supported peripherally by a harder inlay wax to prevent distortion at the limits of excursion.

A   B

Fig. 210. Articulated casts providing both anatomic and functional registrations of the opposing teeth on the same articulator. **A,** A conventional mounting to an occluding cast obtained on a wax interocclusal record. The correct vertical relationship is maintained by natural tooth contact anteriorly; otherwise a stone stop should be provided rather than depend on the vertical stop of the articulator alone. **B, A**n occluding stone template formed from a functional occlusal registration is interposed between the two casts for the purpose of establishing functional occlusal surfaces on the restorations. This removable template overlays the opposing anatomic cast and is extended anteriorly and posteriorly to provide vertical stops when the template is in use.

Patterns are waxed to occlude with the opposing template. Generally, occlusal relations with the opposing teeth will not be jeopardized from an esthetic standpoint by carving restorations to a template alone. However, where interdigitation or the correct horizontal overlap might be difficult to ascertain when a template alone is used, another procedure may be followed. In this procedure, a conventional mounting to an occluding cast is made first, using an occluding stone cast which has been poured directly into a wax or some other centric "bite." (Fig. 210, *A.*) This provides an anatomic opposing cast for the purpose of establishing interdigitation and the desired amount of horizontal overlap. This is frequently desirable from an esthetic standpoint and to avoid a cusp-to-cusp occlusion on the completed restoration.

An occlusal registration made on an acrylic frame is then positioned on the working cast as described previously and a clay matrix formed around it, leaving stone exposed at either end for a vertical stop. The opposing anatomic cast is then lubricated or treated with some separating medium such as a solution of sodium silicate, the occlusal registration filled with stone, and the anatomic cast seated into the stone (Fig. 210, *B*). Sufficient thickness of stone must remain for strength.

After the occlusal template has set, it may be separated and trimmed. Two articulator mountings are thus obtained; one is an anatomic opposing cast, and the other is a removable stone template complete with vertical stops to which a functional occlusion may be perfected that will be free of eccentric interference. The same degree of occlusal harmony is possible by this method as with the functional occlusal record alone, with the added advantage of assuring an acceptable esthetic relationship with the opposing teeth. Occlusal surfaces may be made as narrow as desired, and occlusal anatomy should be added for masticating efficiency. Finished castings and the assembled bridge should then be

Fig. 211. The Hanau twin-stage occluder. An anatomic occluding cast is attached to one upper arm and an occlusal template to the other. Better esthetic results are made possible by occluding the wax patterns to both a functional and an anatomic cast. (Courtesy Hanau Engineering Co., Buffalo, N. Y.)

reoccluded to the template to eliminate discrepancies caused by spruing and soldering.

Fig. 211 illustrates an articulator made by the Hanau Company, called the twin-stage occluder, which further facilitates the use of both a functional and an anatomic cast when occluding wax patterns to a functional bite record. Fig. 212 shows an improved version of the Verticulator made by the Jelenko Company for use with either full arch or sectional casts, which also permits the use of dual opposing surfaces. Two upper arms are provided, both machined to fit a single lower arm. An anatomic bite record may be attached to one arm and a functional bite record to the other and the two can be interchanged at will.

One disadvantage of using a simple crown and bridge articulator as illustrated in Fig. 210 is the small arc of closure dictated by the proximity of the hinge to the occlusal surface. An occluding template is most effectively used when vertical or nearly vertical closure is possible. When an instrument such as the Hagman Balancer is used, the arc of closure is sufficiently great that it may be considered nearly vertical at the plane of occlusion. Otherwise it is best that an instrument such as the Jelenko Verticulator (Fig. 212), which permits only vertical closure, be used in conjunction with an occluding template. The Verticulator has a further advantage of providing a spring-loaded metal-to-metal stop which positively prevents possible abrasion of the occluding surfaces and loss of the established vertical dimension.

A bridge restoration made with functional occlusal surfaces should have a

Fig. 212. Two models of the Jelenko Verticulator. Designed for use with the Pankey-Mann technique, they are suitable for use with either an anatomic occluding cast or a functionally generated path. However, since only vertical movement is permitted, with positive metal-to-metal vertical limitation, the instrument is best suited for use with the functionally generated path. The dual model permits an interchange between a functional cast and an anatomic cast by substituting two matched and identical upper members. (Courtesy J. F. Jelenko & Co., New York, N. Y.)

harmonious occlusion in centric and in all voluntary eccentric positions. As with a single crown, any remaining eccentric interference must be eliminated in the mouth. Since these are not caused by voluntary movements, it is best that the patient wear the restorations with dull occlusal surfaces (preferably sandblasted surfaces) for a period of twenty-four hours or more. Any remaining interference may then be identified by shiny areas in eccentric position, and these may be eliminated before final polishing. Indeed, it may at times be esthetically desirable to leave occlusal surfaces unpolished, with only a satin finish created by sandblasting.

Establishing Jaw Relations for a Mandibular Partial Denture Opposing a Maxillary Complete Denture. It is not uncommon for a mandibular partial denture to be made to occlude with an opposing maxillary complete denture. The maxillary denture may already be present or it may be made concurrently with the opposing partial denture. In any case, the establishment of jaw relations in this situation may be accomplished by one of several methods previously outlined.

If an existing maxillary complete denture is satisfactory and is not to be replaced, that arch is treated as an intact arch as though natural teeth were present. A face-bow transfer is made of that arch and the cast mounted on the articulator in the usual manner. Maxillomandibular relations may be recorded on accurate record bases attached to the mandibular partial denture framework, using one of the recording mediums previously outlined, such as wax, modeling plastic, quick-setting plaster, impression paste, or quick-curing acrylic resin. Centric relation is thus recorded and transferred to the articulator. A protrusive record is rarely used, and the articulator is set to coincide with the existing tooth relationship.

In rare instances, where the mandibular partial denture replaces all of the posterior teeth and the anterior teeth are noninterfering, a central bearing point tracer may be mounted in the palate of the maxillary denture and centric relation recorded by means of an intraoral stylus tracing against a stable mandibular base.

If the relationship of the posterior teeth on the maxillary denture to the mandibular ridge is favorable and the complete denture is stable, jaw relations may be established by recording occlusal pathways in the mandibular arch the same as for any opposing intact arch. This method is the most satisfactory of all, because the opposing complete denture becomes fully seated during the establishment of functional pathways, the mandible may become repositioned to correct for bilateral or unilateral overclosure, the heads of the mandibular condyles may be repositioned, and occlusal harmony in eccentric positions is assured. The success of this method depends upon the stability of the denture bases, the quality of tissue support, the relation of the opposing teeth to the mandibular ridge, and the interrelation of existing artificial and natural teeth.

More times than not, the existing maxillary complete denture will have been made to occlude with malpositioned mandibular teeth, which have since been lost, or the teeth will have been set without consideration for the future occlusal relation with a mandibular partial denture. Too frequently one sees a maxillary denture with posterior teeth set close to the residual ridge without regard for interarch relationship and with an occlusal plane that is too low. In such case, the least that can be done is to reposition the posterior teeth on the maxillary denture before establishing maxillomandibular relations. This can only be justified where the maxillary denture is otherwise satisfactory as to fit, appearance, and occlusion elsewhere in the arch. Usually, however, a new maxillary denture must be made concurrently with the mandibular partial denture. In such case, jaw relations may be established in one of two ways.

If the mandibular partial denture will be tooth supported (a Kennedy Class III arch accommodating a bilateral removable bridge prosthesis), that arch is restored first. The same applies to a mandibular arch being restored with fixed bridges. In either case, the mandibular arch is completely restored first and jaw relations are established as though to a full complement of opposing teeth. Thus the maxillary complete denture is made to occlude with an intact arch, and the procedure for doing so need not be included here.

On the other hand, as is more frequently the case, the mandibular partial denture may have one or more free-end bases. The situation then requires that either the occlusion be established on both dentures simultaneously or the maxillary denture be completed first.

Following the making of final impressions, which includes the correction of the mandibular cast to establish optimal support for the free ends of the partial denture (the denture framework must be made previously if a wax correction method is used), the maxillary bite rim is contoured, vertical relation against the remaining lower teeth is established, and a face-bow transfer of the maxillary arch is made. Maxillomandibular relations may then be recorded by any one of the several methods previously outlined and the articulator mounting completed. Occlusion may be established as for complete dentures, taking care to establish a favorable tooth-to-ridge relationship in both arches, an optimal occlusal plane, and cuspal harmony between all occluding teeth.

After try-in, either of two methods may be used. Both dentures may be processed concurrently and remounted for occlusal correction, or the maxillary denture may be processed first and, after remounting, the teeth, still in wax on the partial denture, adjusted to any discrepancies occuring. The latter method is preferable, as it is any time that two opposing dentures are being made on the same articulator mounting.

While the above procedure is commonly used for an opposing complete and partial denture combination, the advantages of establishing a functional occlusion are as great in this situation as when a single partial denture or two opposing partial dentures are being made—perhaps even more so, since the stability of a complete denture and the health of the supporting tissues depend to a large extent upon the occlusal harmony present. A maxillary complete denture may be completed first, and, if the posterior teeth are favorably positioned, the occlusion on the opposing partial denture may be established by recording occlusal pathways the same as to any opposing intact arch.

Up to the point of establishing the final occlusion on the partial denture, jaw relations, articulator mounting, and try-in are accomplished as though both dentures were to be completed at the same time. The teeth on the mandibular partial denture are set in wax so that a favorable ridge relationship and occlusal plane will have been established. The maxillary denture alone is then remounted to adjust the occlusion to the remaining natural teeth and is inserted in the mouth as a completed restoration.

The teeth in wax are removed from the partial denture base and replaced with hard inlay wax occlusion rims secured to acrylic resin bases which are attached to the denture framework. A functional occlusal record by registering occlusal pathways is then accomplished, treating the opposing complete denture as an intact arch. The occlusal registration thus obtained is placed back on the master cast, boxed with clay, and an occluding template formed complete with stone-to-stone vertical stops. The same articulator may be used, replacing the original upper cast with the template, or the mandibular cast and the template may be mounted on a simple hinge-type articulator.

It is necessary that the acrylic resin record base be removed by softening it over a flame before the teeth are reset to occlude with the template. The teeth that were formerly set to occlude with the maxillary denture are then modified to fit the template, and the denture bases are waxed and processed. Investing must be done in such a manner that the cast may be recovered intact and remounted for occlusal refinement to the template.

Occlusion thus established on a mandibular partial denture opposing a maxillary complete denture provides occlusal harmony and efficiency superior to that obtained by the more commonly used methods. Not only does greater stability of both dentures result, but trauma conducive to tissue changes beneath both dentures is held to a minimum. The harmony of occlusion thus established more than justifies the added steps necessary to accomplish such results.

Chapter 17

Laboratory procedures

This chapter will cover only those phases of dental laboratory procedure that are directly related to partial denture construction. Familiarity with laboratory procedures relative to the making of fixed restorations and complete dentures is presumed. Such information is already available in the numerous excellent textbooks on those subjects and will not be duplicated here. For example, the principles and techniques involved in the waxing, casting, and finishing of single inlays, crowns, and fixed bridges are adequately covered in lecture material and textbooks and in manuals available to the dental student, the dental laboratory technician, and the practicing dentist. Similarly, knowledge of the principles and techniques for mounting casts, articulating teeth, and waxing, processing, and polishing complete dentures is presumed as a necessary background for the laboratory phases of partial denture construction. Therefore, this chapter will be directed specifically toward the laboratory procedures involved in the making of a partial denture.

Following is a list of the subjects that will be considered in this chapter. It will be noted that some have been covered previously. These will not be repeated in this chapter but may be found as noted.

The making of a cast from an elastic impression (see Chapter 14, Impression Materials
   and Procedures for Partial Dentures)
Duplicating a stone cast
Waxing the partial denture framework on an investment cast
Adapting wrought-wire retentive clasp arms
Anatomic replica plastic patterns (Tru-Rugae technique)
Spruing, investing, casting, and finishing the partial denture framework
The making of impression trays and bases
Correcting the master cast to the functional form of the ridge (see Chapter 15, Support
   for the Free-End Denture Base)
Occlusion rims
Making an occlusal template from a functional occlusal registration

DUPLICATING A STONE CAST

The duplication of a stone cast may be for one or two purposes. One is the duplication in stone of the original or corrected master cast for the purpose of preserving the original. Upon this duplicate cast the denture framework may be fitted without danger of abrading or fracturing the surface of the original master cast. Most of the better commercial dental laboratories have adopted a policy of doing all of the work on a duplicate cast, including the fitting procedures. The finished casting is then returned to the dentist on the master cast after all fitting has been completed on the duplicate cast.

The student or the dentist doing his own laboratory work should likewise follow the policy of making a duplicate cast for the purpose of fitting the denture framework. While some dental laboratories may also use the duplicate cast for surveying and blockout, it is preferable to do the blockout on the master cast just prior to a second duplication rather than to use the duplicate cast for this purpose.

Following blockout of the master cast, a second duplication is done for the purpose of making an investment cast. Upon this investment cast the wax and/or plastic pattern is formed, and the metal framework is ultimately cast against its surface.

While both the fitting cast and the investment cast must be an accurate reproduction of the original, the fitting cast is made of a hard stone and is not directly involved in the making of the metal framework. The investment cast, on the other hand, must possess the properties of a casting investment, such as the ability to withstand burnout temperatures while providing the necessary mold expansion. Gold alloys and also Ticonium are cast to plaster-bound silica investments, whereas the higher melting stellite alloys are cast to investments containing quartz held together by a suitable binder so that they will withstand the higher casting temperatures necessary with these alloys. Although the latter are generally harder than gypsum investments, any investment cast may be easily abraded and must be handled carefully to preserve the accuracy of its surface. The practice of treating the dried investment cast by dipping it in melted rosin and beeswax reduces considerably the danger of its becoming abraded during subsequent handling.

The use of pre-formed plastic patterns eliminates some of the danger of altering the surface of the investment cast in the process of forming the pattern. With free-hand waxing, considerable care must be taken not to score or abrade the investment cast. The student, however, needs the experience of free-hand waxing to give him a better comprehension of the bulk and contours necessary to produce an acceptable denture framework. A continuation of this practice is recommended. For the same reasons, it is also recommended that the laboratory technician be experienced in the use of wax shapes and free-hand waxing before he is allowed to use pre-formed patterns.

Dulicating Materials and Flasks. Duplicating materials are colloidal materials which are made fluid by heating and return to a gel upon being cooled.

The cast to be duplicated must be placed in the bottom of a suitable flask called a duplicating flask. This flask is necessary to contain the fluid material, to facilitate cooling, to facilitate removal of the cast from the mold without permanent deformation or damage to the mold, and to support the mold while it is being filled with the cast material. There are numerous duplicating flasks on the market. (Fig. 213.) One type is a metal bell with holes in the top for pouring. Another is a simple metal ring with removable bottom and top, the latter having a center hole for pouring. Still another has the top and bottom secured with thumb screws.

More recently a new style of duplicating flask has been designed by Dr. N. G. Wills. To Dr. Wills is due much credit for his untiring efforts in furthering the development of accurate cast duplication equipment. Two of these duplicating flasks are illustrated in Fig. 213. They consist of a machined metal top and bottom fitting onto a formica ring 2 or 2¼ inches high. Formica instead of metal is used for the ring because formica acts as an insulator to prevent too rapid cooling through the sides of the flask. The center hole in the top of each type is provided with a filling reservoir, or "feeder ring." While not all duplicating flasks provide for a filling reservoir, it is most desirable that a ring superstruc-

Fig. 213. Five types of duplicating flasks. Upper left, the Wills flask, type E; upper right, the Wills flask type F. Both of these flasks have a formica ring, 4 inches inside diameter and 2 inches wide, but may be ordered wider, if desired, for additional height. The formica is used for its non-heat-conducting property and is machined with a 5-inch inside taper. In the center is a bell-shaped flask; lower left, the Kerr duplicating flask; lower right, a light-weight brass flask in common usage.

ture be provided to serve as a reservoir for feeding the warm material into the mold. Thus as cooling and subsequent shrinkage occur, additional fluid material is fed into the mold from the reservoir above. This is similar to the cooling of dental gold after casting. Gold requires an additional bulk of metal so that upon cooling the piece being cast can draw upon additional metal from the reservoir which we call the "button." Without the additional bulk of metal the casting would likely show porosity. In duplication, cooling from the bottom of the flask causes the duplicating material to shrink, which has a tendency to draw the chilling solution into closer adaptation to the cast.

The metal bottom of one of the types is provided with legs to hold it off the bottom of the cooling tank, thus allowing circulation of water beneath. While initially the flask should not be immersed completely in running water, any depth short of the metal top is permissible because of the insulating properties of the formica ring.

Fig. 214. The underside of the lids from two types of Wills duplicating flasks. Type E on the left is undercut for locking the duplicating material to the lid, whereas the type F (right) is keyed to permit complete removal of the mold from the flask and later repositioning.

Fig. 215. The Wills type D flask, made entirely of aluminum, with a ring 1¾ inches high. The upper portion of the top lid has a depressed surface for holding surplus duplicating material, thus serving as a reservoir. This flask is competitively priced because the costlier formica ring is not used.

The principal difference in the two types is in the disassembly of the flask for the purpose of removing the cast from the mold (Fig. 214). One type has a lid that is machined to provide a definite undercut for the purpose of securing the mold to the lid. The bottom and the formica ring may be removed to permit flexing the mold while the cast is being removed, but the mold remains securely attached to the lid at all times. The tapered ring may then be placed back over the mold to support it while it is being filled. While this type provides support for the mold at all times, any accidental dislodgment from the undercut metal top would lead to permanent deformation of the mold. This hazard is eliminated in the second type, which permits complete disassembly of the mold from the flask to facilitate removal of the cast from the mold. The inside of the ring is tapered and every part is keyed to facilitate the return of the mold to its original relationship with the flask. This type is preferred for school use.

The technique for duplicating is the same for any cast, whether or not blockout is present. However, if wax or clay blockout is present, the temperature of the duplicating material must not be any higher than that recommended to avoid melting and distorting the blockout material.

Any clay used for blockout prior to duplication must be of the insoluble type (see Chapter 5, Surveying). Therefore, only an oily base clay may be safely used for this purpose.

While ordinary baseplate wax may be used for paralleled blockout and ledges, care must be taken that the temperature of the duplicating material is not high enough to melt the wax. The use of prepared blockout material may be preferred, such as Ney blockout wax or Wills undercut material. A formula has been given in Chapter 5 for those preferring to prepare their own blockout material.

Duplicating Procedure. The equipment needed for duplication is as follows (Fig. 216):

Bunsen burner and tripod
Enamel or stainless steel double boiler
   (aluminum utensils should not be
   used, as aluminum seems to have a
   deleterious effect on the composition
   of the duplicating colloid)
Duplicating flask

Plaster bowl (600 ml.)
Stiff spatula (Kerr laboratory spatula or
   Buffalo Dental No. 4 R)
Vibrator
Rubber suction cup
No. 7 spatula

Step-by-Step Procedure (Fig. 217, A-J). While the procedure given describes the use of the Wills late-model flask, it applies as well to the use of any duplicating flask.

1. New hydrocolloid duplicating material is usually packaged in a semidried state. It may be in the form of a crumbled meal. In such case, further chopping is unnecessary. If in bulk form, it must be chopped into fine particles. This is greatly facilitated by running it through a kitchen meat chopper. Any duplicating material being reused should similarly be reduced to small pieces before heating.

Heat the duplicating material in the top of the double boiler, stirring to dissipate lumps. New material must be diluted with water in the proportions recommended by the manufacturer; material being reused may be diluted if needed to

Fig. 216. Armamentarium for preparing material for duplicating: double boiler, ring stand, Bunsen burner, stiff laboratory spatula for stirring the duplicating material and for mixing the cast material in the plaster bowl, No. 7 wax spatula for directing the stream of fluid duplicating material over critical areas of the cast, vibrator, duplicating flask with feeder ring, and rubber suction cup for extracting the cast from the chilled mold.

replace water lost by evaporation. Remember that duplicating material may be further thinned with warm water during preparation as it becomes necessary, but the incorporation of dry material into a mix that is too thin is as much more difficult to accomplish. Therefore, it is best that any thinning be done by adding water slowly until the right consistency has been obtained.

When a smooth, creamy mix has been obtained, remove the upper pan of the double boiler from the burner and *continue stirring* until the temperature has dropped to 125° to 130° F. At this temperature, which is just low enough not to burn a finger immersed in it, the duplicating material is ready to pour.

2. For ten minutes just prior to duplication, immerse the cast in water at about 85° F., preferably in water that has lost its ability to etch the surface of the stone. Do this while the duplicating material is being cooled to a usable temperature. Immerse the cast upside down to allow the escape of any air trapped beneath sheets of wax placed on the master cast for relief.

Water which has been allowed to stand for some time with pieces of dental stone or plaster in it will have lost its ability to etch the surface of a stone cast. Therefore, any soaking of a stone cast should be done in water prepared for that purpose rather than in tap water.

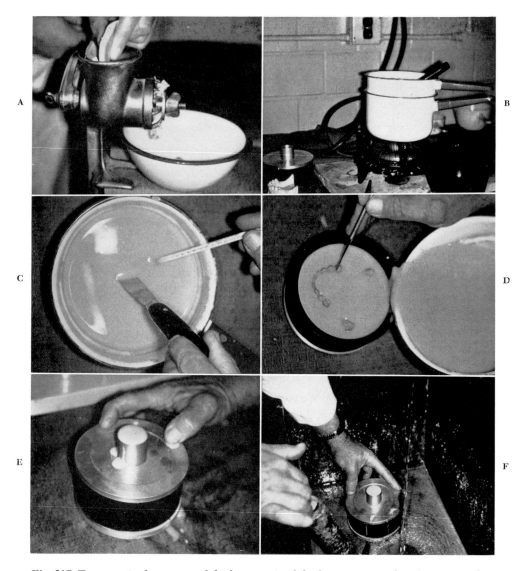

Fig. 217. Ten steps in the process of duplication. **A,** If duplicating materials is being reused, it should be ground into small pieces before being heated, to avoid lumps and uneven consistency. **B,** The material is then placed in the top of a double boiler and stirred well with a spatula until it has reached a smooth, creamy consistency. Warm water may be added sparingly to dilute it if necessary, but avoid overdilution. **C,** Remove the pan from the double boiler and continue stirring until the temperature has dropped to about 130° F. This is a temperature at which the finger may be immersed without burning, but it is more accurately checked with a thermometer. **D,** The cast to be duplicated, which has been immersed in water just prior to duplication, is placed in the bottom of the duplicating flask, over a small pellet of clay. A small continuous stream of duplicating material is poured in at the heel of the cast while the material is guided over critical areas with a No. 7 spatula held in the other hand. **E,** After filling the flask, the top and feeder ring are positioned, and duplicating material is added to completely fill the feeder ring. **F,** The flask is placed in running tap water about 1 inch deep until the material in the feeder ring has completely gelled, with a depression in its center to show that shrinkage has occurred. The flask may then be completely immersed in running tap water for an additional thirty minutes, *Continued on opposite page.*

When pieces of plaster or stone have been previously placed in tap water, solution will occur until the water becomes saturated with calcium sulfate. Once the water has become saturated, an equilibrium occurs with no further dissolution taking place. A stone cast placed in such water will not become etched because the water already contains all of the calcium sulfate it can hold. A container of such water should be available in the laboratory for use any time a cast needs to be soaked, such as prior to duplication or prior to repouring a portion of the original cast.

The broken pieces of plaster or stone should be small to medium in size but

Fig. 217 (cont'd). G, The feeder ring is removed and the projecting material cut off flush with the top of the flask. H, the flask is inverted and the bottom of the flask removed, exposing the base of the cast. In this position, the open end now becomes the top of the mold and the original top of the flask becomes the bottom. Excess duplicating material is then removed around the base of the cast. I, A rubber suction cup is applied to the base of the cast *under water*. The mold is then removed from the flask and flexed gently around the sides as the cast is removed with the suction cup acting as a handle. J, The *mold* is dried gently with compressed air and inspected for defects. It is then returned to the flask precisely in its original position, the original lid placed on the bottom for support, and the stone or investment, properly proportioned and spatulated, is slowly vibrated around the arch, tooth by tooth, to avoid trapping air or diluting the material with moisture. The mold is then completely filled and either immersed in still water or covered with a wet towel or a bell jar to prevent dehydration of the mold at the expense of the water of crystallization of the cast material. While a duplicating mold will not be poured a second time, its dimensional accuracy must be preserved until the cast material has completely set.

not fine enough to remain suspended in the water when it is agitated. These pieces should remain in the water at all times to maintain the equilibrium of the calcium sulfate. When used, the water should be clear.

Blow surface moisture off of the cast with compressed air, and center the cast in the bottom of the duplicating flask over a small pellet of clay. Press the base of the cast firmly against the bottom of the flask.

3. With one hand, slowly pour the duplicating material into the flask just behind one heel of the cast. A stream of duplicating material about $\frac{1}{8}$ inch in diameter should be poured continuously at this point until the base of the cast has been completely covered. At this time, with a No. 7 spatula in the other hand, guide the material around the teeth, into interproximal spaces, and upon critical tooth surfaces. This prevents trapping air bubbles in critical areas.

After the teeth have been completely covered, fill the flask within $\frac{1}{8}$ inch of the top. Then interrupt the pouring while positioning the metal top and feeder ring, after which completely fill the mold to the top of the feeder ring.

4. Now place the flask in about 1 inch of cold (preferably running) water. The water should cover no more than the metal base and the lower $\frac{1}{2}$ inch of the formica ring, so that initial cooling will occur only through the metal bottom.

While cooling *must* be done slowly and from the bottom to control shrinkage and avoid distortion, it is not absolutely necessary that cooling be hastened by using cold water. Time permitting, a hydrocolloid mold may be bench cooled without affecting its accuracy, whereas too rapid cooling may cause distortion. With this in mind, allow the mold to set completely in a shallow water bath. However, to facilitate early separation of the mold, when the feeder ring has gelled, immerse the flask in cold running water, where it should be left for at least thirty minutes to assure chilling throughout.

5. After thorough chilling, remove the flask from the water bath and remove the feeder ring. Cut off the hydrocolloid projecting above the lid flush with the top of the lid. Then invert the flask and remove the bottom, exposing the base of the cast. Remove any hydrocolloid covering the base of the cast and the flattened piece of clay, leaving the smooth base of the cast exposed.

The inside of the formica ring is tapered; therefore it may be removed by sliding it away from the top, leaving the mold attached only to the top. In the inverted position, the top now has become the bottom and will remain so during the subsequent procedures. The original bottom, now removed, will not be replaced on the mold, as this becomes the open end into which the cast material is poured.

If the top of the flask is undercut, the mold is not removed from it, and it becomes the base for supporting the mold. If the flask has a top that is keyed but not undercut, the mold is removed from it also to facilitate flexing as the cast is being removed from the mold. In either case, removal is best accomplished by applying a rubber suction cup to the base of the cast under running tap water and lightly flexing the mold while extracting the cast.

The suction cup is used as a convenient handle. Without it, the mold would have to be cut away to expose enough of the sides of the cast for a finger grip. After pouring and removing the duplicate cast, an excess would result where the mold has been cut away. While this may be trimmed on the model trimmer, it must be remembered that the base of the cast has been scored in three places to facilitate repositioning on the surveyor. If this is inadvertently trimmed away, there will be no record of the path of insertion on the duplicate cast to aid in positioning it on the surveyor for locating contour lines. This necessity does not exist where clasp ledges were formed on the master cast. But where waxing is to be done in relation to a survey line only, it is necessary that the original cast position be recorded on the duplicate cast. On the other hand, such a record must always be preserved on a duplicate stone cast to be used for fitting. This is particularly true where wrought-wire clasp arms must be accurately adapted in relation to the height of contour of the abutment teeth.

6. After removing the cast, replace the mold in the flask in exactly the same position as before. This is made possible by the keyed relationship of the parts of the flask. Reposition the hydrocolloid in the tapered formica ring so that the longer of the three grooves in the hydrocolloid mold points to the centering screw on the outside of the ring. Replace the keyed top which is to become the bottom and invert the ring so that the open end of the mold is up. If the reassembly has been properly done, the mold is in exactly the same relation to the flask as before; otherwise distortion of the mold may result.

Remove any free moisture from the mold by inverting it and blowing it out with compressed air. Care must be taken not to hold the stream of air on any area long enough to cause dehydration of that area.

With the correct amount of water in the plaster bowl, add a measured amount of stone on investment, following the manufacturer's recommendations. The corrected water-powder ratio is given by the manufacturer for each 100 grams of powder.

Mix thoroughly with a stiff spatula or a mechanical mixer. Vacuum mixing is always preferable, to eliminate entrapped air. If this equipment is not available, knead the mixture on the vibrator to remove as much air as will come to the surface. Many of the small air voids in a cast are due to air bubbles being carried into the mold in the mix rather than to air trapped in the mold during pouring.

Fill the hydrocolloid mold in much the same manner as an impression of the mouth. With the No. 7 spatula, add small amounts of material at one heel only while using the vibrator. The material is thus made to flow around the arch by the weight of the material behind it. Add material at the original site only until all of the critical areas of the mold have been filled. In this manner, excess moisture is pushed ahead of the material until it reaches the extreme opposite end of the mold, where it should be expelled and discarded. This avoids any dilution of the mix by the moisture remaining in the mold, minimizes the chances of trapping air, and results in a uniformly dense cast.

7. Immediately upon filling the mold immerse it in still water and allow it to set for about forty-five minutes. Immersion supplies the cast material with needed water of crystallization, some of which may otherwise be taken up by the hydrocolloid, resulting in a chalky cast surface. On the other hand, immersion should not be for longer than an hour or so, and never overnight, or etching of the surface of the cast may result.

After the cast material has set, remove the flask from the mold and *break the mold away from the cast* rather than attempt to remove the cast from the intact mold. The mold should not be poured a second time anyway, and fresh surfaces of the cast may be rubbed off in withdrawing it from the mold. Therefore, the mold should always be broken away from the cast.

Duplicating material may be washed and placed in water in a covered jar for reuse, especially where it will likely be reused in the near future. However, if there is any doubt as to its texture, it should be discarded. One should not attempt to revitalize old duplicating material by replenishing with new. Instead, any questionable material should be discarded and a new batch of material mixed as needed.

A freshly duplicated cast should not be handled unnecessarily, particularly one made of investment material, until it has been allowed to dry in air or in an oven. An investment cast should not be trimmed on a model trimmer, as this causes a slurry of investment to splash over the cast, which may not then be entirely removed by rinsing. For that matter an investment cast should not be rinsed at all. Instead, any necessary grinding should be done with a dry stone on a lathe and any powdered investment blown off with compressed air.

After initial drying and trimming, an investment cast should be dried in an oven at 180° to 200° F. for one to one and one-half hours, depending upon the size of the cast. It should then be dipped in a rosin-beeswax preparation as follows:

Melt the beeswax in a pan to a temperature of near 300° F. or just when the beeswax begins to smoke. This temperature is approximately 100° F. above that of the cast when it is removed from the drying oven.

Remove the cast from the oven and immerse it in the beeswax for approximately ten seconds. Then remove and stand the cast on a piece of absorbent paper until it has cooled.

Some of the advantages of dipping an investment cast in a rosin-beeswax preparation are (a) it eliminates the necessity for soaking the investment cast prior to painting on the outer investment; (b) it provides a smooth dense surface on the investment cast; and (c) the combination of drying and dipping eliminates any excess moisture in the cast.

WAXING THE PARTIAL DENTURE FRAMEWORK

Experience with free-hand waxing and the use of ready-made wax shapes is recommended as a prerequisite to the use of pre-formed plastic patterns. Unless plastic patterns are selected and used with care, they are better not used at all. The fact that they facilitate rapid production of partial denture castings has led to their widespread use in commercial and military service laboratories, but this alone does not justify their use. Even where plastic patterns are used, parts of the denture framework must be waxed free-hand to avoid excessive bulk and to create the desired contours. (Fig. 218, *A-C.*)

The use of ready-made wax shapes facilitates free-hand waxing to the point where an experienced operator can complete a wax pattern in little more time than is necessary when plastic patterns are used. Much of the speed with which a wax pattern may be produced depends upon how well the step-by-step procedure is organized so as to take fullest advantage of the wax shapes.

Fig. 218. Three steps in the making of a denture framework using blockout ledges and ready-made pattern forms. **A,** The master cast with shaped blockout ledges for the location of retentive and nonretentive clasp arms. **B,** The completed pattern using a Tru-Rugae palatal pattern, plastic clasp forms resting on investment ledges, and retention mesh anteriorly. The pattern is then waxed to completion. **C,** The finished casting returned to the master cast. The blockout ledges may be seen below the three lingual clasp arms.

The student in the technique laboratory should begin his waxing experience on a stone cast rather than on the softer investment cast, so that he may be free to modify and correct his errors as they are pointed out to him. Only after having a clear understanding of the location, bulk, and contours of the various parts of the wax pattern being done should he be allowed to wax on the investment cast. Since corrections on the investment cast may result in a rough casting, it is imperative that the waxing on the investment cast be done in a positive manner with a minimum of changes and corrections.

The same applies to the making of a partial denture framework in the undergraduate dental clinic. Although the typical dental student will probably not fabricate his own partial denture castings after graduation it is essential that he has a background and experience in dental laboratory procedures which will enable him to design the denture framework and prescribe how it is to be fabricated (Fig. 219). Not only this, but he must also be capable of evaluating the finished product to the end that the quality of dental laboratory services is maintained.

Fig. 219. The technician should receive from the dentist a master cast that has been surveyed and had reference lines scratched on the two sides and dorsal aspect of the base of the
cast. Upon this cast, the outline of the denture framework should be drawn precisely where
the component parts of the framework are to be placed and their dimensions be indicated.
In addition, written instructions should be included. From such a prescription, the technician
may be expected to return a polished casting that conforms to the penciled design.

With this in mind, it is desirable that two or more partial denture frameworks
be waxed to completion, if not cast and finished, by the clinical student himself.
In order to avoid discrepancies occurring as a result of inept waxing and subsequent corrections on the investment cast, it is most desirable that the student
first do a practice wax pattern on a duplicate stone cast. After all corrections have
been approved by his instructor, waxing on the investment cast may be done with
confidence and dispatch, resulting in a casting of high quality. While this policy
may be criticized as time-consuming, the total time spent should be little more
than that required when it is done on the investment cast alone with numerous
corrections. A higher percentage of satisfactory castings and fewer remakes will
result when this policy is followed in the undergraduate clinic. The quality of the
finished product and the knowledge and experience gained by the student more
than justify the additional time spent.

Waxing a Lower Class I Partial Denture Framework. One waxing exercise
will be given which embodies many of the essentials of waxing a partial denture
framework. Perhaps the most basic of all partial denture designs is the mandibular
bilateral free-end denture framework. The following technique is given for an
arch with second premolars remaining and bilateral edentulous molar areas:

1. On a suitable cast, outline lightly in pencil the inferior border of the
lingual bar major connector in relation to the moving tissues of the floor of the
mouth. Outline similarly the superior border located at least 2 mm. and preferably
3 mm. below the gingival margins. Some compromises may be necessary where
mucogingival junctions are high or gingival margins low, but interference with
either must be avoided. Generally, the lingual bar should be as low as possible
without danger of impinging moving tissues. Parallel the two lines about 4 mm.

Fig. 220. Design and finished casting for a lower Class I partial denture. The laboratory should be expected to follow such a design explicitly if done with the aid of a surveyor and with a specific path of insertion in mind.

A B

Fig. 221. A, The design of the partial denture framework is outlined on the master cast for the technician to follow in waxing and casting the framework. **B,** The cast framework as returned from the laboratory, superimposed upon the penciled design. Note the contouring of the thin lingual apron continuous with the half-pear-shaped lingual bar major connector. In the modification space a metal base is used with undercut finishing lines and nailhead retention for the attachment of denture teeth later with a resin base material. (From Mc-Cracken, W. L.: Contemporary Partial Denture Designs, J. Pros. Den. 8:71-84, 1958.)

apart and extend them distally to just below the distal aspect of the abutment teeth.

2. Adapt one thickness of 28-gauge sheet wax, either green casting wax or adhesive wax, over the entire lingual surface from the gingival margins to the floor of the cast. Be careful not to stretch the wax, thereby altering its thickness.

3. Adapt a piece of 6-gauge half-pear-shaped wax over the sheet wax so as to conform to the paralleled pencil lines showing through the sheet wax. The greater bulk of the half-pear shape must be at the lower border, with the tapered edge along the top pencil line. The thickness of the wax shape plus the sheet

wax previously adapted will be the thickness of the major connector before polishing.

4. Cut away the sheet wax extending above and below the wax shape which has now become the lingual bar, and cut off both the bar and the sheet wax even with the distal aspect of the abutment tooth. Use a dull instrument for this purpose to avoid scoring the cast.

5. Seal the inferior and superior borders of the bar to the cast. It is important that the wax be sealed to the cast throughout its course, yet that the original half-pear shape be preserved. Should any part of the wax pattern not be sealed to the cast, the pattern may become dislodged during the application of the outer investment, resulting in the investment seeping under the pattern. This would result in a false undersurface on the casting.

6. Beginning at the distal end of the major connector, from its superior border adapt a piece of *14-gauge round* wax up to and along the guiding plane surface of the abutment tooth. Continue this piece of round wax over the marginal ridge and onto the occlusal rest area. Seal this wax to the cast and to the superior border of the major connector. All junctions with the major connector should be reinforced and blended smoothly into its contour.

In the process of sealing the 14-gauge round wax, a half-round shape should result. Additional wax may then be added to provide the greatest bulk toward the lingual surface. The minor connector thus established should be tapered to the buccal surface to provide the least interference with the placement of the adjacent denture tooth.

As the wax in the occlusal rest area is sealed, the form of the occlusal rest lug will be established. This should not be allowed to extend beyond the rest preparation but rather should conform to its outline. Some additional wax may need to be added to prevent weakness at the marginal ridge.

7. Adapt a piece of *14-gauge round* wax on and above the height of contour of the lingual surface of the abutment tooth, extending mesially from the minor connector just below the marginal ridge. (This area is called the "body" of the clasp, from which the occlusal rest, retentive clasp arm, and reciprocal clasp arm originate.) In this particular case, the retentive clasp arm will be on the buccal surface, and the lingual clasp arm now being waxed is the nonretentive reciprocal arm.

Seal the wax shape to the cast, thus converting it to a half-round form. Taper the margins slightly to the tooth surface, and trim the inferior margin continuous with the height of contour. Add sufficient wax throughout its course to assure uniform bulk and rigidity. This clasp arm should be nonretentive and therefore should not be tapered except to avoid abruptness and irritation to the tongue at its terminal end.

8. Adapt a piece of *14-gauge wax* from the superior border of the lingual bar up the embrasure between the canine and first premolar tooth, then over the marginal ridge, and onto the rest area prepared in the first premolar for indirect retention. This minor connector should pass perpendicularly from the lingual bar up the interdental embrasure. A rule previously stated is that *any crossing of gingival tissues by the denture casting should be abrupt and definite.* A second

rule to be followed is that *minor connectors should conform to interdental embrasures whenever possible and should be shaped to present as little bulk to the tongue as possible.*

Seal the wax shape to the cast, thus converting it to a half-round form, and wax the occlusal rest to conform to the outline of the rest preparation. Strengthen the wax at the marginal ridge if necessary.

Should an extention of the indirect retainer onto the lingual surface of the canine be desired, a short piece of 14-gauge round wax may be extended mesially from the indirect retainer, which is then sealed and formed as a finger extension onto the canine tooth.

9. Perfect the waxing done thus far by smoothing and adding to weak points. *Smoothing* does not mean *polishing* or *flaming* the wax pattern, either of which affects only the highest part of the convex surfaces and serves only to flatten and alter the shape of the wax. Rather, smoothing should be done by gentle carving which preserves its original form. Therefore, as weak areas become evident, reinforce them by flowing on additional wax and blending it into the original waxing with a hot spatula and by carving. In the process of smoothing, gently trim away all excess wax around the borders of the pattern.

10. Retention for the attachment of resin bases is added next. This consists of two parallel pieces of round wax connected with cross rungs to form a ladder-like framework.

Beginning at the base of the vertical minor connector, adapt a piece of *16-gauge round* wax along the lingual surface of the residual ridge at the ridge crest. Extend this piece of wax approximately two thirds the length of the edentulous area. Seal and blend the proximal end of the wax into the minor connector at its point of origin and just tack the distal end to the cast. The retentive frame is *not* sealed to the cast throughout its course.

Beginning also at the minor connector 2 to 3 mm. below the first, adapt a piece of *18-gauge round* wax. Extend this second piece parallel to but 2 to 4 mm. below the first. At the same length as the first, cut it off and tack it to the cast at its distal end only. At its point of origin, add wax to reinforce and blend it into the minor connector.

At equally spaced intervals of about 4 mm. join the two longitudinal pieces with connecting bars of *18-gauge round* wax. This forms the rungs of the ladder-like construction. Each end of each rung must be attached securely to the longitudinal pieces with additional wax, so that reinforcement rather than weakness will exist at each point of junction. None of these crossbars should be sealed to the cast.

From one rung of the ladder, usually the third from the end, curve a piece of *18-gauge round* wax over the buccal side of the ridge to join the most distal rung at the end of the framework. This is for the purpose of providing additional support to the buccal flange of the resin denture base. To facilitate casting from lingually placed sprues, this buccal loop should be continuous with any two cross rungs. Attach the buccal loop securely with additional wax but do not seal it to the cast. In a long span, such as a distal extension from a canine abutment, two such buccal loops should be used; otherwise one will usually suffice.

Some mention must be made of the use of a supporting "foot" on the distal end of the retentive frame. The purpose of such a foot is to support the retentive framework during the processing of the resin base. It may be utilized only if the resin base is to be processed to the original surface of the cast, such as was recorded with an elastic impression material (or if the cast has been corrected previously to the supporting form of the ridge, using a resin tray impression technique). Where a wax impression of the supporting ridge form is to be made later by using the casting to support the impression base, a foot made to contact the original cast surface serves no purpose. Support for the retentive frame must be accomplished by other means, which will be discussed under Processing the Denture.

If, however, a usable foot is to be incorporated in the denture framework, this must be known prior to blockout and duplication so that the relief over the ridge area may be either cut out, exposing the surface of the cast, or ended at the point where the foot will be placed. In either case, some area at the distal end of the retentive framework must be waxed directly to the surface of the cast to provide distal support to that portion of the framework.

The wax pattern is now completed except for the adding of wrought-wire retentive clasp arms and the finishing line for the resin base.

Forming the Retentive Clasp Arm. The waxing has now been completed up to the point of adding the necessary retentive clasp arms. These have been classified in Chapter 9, Direct Retainers. Where a cast retentive clasp of any type is to be used, it must be waxed in relation to the height of contour with the terminal one third of the tapered clasp arm engaging a retentive undercut.

The location and extent of the undercut to be utilized are established first on the master cast and the clasp arm outlined from its origin to its terminus. If a wax ledge is used, the ledge is carved so as to establish the location of the inferior border of the clasp arm. This ledge is duplicated on the investment cast and the clasp is waxed or the plastic pattern placed with its inferior border along the ledge.

A second method utilized by some laboratories is to score the master cast lightly at the center of the retentive clasp as outlined, from its origin to its terminus. On the investment cast, the pattern is then centered over the scored line. The embossed line resulting on the casting is then removed during finishing.

When neither method is used, the height of contour must be lightly outlined in pencil on the investment cast by positioning the cast on the surveyor for that purpose. As mentioned previously, it is necessary that the scoring on the base of the master cast be reproduced and preserved on the investment cast so that the original path of insertion may be maintained. A light pencil line is all that is needed to identify the height of contour. Having outlined the clasp previously on the master cast, it may then be waxed on the investment cast without the aid of ledges and without scoring the tooth surface.

Although plastic forms may be used satisfactorily for this purpose, student and technician alike should have had experience in free-hand waxing and in the use of wax shapes. *Fourteen-gauge round* wax is used to form the outline of the clasp which is then sealed to the cast and converted to a half-round tapered form with the wax spatula. Some reinforcement at the point of origin and some trimming along the sealed margins will be necessary. The finished clasp pattern should have a uniform taper throughout its course, terminating in a predetermined infrabulge area. With a circumferential clasp, the height of contour is crossed at about two thirds of its length as the diameter of the clasp decreases and the terminal third engages the tooth undercut. With a bar clasp, the height of contour is not always crossed by the clasp arm, but the clasp must have a uniform taper from its point of origin to its termination in the undercut area. The point of origin of a bar clasp is at the denture base or where it emerges from the denture base. Its taper, therefore, should begin at this point rather than at its attachment to the denture framework. Any portion thereof which will be embedded in a resin base must be considered a rigid connector and not part of the retentive clasp; therefore, only the exposed part is tapered to form clasp arm.

A cast clasp arm should not be indiscriminately polished and then "pliered" to place. Rather, waxing should be done in such a manner that a minimum of finishing is necessary and its intended relationship to the abutment tooth is maintained.

Forming Wrought-Wire Retentive Clasp Arms. The design for the mandibular partial denture framework waxed thus far calls for the use of wrought-wire retentive arms. The wrought wire used is *18-gauge round* Ticonium wire. Other wrought-wire materials may also be used, but the Ticonium wire is preferred for its toughness and its resistance to accidental deformation. Gold or Ticonium may be cast directly to it and it may be soldered to higher fusing chrome alloys without crystallization.

Any wrought wire may be fatigued by repeated straightening and bending,

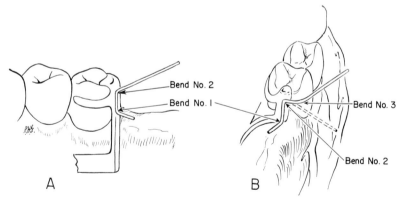

Fig. 222. Three steps in the shaping of a wrought-wire retentive clasp arm prior to attaching it to the wax pattern. **A,** A lingual view of bend No. 1 which forms a right-angle "foot" to be embedded in the casting lingual to the crest of the ridge. **B,** A distal view of bend No. 2 which is an acute bend just below the occlusal rest area toward the retentive side of the abutment tooth. Bend No. 3, which forms the beginning of the contoured portion of the clasp arm, should be adapted to the abutment tooth to the point where the clasp arm will eventually cross the height of contour. From this point the wire is left straight, breaking contact with the abutment at the height of contour and projecting downward and away from the surface of the cast. This portion will be adapted later into a retentive undercut.

and prolonged manipulation with pliers causes nicks in the wire. Either may result in early failure of the clasp arm through no fault of the material itself. To avoid having to correct mistakes by rebending, the student should practice first with paper-clip wire of similar gauge. When the student has learned to contour the wire with a minimum of manipulation he may then proceed to adapt the tougher wire.

Pliers which may be used most effectively for clasp wire–bending purposes are those designated by the numbers 53G (Dixon), 200 (three-pronged), 107 (round nose), and 137 (contouring).

The step-by-step procedure for forming wrought-wire clasp arms is as follows:

1. *Determine the length* of wire needed by adapting a piece of 14-gauge round wax to the abutment tooth, following the outline of the clasp as penciled on the master cast. Extend the wax down the guiding plane surface and 4 mm. onto the ridge area. Straighten this wax form and cut a piece of 18-gauge wire to the same length.

2. With No. 200 pliers *make a right-angle bend* approximately 3 mm. from one end of the wire. This forms the right-angle "foot" which will be embedded in the casting just lingual to the crest of the ridge (Fig. 222, *A*). Since there will be only mechanical attachment to the casting alloy, the "foot" is necessary to secure the wrought wire in the casting. Mechanical attachment may be enhanced by roughening this part of the wire with a file or stone.

3. Lay this "foot" on the ridge area of the cast just lingual to the crest and against the minor connector, leading up to the marginal ridge and occlusal rest area. Make a pencil mark just below the marginal ridge.

4. With No. 200 pliers *make an acute bend toward the retentive side of the abutment tooth* (Fig. 222, *B*). In this instance it will be toward the buccal side of the abutment tooth, but frequently lingual retention is preferred on mandibular teeth. The latter has the advantage of preventing possible distortion of the clasp by the patient during removal, since the accessible clasp arm is then the rigid cast reciprocal arm. However, esthetics is somewhat less favorable when the buccal arm is cast. On some unrestored mandibular abutment teeth, retention may be available only on the lingual side of the tooth. In such case, the bend is made toward the lingual side.

After making the second bend, lay the wire against the minor connector to make sure that the *angle* of the bend lies just below the marginal ridge.

5. The *third bend* is now made which forms the beginning of the contoured portion of the clasp arm (Fig. 222, *B*). It should be adapted to the abutment tooth from the minor connector to the point where the clasp arm will cross the height of contour. From this point, the wire is left straight, breaking contact with the abutment at the height of contour and projecting downward and away from the surface of the investment cast. It will eventually be secured by the outer investment, thereby maintaining the position of the wrought wire during the casting process. The reason for carefully adapting the wire along its suprabulge course is to avoid difficulty in contouring that portion later due to its proximity to the casting.

6. Lightly warm the wire and embed it into the minor connector and against the guiding plane surface of the abutment tooth. The wire must not be heated enough to cause the wax to flow. If this should happen, a film of wax may flow beneath the wire, which will result in a thin shim of cast metal between the wire and the abutment tooth. This would interfere with later contouring of the clasp arm.

If the casting is to be made of gold or Ticonium, all of the wrought wire but the clasp proper must now be covered with a film of wax so that the origin of the clasp will be embedded in the casting. If the casting is to be made of a higher fusing chromium-cobalt or stellite alloy, such as Vitallium, Nobilium, Retentaloy, Durallium, and others, the wrought wire must be removed from its waxed bed and later attached to the casting by soldering.

The wrought-wire clasp is now added similarly to the opposite abutment.

One step remains to be done before spruing and investing the pattern. This is the forming of a definite undercut finishing line where the resin will meet the connectors lying anterior to it and has purposely been deferred until all waxing has been completed.

With a sharp blade, cut a right-angle step in the lingual aspect of the vertical minor connector from just below the marginal ridge to the bottom of the lingual bar. This step is present in pre-formed plastic patterns but is usually curved arbitrarily and is not undercut sufficiently, if at all. Rather, the finishing line should include not only the lingual bar but also the minor connector and should be undercut sufficiently to afford a definite mechanical lock at the point of junction between the resin and the metal. If the bulk of wax is insufficient to permit the formation of such an undercut finishing line, add enough wax and blend it into the pattern to permit the formation of a definite undercut. It is highly desirable that the finishing line on any partial denture wax pattern be treated in this manner, to avoid seepage and separation at the junction of the resin with the metal framework.

The wax pattern is now completed and ready for spruing and investing (Figs. 223 and 224).

Waxing Metal Bases. A technique for forming the retentive framework for the attachment of resin bases has been given. There are two basic types of metal

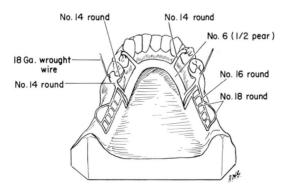

Fig. 223. The completed wax pattern for a lower Class I partial denture framework.

Fig. 224. A completed lower Class I pattern with bilateral indirect retainers and wrought-wire retentive arms in place. These will be shortened and adapted into the retentive undercut after the casting is polished and fitted. The vertical portion and right-angle "foot" of the wrought wire are embedded in wax, while the projecting portion will be held by the outer investment during casting.

bases that may be used instead of the resin base. The advantages of using cast metal bases over resin bases has been discussed previously in Chapter 11, under Denture Bases and Stress Breakers.

The type of base to be used must be known prior to blockout and duplication so that the relief over each edentulous ridge may be provided or eliminated as required. For a resin base, full relief for the retentive frame must be provided. For a full metal base, no relief over the ridge is used. For a partial metal base, the junction between metal and resin must be clearly defined by trimming the relief along a definite, previously determined line.

One type of metal base is the full base with metal periphery, to which tube teeth, cast copings, or a resin superstructure may be attached. If porcelain or plastic tube or grooved teeth are used they must be positioned first and the pattern waxed around them to form a coping (Figs. 225 and 226, A-D). The teeth are then attached to the metal base by cementation or, with the use of resin teeth, attached with additional acrylic resin under pressure, a so-called "pressed-on" method of attaching resin teeth to a metal base. Another method of attaching teeth is to wax the base so as to form a coping for each tooth, either by carving recesses in the wax or by waxing around dummy teeth. Instead of attaching a ready-made tooth, the full tooth may be waxed into occlusion, the base invested, and the wax patterns replaced with a processed acrylic resin tooth. This method permits some variation in the dimension and form of the supplied teeth not possible with ready-made teeth. It is particularly applicable to abnormally long or short spaces or where a stock tooth of desired width is not available. With modern cross-linked acrylic resins, such processed teeth are durable, and yet if they do wear down they may be added to successfully.

Fig. 225. A ready-made porcelain or resin tube tooth, or a denture tooth used as a tube tooth, should be ground to accommodate a cast coping as illustrated. A hole is drilled from the underside of the tooth, or if one is already present it is made larger. Then the tooth is ground to fit the ridge with enough clearance for a minimum thickness of metal. A 45-degree bevel is then formed around the base of the tooth, and finally a collar is created on the lingual side, extending to the interproximal area. The tooth is then lubricated and the wax pattern for the denture base formed around it.

Wax patterns of the teeth to be supplied may be waxed directly onto a metal base and then cast in gold and attached to the base by soldering. In this method, the denture teeth are carved as for resin veneer bridge pontics. After attachment to the metal base, resin veneers are then processed to match any adjacent veneered abutment crowns. Teeth visible are usually abutted to the ridge and cast flanges are used only in the posterior part of the mouth. This method is generally used only in conjunction with full mouth reconstruction. Both the denture framework and the cast pontics are usually made of gold to facilitate assembly by soldering.

When denture teeth are to be set to occlude with an opposing cast or an opposing template, the metal base must be formed with a boxing for the attachment of the tissue-colored denture resin supporting the teeth. This is the most common method of attaching teeth to a metal base. The wax pattern for the base is formed from one thickness of 26-gauge casting wax, which is then reinforced at the periphery, and a boxing is formed for the retention of the resin superstructure. Since metal peripheries are more difficult to adjust than resin, they are usually made somewhat short of the area normally covered with a resin base. Also, since peripheral thickness adds objectionable weight to the denture, it is made with only a slight peripheral roll. This is one disadvantage of the full metal base, in that the peripheral accuracy of the impression registration

Fig. 226. A, A wax pattern for a lower Class II, modification 1, partial denture using tubed teeth and metal bases throughout and two wrought-wire retentive clasp arms. **B,** Close view of the free-end metal base. Note the convex surface with rolled periphery and the location of the 18-gauge wrought wire in relation to the height of contour of the abutment tooth. **C and D,** Profile and occlusal views of the completed denture. Wrought-wire retentive arms have been contoured and tapered at their terminal end.

cannot be used to fullest advantage, and the contouring of facial and lingual surfaces cannot be as effective as with a resin base where added bulk can sometimes be used to advantage.

The periphery is first penciled lightly on the investment cast, and then the 26-gauge sheet casting wax (adhesive type) is smoothly adapted. Considerable care must be taken not to stretch and thin the sheet wax in adapting it to the cast. To avoid wrinkling, the wax should be adapted in at least two longitudinal pieces and joined and sealed together at the ridge crest. The wax is then trimmed along the penciled periphery with a dull instrument to avoid scoring the investment cast.

A single piece of *14-gauge round* wax is now adapted around the periphery *over* the sheet wax. With a hot spatula this must be sealed to the cast along its outer border. The inner half of the round wax form remains untouched. Then, sufficient wax is flowed onto the round wax to blend it smoothly into the sheet wax, thus completing a peripheral roll. Wax is added where needed to facilitate carving without trimming the original 26-gauge thickness. The result should be a rounded periphery blending smoothly into the sheet wax.

The boxing for the resin, which will in turn support the denture teeth, is now added, again using *14-gauge round* wax. The proposed outline for the boxing is identified by lightly scoring the sheet wax. Upon this scored line, the 14-gauge round wax is adapted, thus forming the outline of the boxing.

With additional wax, the ditch between the sheet wax and the outer border of the round wax is filled in and blended smoothly onto the sheet wax. This is done in the same manner as the periphery, adding sufficient wax to allow for smoothing and carving. As mentioned previously, the pattern should not be flamed or polished with a cloth. Instead, the pattern must be smoothed by carving or by using the tip of the finger as an abrasive.

The result thus far should be a pattern reinforced at the periphery and at the boxing and slightly concave in between, with some of the original sheet wax exposed. The inside of the boxing is not sealed to the sheet wax, thus leaving a slight undercut for the attachment of the resin. With a sharp blade, the margins of the boxing are then carved to a knife-edge finishing line. Using the back side of the large end of the No. 7 wax spatula, this margin may be lifted slightly, further deepening the undercut beneath the finishing line.

In addition to the undercut finishing line, retention spurs, loops, or nailheads are added for retention of the resin to be added later. Spurs are usually made of 18-gauge or smaller round wax attached at one end only at random acute angles to the sheet wax. Loops are small-gauge round wax circles attached either vertically or horizontally with space beneath for the resin attachment. Nailheads are made of short pieces of 16-gauge round wax attached vertically to the sheet wax, with the head flattened with a slightly warmed spatula. Any method of providing retention is acceptable as long as it permits positive attachment of the resin and will not interfere with the placement of denture teeth.

A metal base waxed as described will provide optimal contours with a mini-

Fig. 227. A Tru-Rugae pattern for an upper Class II, modification 1, partial denture. Note the uniformity of the pattern over the palatal torus. This is waxed for a partial metal base, with diagonal spurs and lingual finishing line for retention of the resin base. The right-angle "foot" of the wrought wire may be seen just above the finishing line distolingual to the abutment.

mum of bulk and weight and with adequate provision for the attachment of denture teeth to the metal base. Properly designed, the more visible portions of the
metal base will be covered with the denture resin supporting the supplied
teeth.

The second type of metal base is the partial metal base, either without any
metal periphery or without a metal periphery in visible areas. The most common
of these resembles a full metal base in all respects except that the buccal periphery is made short and ends abruptly without a finishing line (Fig. 227). Or
it may be made without any finishing line, with both buccal and lingual peripheries to be completed with resin. Esthetically and physiologically, a metal base
with resin peripheries offers some advantages over the full metal base in that
the thickness and contour may be made similar to a full resin base, yet with many
of the advantages of a cast metal base.

Ordinarily no relief on the master cast is necessary where a metal base is to
be used. In some instances, however, only the lingual portion of the base is made
of metal. This is more often done in the maxillary arch where some changes in
buccal ridge contours are anticipated. In such case, relief is used on the buccal
half of the ridge only and a retentive frame to support the resin flange is necessary. This permits later relining of the buccal flange to compensate for ridge
changes. Any time such a combination is used, relief should be trimmed sharply
along a definite line to provide a definite finishing line between the metal and the
resin base. This eliminates any unsupported flash of resin which would later become loosened to permit seepage, resulting in an unclean denture. Since definite
undercut finishing lines are not present on partial metal bases, other means of
providing mechanical retention must be used. These are usually in the form of
numerous spurs at random angles, although numerous small nailheads or loops
may be used if preferred. Marginal seepage between the resin and partial metal
bases is much more likely to occur over a period of time than where a full metal
base with undercut finishing lines is used. Therefore, every precaution must be
taken to provide the best possible mechanical retention.

Where a partial metal base or a full metal base without metal peripheries is
used, teeth are set up in wax, and subsequent steps are completed as for a full
resin base. The metal base is visible from the tissue side of the denture only,
thus combining the advantages of a metal base and with those of a resin base.

ANATOMIC REPLICA PATTERNS

A technique for obtaining a duplication of the palatal portion of a maxillary
cast was developed orginally by William Thompson as an aid to phonetics. This
was called the *Thompson Tru-Rugae technique.* It was soon discovered that many
other advantages as well resulted from anatomic replica patterns. It was found
that patients became accustomed to an anatomic replica palate much more
readily than to a smooth highly polished surface or to the concentrated bulk
of palatal bars. It has been claimed that an irregular palatal surface seems to improve mastication by giving the tongue a "washboard" surface against which to
press out the softer food particles and thereby separate them for mastication by
the teeth.

The appearance of the denture is improved by its anatomic form and by the fact that the surface is never highly polished. This fact is readily recognized by the tongue, which makes the patient aware of the fact that it is a personalized reproduction of his own palate rather than a foreign body to be tolerated.

The irregular contour of the anatomic replica palate adds rigidity to the casting by it corrugated shape, thus permitting the use of the thinner castings than would be permissible with a smooth, uncorrugated surface. This adds to patient acceptance and comfort by decreasing both weight and bulk.

To the laboratory, the anatomic replica palate means a saving in polishing time and in finishing and polishing materials.

The original Thompson technique was cumbersome but worthy of note because it led to later developments in anatomic replica techniques. Walker and Orsinger are credited with originating the present technique for palate reproduction, a description of which appeared in 1954. It is now almost a universally accepted technique for making full and partial palate reproductions.

The material is available as a Tru-Rugae kit and contains all the materials needed to make anatomic replica palates for complete and partial dentures. Whether used as a pattern to be burned out and cast or, in slightly thicker form, as an anatomic pattern of the palate to be discarded when boiling out a flasked denture, the technique is essentially the same. Walker and Orsinger listed the equipment and materials required as follows:

Cardboard box approximately 6 by 6 by 2 inches deep [to permit reuse of the polymer]
Camel's-hair brush, large water coloring size, or larger
Small nasal atomizer (DeVilbiss Economy Atomizer No. 182 is satisfactory)*
Wax spatula
Iris or cuticle scissors
Powder: Ethyl methacrylate powder, Dupont Lucite HG-24 or equal
Liquid: Methyl methacrylate monomer, or any denture base liquid acrylic resin
Coloring material for liquid: Prussian blue, artist's color ground in oil
Pattern cement: Preformed plastic pattern scraps dissolved in acetone
Plasticizers: Methyl salicylate, camphor, rosin, or suitable commercial plasticizers such as Dow Resin 276 . . . [The plasticizer is added to the liquid in the atomizer or spray gun only, about six drops to the small atomizer, correspondingly more to the larger spray gun.]†

Procedure for Making an Anatomic Replica Pattern. The procedure for making the anatomic replica pattern (or wafer) is as follows:

1. Either save the hydrocolloid mold after removing the investment cast or make an alginate impression of the master cast. The sides of the mold should be cut down to provide better access to the impression. Rinse the mold to remove

---

*Instead of using the hand-operated atomizer, experience has shown that compressed air-operated spray guns give a much finer and more uniform spray and are not subject to clogging. Two of these are the Thayer Chandler air brush and the Dupli-Color touch-up spray gun, model A, both of which require compressed air for operation.

†From Walker, T. J., and Orsinger, W. O.: Palate Reproduction by the Hydrocolloid-Resin Method, J. Pros. Den. 4:54-66, 1954.

any loose particles, and remove any excess moisture with compressed air. Leave the surface damp but free of surface moisture.

2. Fill the mold with powder from the cardboard box. (It is suggested that only enough powder be kept in the box to completely fill a hydrocolloid mold rather than to reuse larger quantities. Since this material becomes contaminated, it can be screened to remove foreign particles and replenished with fresh powder from the original container.)

3. Invert the mold over the cardboard box and dump out the surplus powder. Give the back of the hand holding the mold three or four slaps to remove more excess powder. This leaves powder layer No. 1 in the mold, which now has a fine sugar-coated appearance.

4. Using the atomizer, or preferably an air gun giving a fine misty spray, spray the face of the mold, as it is held in the other hand, with monomer. In this manner, the liquid is prevented from building up in deeper areas of the mold. The monomer should contain several drops of plasticizer, depending upon the size of the container.

5. Immediately fill the mold again, and again dump and tap out the excess powder. This is powder layer No. 2, which is then sprayed with monomer as before. Use sufficient liquid to saturate the powder particles.

Ordinarily, three layers of powder are sufficient to make a pattern thick enough for casting. (For palate reproductions on complete dentures, five or six layers may be necessary.) The thickness will be determined by how hard the operator knocks out the excess powder from the mold and also by the length of time the second and third applications of powder are left on the mold before they are knocked off. The longer they remain on the mold, the thicker the wafer will be, because the powder picks up more liquid as it stands.

6. Set the mold under an inverted container or in a bell jar to prevent evaporation of the monomer and to allow the liquid to more thoroughly penetrate the grains of powder. This results in a finer surface and a more uniform thickness after cementation on the refractory cast. (This precaution applies equally well to any procedure where denture bases are made by a sprinkling method. An inverted bowl or glass refrigerator jar serves the purpose of preventing evaporation and allows more thorough penetration of the monomer during polymerization.

7. When the plastic wafer has reached a flexible polymerized state (in about thirty minutes), strip it out of the mold completely. With fine iris scissors, trim the wafer to correspond to the outline of the palatal coverage previously penciled lightly on the refractory cast. Discard the cuttings, leaving only the wafer to be cemented to the refractory cast. If a definite ledge for a finishing line was established on the master cast with relief wax, the plastic wafer should extend about 2 mm. beyond the platform that has been reproduced on the investment cast. This establishes the finishing line on the tissue side of the casting. (The undercut finishing line on the exposed side will be waxed on the plastic wafer about 2 mm. in from its trimmed edge.)

8. With a fine camel's-hair brush, paint a uniform layer of the Tru-Rugae cement on the investment cast inside the penciled outline. If preferred, this

cement can be made up by dissolving plastic pattern forms in acetone. If it becomes too thick it may be thinned with monomer. Excess cement should be avoided as it will cause irregular borders to be reproduced in the casting. Press the plastic wafer to place on the cast, making sure it conforms to the penciled outline. Make sure that the mold is free of debris, and invert the investment cast into it. Add some weight to the base of the cast to assure close contact with the mold while the cement is hardening. In about one hour, the cast with the plastic wafer cemented to it may be removed. The remainder of the denture pattern may then be completed in the usual manner. Should it be necessary to store the wafer overnight before completing the pattern, it should be covered with an inverted glass container or placed under a bell jar to maintain its plasticity.

In making cast palate reproductions for a complete upper denture the method is essentially the same as that for a partial denture. For resin palate reproductions, an alginate hydrocolloid impression of the master cast is used rather than a duplication mold, since no refractory cast is involved. The wafer is sprayed into the mold somewhat thicker than for a metal casting, then removed after polymerizing and trimmed as above. The wafer is not cemented to the master cast but merely waxed to place to form the palate of the denture. This is done after the denture try-in has been completed. The palate of the original base is then cut out and replaced with the anatomic palate wafer. This is discarded during boilout, leaving a mold which results in an anatomic replica palate on the completed denture.

SPRUING, INVESTING, CASTING, AND FINISHING THE PARTIAL DENTURE FRAMEWORK

Brumfield has listed some of the factors that influence the excellence of a dental casting:

1. Care and accuracy with which the model [cast] is reproduced.
2. Intelligence with which the case is designed and proportioned.
3. Care and cleanliness in waxing up the model [cast].
4. Consideration of the expansion of the wax due to temperature.
5. The size of the sprues.
6. The length of the sprues.
7. The configuration of the sprues.
8. Points of attachment and manner of attachment of the sprues to the cast.
9. Choice of investment.
10. The location of the pattern in the mold.
11. The mixing water; amount, temperature, and impurities.
12. The spatulation of the investment during mixing.
13. The restraint offered to the expansion of the investment, due to the investment ring.
14. Setting time.
15. Burn-out temperature.
16. Burn-out time.
17. Method of casting.
18. Gases: adhered, entrapped, and absorbed.
19. Force used in throwing the metal into the mold.
20. Shrinkage on cooling.
21. Removal from the investment after casting.

22. Scrubbing, pickling, etc.
23. Polishing and finishing.
24. Heat handling.*

Spruing. Brumfield describes the function of the sprues as follows:

> The sprue channel is the opening leading from the crucible to the cavity in which the appliance is to be cast. Sprues have the purpose of leading the molten gold from the crucible into the mold cavity. For this purpose, they should be large enough to accommodate the entering stream, and of the proper shape to lead it into the mold cavity as quickly as possible, but with the least amount of turbulence. The sprues have the further purpose of providing a reservoir of molten metal from which the casting may draw during solidification, thus avoiding porosity due to shrinkage. The spruing of the cast may be roughly summarized in three general rules.
>
> 1. The sprues should be large enough that the molten metal in them will not solidify until after the metal in the casting proper has frozen. (8 to 12 gauge round wax is usually used for multiple spruing of partial denture castings.)
>
> 2. The sprues should lead into the mold cavity as directly as possible and still permit a configuration which will induce a minimum amount of turbulence in the stream of molten metal.
>
> 3. Sprues should leave the crucible from a common point and be attached to the case at its bulkier sections. That is, no thin sections of casting should intervene between two bulky, unsprued portions.
>
> The configuration of the sprues, from their point of attachment at the crucible, until they reach the mold cavity may be influential in reducing turbulence. One of the more important sources of difficulty in casting is the entrapment of gases in the mold cavity, before they have a chance to escape. If the sprue channels contain sharp right angle turns, great turbulence is induced which is calculated to entrap such gases and so lead to faulty castings. Sprue channels should make long radius, easy turns and also enter the mold cavity from a direction designed to avoid splashing at this point.
>
> As pointed out, the sprues should be attached to the bulky points of the mold. If two bulky points exist with a thin section between them, each of the bulky spots should be sprued. The points of attachment should be flared out and local constrictions avoided. If this practice is followed, the sprue, being bulky enough to freeze after the case has frozen, will continue to feed molten metal to the case until it has entirely solidified, thus providing sound metal in the casting proper with all shrinkage porosity forced into the sprue rod, which is later discarded.*

There are two basic types of sprues: multiple and single (Figs. 228 and 229). The majority of partial denture castings require multiple spruing, using 8- to 12-gauge round wax shapes for the main sprues and 14- to 18-gauge round wax shapes for auxiliary sprues. Occasionally, however, a single sprue is preferred for full cast palates and cast metal bases for the mandibular arch when these are used as complete denture bases. With partial dentures, the use of a single sprue is limited to those maxillary cases where, because of the presence of a palatal plate, it is impossible to locate multiple sprues centrally. In such cases, the single sprue may be used advantageously. A single sprue must be so attached to the wax pattern that the direction of flow of the molten metal will be parallel to the long axis of the single sprue. In some instances, the investment cast may

---

*From Brumfield, R. C.: Dental Gold Structures, Analysis and Practicalities, New York, 1949, J. F. Jelenko & Co., Inc.

Fig. 228. View of a sprued wax pattern. Three 10-gauge sprues attached to the lingual bar and two 16-gauge sprues attached to the retention form are joined at the central sprue hole in the investment cast.

Fig. 229. Full cast denture bases and broad palatal coverage are best sprued with a single sprue located posteriorly. Where a cast denture base for a completely edenulous arch is being sprued, the single sprue may be located anteriorly. (Courtesy Ticonium, Division, CMP Industries, Inc., Albany, N. Y.)

have to be cut away anteriorly to make room for the attachment of the sprue; in others, the sprue may be attached posteriorly. One disadvantage of using a single sprue for large castings is that an extra long investment ring must be used.

Some important points to remember in multiple spruing are as follows:

1. Use a few sprues of larger diameter rather than a number of smaller sprues.

2. Keep all sprues as short and direct as possible.

3. Avoid abrupt changes in direction; avoid T-shaped junctions.

4. Reinforce in all junctions with additional wax to avoid constrictions in the sprue channel and to avoid V-shaped sections of investment which might break away and be carried into the casting.

Step-by-Step Procedure. The laboratory procedure for multiple spruing is essentially the same for all mandibular castings and maxillary castings except those with a palatal plate. The following technique is given for a typical mandibular Class I partial denture casting:

1. Reduce the base of the cast to about ½-inch thickness. Trim all edges of the cast until it is slightly larger than the wax pattern and tapers from the occlusal aspect toward the base.

2. Cut a ⅜-inch hole through the cast centered on a line joining the distal end of the major connector on each side. This hole must be large enough to accommodate the main sprue from which other sprues will lead to the framework. (Stainless steel sprue cones may be purchased for the purpose of forming the main sprue hole. These are available in several sizes and shapes and are used to form the hole in the investment cast at the time the cast is poured into the duplication mold.)

3. Roll one-half sheet of softened pink baseplate wax into a rod of such diameter that it will just pass through the hole cut in the base of the cast when it is inserted from the bottom. Allow the wax rod to protrude slightly on the wax pattern side of the cast. Seal this portion to the cast all around its periphery. The long portion protruding from the underside of the cast will serve as a handle during investment. The slight projection on the wax pattern side serves as an overjet, with the sprue leads attacked approximately 3/16 inch below the tip of the main sprue. By using this overjet principle of spruing, the initial thrust of molten metal is directed against the tip of the main sprue reservoir and the turbulence that is created is confined to this area rather than at the entrance to the pattern mold cavity.

4. From this main sprue, attach three pieces of 8-gauge round wax extending radially to the lower border of the lingual bar major connector. Direct one piece to the central portion of the connector and the other two to just anterior to the finishing line where the major connector joins the base retention on either side. Thus the molten metal is fed to the clasp assembly as well as to the bar itself. Attach these sprues to the bulkiest part of the major connector, being careful not to involve any critical margins. In spruing a tooth-borne partial denture framework consisting of four clasp assemblies, four such sprues should be used, each attached to the major connector just below the clasp assembly.

5. In a similar manner, using pieces of 14-gauge round wax, connect the main sprue to the retentive framework or to any metal bases about two thirds of its length. In attaching to a retentive framework, make sure this is at the junction of a crossbar, thus assuring a free flow of metal with a minimum of changes in direction.

6. Reinforce all points of junction between the sprues and the denture framework with additional wax. The spruing is now completed (Fig. 230).

Investing the Sprued Pattern (Fig. 231). The investment for a partial denture casting consists of two parts: the investment cast upon which the pattern is formed and the outer investment surrounding the cast and pattern. The latter is confined within a metal ring, which may or may not be removed after the outer investment has set. If the metal ring is not removed, it must be lined with

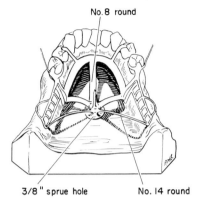

No. 8 round

3/8" sprue hole   No. 14 round

Fig. 230. The wax pattern is sprued as illustrated.

Fig. 231. The trimmed investment cast and sprued pattern are secured to the sprue former with the threaded sprue, approximately half of which is threaded into the sprue former and half into the investment cast. The elevation of the pattern in the ring may be adjusted by applying a screwdriver through the hole in the base of the sprue former.

a layer of asbestos to allow for both setting and thermal expansion of the mold in all directions.

The investment must conform accurately to the shape of the pattern and must preserve the configuration of the pattern as a cavity after the pattern itself has been eliminated through vaporization and oxidation. Brumfield has listed the purposes of the investment as follows:

1. Investment provides the strength necessary to hold the forces exerted by [the] entering stream of molten metal until this metal has solidified into the form of the pattern.
2. It provides a smooth surface for the mold cavity so that the final casting will require as little finishing as possible and in some cases a de-oxidizing agent to keep surfaces bright.

3. It provides an avenue of escape for most of the gases entrapped in the mold cavity by the entering stream of molten metal.
4. It, together with other factors, provides necessary compensation for the dimensional changes of the gold [alloy]* from the molten to the solid, cold state.†

The investment for casting gold alloys is a plaster-bound silica material, so compounded that the total mold expansion will offset the casting shrinkage of the gold, which varies from 1 to 1.74 per cent (the highest figure being the shrinkage of pure gold). Generally, the higher the percentage of gold in the alloy, the greater the contraction of the casting upon solidifying.

Only one chromium-cobalt alloy has a sufficiently low melting temperature to be cast into a plaster-silica investment mold. According to Peyton, for the others having a higher melting temperature, an investment containing quartz powder held together by an ethyl silicate or sodium silicate binder is usually used. Expansion to offset casting shrinkage for the chromium-cobalt alloys is accomplished primarily through thermal expansion of the mold and must be sufficient to offset their greater casting shrinkage, which is in the order of 2.3 per cent. For this reason, the metal ring is usually removed after the mold has hardened, to allow for the greater mold expansion necessary with these alloys.

Since the investments for chromium-cobalt alloys are generally less porous, there is greater danger of entrapping gases in the mold cavity by the molten metal. Spruing must be done with greater care and, in some cases, provision for venting the mold is necessary to avoid defective castings.

Step-by-Step Procedure. The technique for applying the outer investment is usually spoken of as "investing the pattern." Actually, the cast upon which the pattern is formed is part of the investment also. The following technique is given as being representative and applicable to all partial denture castings:

1. Just before mixing the investment, line the ring with one layer of sheet asbestos. The asbestos should be 1/4 inch shorter than the ring at the crucible end. The asbestos permits hot gases to escape at the back through the asbestos, yet some investment in contact with the ring at the crucible end prevents the investment from falling out when handling the ring after heating. Wet the asbestos after it is in place, but do not pack it tightly against the walls of the ring. (Step 1 is omitted if a split-type forming flask is used that will be opened and removed as soon as the investment has set.)

2. Unless the investment cast has been dipped in beeswax, which prevents it from absorbing water from the painting investment, it must be soaked in water before painting. In such case, immerse the cast with the sprued pattern in a pan of water at about 85° F. Water saturation of an untreated investment cast assures a good bond between the old investment and the new, but cold water must not be used for fear the pattern will shrink and be loosened from the cast.

---

*Note the substitution of the word *alloy*, as the same principles apply whether the metal be a precious metal alloy or a chromium-cobalt alloy. In some of the latter alloys, the cobalt is partially replaced by nickel; such alloys are sometimes described as "stellite" alloys.

†From Brumfield, R. C.: Dental Gold Structures, Analysis and Practicalities, New York, 1949, J. F. Jelenko & Co., Inc.

3. Mix 100 grams of investment, using 2 ml. more water than was used to make the investment cast. (If the investment for the cast required 28 ml. of water per 100 grams of powder, the painting mix should be 30 ml. of water per 100 grams.) Spatulation must be thorough and should continue for about thirty seconds to distribute water throughout the mix. Remember that a well-spatulated mix gives greater expansion.

Paint the pattern with a wetting agent just prior to applying the investment. With a brush carrying the mixed investment, start at one end of the cast and work the investment under the sprues. Use only indirect vibration, the hand supporting the cast being between it and the vibrator. Keep working the investment under the wax sprues, working from one side of the cast around to the other. Proceed to invest the remainder of the pattern in the same manner. Wrought-wire retentive clasp arms must also be covered with investment. The entire pattern should be covered with about $\frac{1}{4}$ inch of investment. An even layer of investment is necessary to assure uniform expansion of the mold. Set the invested pattern aside until the investment has set. (Unless the vibrator will remain off, do not set pattern on the same bench or vibration transferred through the bench will cause the investment to pull away from the pattern.)

4. After the painting investment has reached its initial set (in about ten minutes), it may be invested in the casting ring or flask former. Just before investing, dip the assembly in water to again saturate, shaking off any excess water. Four hundred grams of powder will be ample, mixed with the same proportion of water as before. *Only hand spatulation for about sixty seconds should be used, as some air in the outer investment is necessary to aid in venting the mold.*

One type of casting ring (Ney partial denture casting ring) has no crucible former and consists of a large heavy metal ring with an opening at one end about the diameter of an inlay casting ring. The other end is open to accommodate the invested pattern. To use this ring, the invested pattern is inserted with its main sprue protruding through the center of the smaller opening. The invested cast in this position should have sufficient space above for an adequate bulk of investment to cover it. In this position, connect the main wax sprue with the sides of the ring at its mouth, thus closing the opening. The main sprue protruding through the wax seal may be held between two fingers while the ring is held inverted in the palm of the hand. The invested cast is now completely covered with investment, filling the ring to the top. A glass slab may be slid over the top of the filled ring, to permit inverting the ring on the bench while the investment sets. The crucible is then cut into the hardened investment at the main sprue.

A second type of ring has a crucible former. Representative of this type are the Kerr and Jelenko partial denture casting rings. This type is perhaps the most frequently used. The invested cast is attached to the crucible former by placing the main sprue into the hole and sealing it to the crucible former. Care must be taken that the invested cast is centered in the ring, with sufficient space all around and at the top for adequate thickness of outer investment. The casting ring is seated onto the crucible former and filled with investment, thus embedding the cast in investment as previously outlined.

Fig. 232. The Wills threaded sprue former and matching casting ring. The base and ring may be either the Kerr or the Jelenko size, but both must match. The projection on the ⅜-inch rod threaded with a No. 16 thread is for positioning the lubricated sprue into the duplication mold prior to pouring the investment cast.

Fig. 233. The threaded sprue being held in the duplication mold by the pointed projection. The sprue is first lubricated with petrolatum or silicone jelly. Note the slotted end to facilitate withdrawal from the cast and, later, for the purpose of adjusting with a small screwdriver the height of the wax pattern in the casting ring.

Dr. Noble G. Wills has recently developed an innovation to the spruing and investing of a partial denture which promises to be a valuable aid in securing the investment cast to the sprue former and in regulating the height of the cast in the ring (Fig. 231).

For a long time, a tapered sprue cone of metal has been used to form the sprue hole in the investment cast, thus eliminating the need for cutting a ⅜-inch sprue hole in the base of the cast later. The sprue is then reinserted into the cast just prior to investment, where it is retained by friction.

The Wills sprue pin is a machined brass untapered screw ⅜ inch in diameter and threaded with a No. 16 thread. This fits into a threaded hole in a metal sprue former made to accommodate the Kerr or the Jelenko partial denture casting ring (Fig. 232). Projecting from the screw is a pin which is used to retain the threaded sprue in the hydrocolloid mold as the investment cast is being poured into it (Fig. 233). The threaded sprue must be lubricated with petrolatum or silicone jelly so that it may be removed from the cast with ease. A screwdriver is then used to remove the sprue from the cast, leaving a threaded sprue hole comparable to that in the sprue former.

After the wax pattern is completed and ready to invest, the brass sprue pin is screwed halfway into the base of the cast and the other half is screwed into the sprue former. Thus, the investment cast is held securely to the sprue former, and by inserting a screwdriver through the hole in the sprue former and engaging the slot in the threaded sprue its height in relation to the ring can be adjusted.

Since there is some probability that the sharp edges of investment making up the threaded sprue channel may become broken off by the force of the molten metal and thus be carried into the mold proper, the threaded sprue hole should be reamed slightly and the particles eliminated just prior to placing the investment in the furnace.

A third type of casting ring is the split-type forming flask which is opened and removed as soon as the investment has set. This flask is available in various diameters and heights, but the medium size will accommodate about 90 per cent of all cases. This type of casting ring does not use a crucible former. Instead, the flask is placed on a glass slab and nearly filled. Then the invested cast (sprue up) is embedded into it, using the sprue as a handle until the investment reaches a consistency sufficient to support the weight of the cast. Sometimes a copper

Fig. 234. Excess investment may be trimmed flush with the rim of the casting ring or flask by rubbing it over a piece of wire mesh or screening material. (Courtesy Ticonium, Division, CMP Industries, Inc., Albany, N. Y.)

screen is used inside the split-type flask to support the investment during heating and casting. This is not necessary if care is taken to avoid too rapid burnout or careless handling of the heated mold.

5. Allow the investment to set for at least an hour. At the end of this time, if the first type of ring was used, cut away the wax and protruding main sprue in such a manner as to form a concavity in the investment with the deepest part at the sprue. If the second type was used, merely remove the crucible former which will leave the investment concaved or funnel shaped. The concavity may be deepened if desired by trimming the walls uniformly smooth, maintaining the funnel shape. If a split-type flask is used, a crucible may be formed by carving a funnel in the mold at the main sprue. Finally, trim the two faces of the mold to be parallel, using the edges of the ring as a guide. This is done by rubbing the mold over a piece of wire mesh screening (Fig. 234). If the split-type ring was used, it is now removed by sliding off the retaining clip which allows the ring to be opened.

Burnout. The burnout operation serves three purposes: it drives off moisture in the mold, it vaporizes and thus eliminates the pattern, leaving a cavity in the mold, and it expands the mold to compensate for contraction of the metal on cooling.

Brumfield has this to say about burnout:

> The time required to drive off the water is mainly a function of the amount of heat available and of the closeness of the heating element to the investment when placed in the furnace. If the furnace is large and a number of molds are burned out at the same time, the burn-out will require more time than would be the case with a single mold in the same furnace. . . .
>
> The temperature of the mold is held down during early stages of burn-out by the vaporization of the water. Water will not rise appreciably above its boiling point until it is all vaporized. At the end of 60 minutes, the water is practically all driven off and the temperature at the inside of the mold will rise fairly rapidly to near the temperature of the furnace. Complete equalization, however, requires another 70 minutes, giving a total burn-out time of about two and one-quarter hours for eliminating the water and raising the temperature of the mold to approximately 1300° F. The so-called soaking period often recommended to be given the mold, after furnace pyrometer shows the full burn-out temperature, is designed to allow time for the water to be eliminated from the mold and the mold temperature to rise to that of the furnace.
>
> During the time the water is being eliminated, the wax is being eliminated through vaporization and oxidation of carbon. Vaporization of wax ordinarily does not require as much time as that for vaporization of the water and will often have been completed when the temperature on the inside of the furnace has risen to about 1000° F. The carbon residue may require more time for elimination. The more oxidizing the atmosphere of the eliminating furnace the better from the standpoint of eliminating wax. . . .
>
> It is essential that the time of burn-out be sufficient to entirely eliminate the moisture. If the moisture is not eliminated, its presence has two bad effects on the casting. The casting made from an incompletely eliminated ring is apt to be porous due to the continued emission of steam by the investment. Second, the venting of the mold cavity is largely accomplished through the interstices of the investment itself. Although the investment is finely ground and these interstices are invisible to the eye, they nevertheless exist in very considerable amounts. Most investments contain

voids (that is, spaces not occupied by investment particles), which amount to as much as 50 per cent of the total volume occupied. It is through these void spaces that the gases entrapped in the mold cavity by the entering stream of molten metal are able to depart with sufficient rapidity to avoid porosity in the casting. If these spaces are already occupied by steam from the incompletely eliminated mold or by finely divided particles of carbon residue from the wax, the entrapped gases cannot escape and porosity results from their inclusion in the casting. It is better to err on the side of too long a burn-out than in the opposite direction.*

In order for the investment to heat uniformly, it should be moist at the start of the burnout cycle. Steam will then carry the heat into the investment during the early stages of the burnout. Therefore, if the investment is not burned out on the same day it is poured, it should be soaked in water for a few minutes before being placed in the burnout furnace.

Just prior to being placed in the furnace, the mold should be placed in the casting machine for the purpose of balancing the weight against the weight of the mold. At this time, the mold should be properly oriented to the machine and its crucible and a scratch line made at the top for later repositioning the hot mold.

The mold should be placed in the oven with the sprue hole down and the orientation mark forward. Burnout should be started with a cold oven, or nearly so. The temperature of the oven should then be increased slowly to a temperature of 1200° to 1300° F. over a period of two and one-half to three hours. This temperature should then be maintained for at least a one-half hour "heat-soaking" period to ensure uniform heat penetration. More time must be allowed for plastic patterns, particularly palatal anatomic replica patterns.

It is important that this temperature not be exceeded during the burnout period. (When a high heat investment is used, the manufacturer's instructions as to burnout temperature should be followed.) For all plaster-bound investments, contraction of the mold occurs beyond 1350° F., and breakdown of the binder begins at about 1450° F. To avoid loss of expansion and possible cracking, the soaking temperature should not exceed 1300° F.

Casting. The method of casting will vary widely with the alloy and equipment being used. All methods use force to quickly inject the molten metal into the mold cavity. This force may be either centrifugal or air pressure; the former is the more commonly used. In any case, either too much or too little force is undesirable. If too little force is used, the mold is not completely filled before the metal begins to freeze. If too much force is used, excessive turbulence may result in the entrapment of gases in the casting. With centrifugal casting machines this is regulated by the number of turns put on the actuating spring. For the Thermotrol casting machine, for example, this is two to three turns.

The metal may be melted with a gas-oxygen blowtorch or by an electric muffle surrounding the metal. In some commercial casting procedures and in some dental laboratories, the induction method may be used, which provides a

---

*From Brumfield, R. C.: Dental Gold Structures, Analysis and Practicalities, New York, 1949, J. F. Jelenko & Co., Inc.

rapid and accurate method of melting the metal. The cost of induction equipment prohibits its widespread use.

The blowtorch method may produce consistently excellent results, but the lack of temperature control leaves much responsibility on the skill and judgment of the operator. Since the temperature at which the metal is thrown into the mold has an important bearing upon the excellence of the casting, the use of controlled melting with an electric muffle, such as the Thermotrol, eliminates many of the variables common to the blowtorch method. Properly adjusted, this machine indicates the temperature of the molten metal at the instant it is thrown into the mold.

Removing the Casting From the Investment. Chromium-cobalt alloys are usually allowed to cool in the mold and are not cleaned by pickling. Finishing and polishing, which are done with special high-speed equipment, require a technical skill in the use of bench lathes not ordinarily acquired by the dental student. The average dentist is more adept in the use of the dental handpiece, whereas the average technician is, by reason of his training, more proficient in the use of bench lathes for finishing and polishing larger castings. The following, therefore, applies specifically to gold alloy castings being completed by the dental student or dentist.

After the casting is completed, allow the mold to cool until the sprue button has changed in color from red to black when viewed in shaded light. This will be about eight to twelve minutes after completion of a large casting. At this time, quench the hot ring in water. With most gold castings, this will produce a fairly soft and ductile condition in the metal. However, the larger the flask and the greater the amount of investment surrounding the casting, the longer the period required for bench cooling prior to quenching. In a recent publication it has been pointed out that when the Ney partial denture flask is used, a cooling period of eight to twelve minutes is sufficient, but that if a flask with straight sides is used, it will hold approximately 60 per cent more investment and therefore requires considerably more time for cooling. For the latter type of flask (such as the Kerr or Jelenko flask) it is suggested that twenty minutes be allowed for bench cooling to avoid the possibility that the casting will be too soft.

The practice of allowing the casting to completely cool in the investment is not recommended for gold alloys. Although it is true that all gold alloys capable of being hardened due to slow cooling will harden if allowed to cool slowly in the investment, the difference between the outside and the center at any given instant may vary 200° F. or more. Heat hardening by this method is not only uneven but shrinkage also is nonuniform, resulting in an inaccurate casting.

After removal of the investment from the casting by brushing under water with a stiff bristle brush, the casting should be further cleaned by *pickling*. Prior to pickling, detergent powder may be used to aid in removing investment particles.

When the casting is clean, it should be pickled in an acid pickling solution. Prevox, Jel-Pac, dilute sulfuric acid, or 30 to 50 per cent hydrochloric acid may be used for pickling. The latter is objectionable because of the fumes and the fact that these fumes corrode laboratory instruments. It is essential that the pickling acid be clean and relatively colorless rather than have the typical green-ish blue color of contaminated acid. Contamination results not only from re-peated reuse of the solution but also from handling the casting with metal tongs during pickling. A contaminated acid contains excessive copper and other salts that will contaminate the surface of the casting, leading to tarnish and discolora-tion in the mouth.

When surface pits and irregularities on the casting become contaminated with foreign salts, later finishing and polishing may fail to remove them com-pletely. When such an appliance comes in contact with sulfur-bearing foods, metallic sulfides are formed which exude from the pits and irregularities. Dark rings of stain and discoloration subsequently spread over a larger area, giving a tarnished appearance to the polished metal. This is the result of using an un-clean pickling bath.

Under no conditions should the casting be heated and plunged into the pickling solution. Pickling is properly done by placing the casting in a clean dish and pouring the clean pickling solution over it to a depth sufficient to cover it. The dish should then be heated over a flame until the surface of the casting brightens. The pickling solution is poured off (flushing generously with water or base solution) and the casting washed with an abundance of water. If the acid solution is fresh and clean, no base metal deposits will occur to cause later discoloration of the polished casting in the mouth.

Finishing and Polishing. Some authorities hold that the sprues should not be removed from the casting until the majority of the polishing is completed. While it is true that this policy may prevent accidental distortion, it is difficult to adhere to and is therefore somewhat impractical. Instead, reasonable care should be exercised to avoid any distortion resulting from careless handling.

Actual polishing procedures may vary widely according to personal prefer-ence for certain abrasive shapes and sizes. However, several rules in finishing the casting are important. These are as follows:

1. High speeds are preferable to low speeds. Not only are they effective but in experienced hands there is less danger of the casting being caught and thrown out of the hands by the rotating instrument.

2. Let the wheels or points and the speed of their rotation do the cutting. Excessive pressure heats the work, crushes the abrasive particles, causes the wheels to clog and glaze, and slows up the cutting.

3. A definite sequence for finishing should be adopted and followed in every case. Such a sequence for finishing a gold casting is given by Berger:

(a) Remove sprues with a jeweler's saw rather than separating discs. This saves gold and prevents accidentally cutting into essential parts of the case.
(b) Grind off sprue stubs with 3/4″ or 7/8″ heatless stones, 1/16″ thick. Rough grind entire case and shape bars, clasps, and saddles. Always grind bars and clasps lengthwise. Cross-grinding can weaken a bar or clasp by grinding it too thin in spots. [If the location of clasps has been properly surveyed, it should not be necessary to grind the insides of the clasps. Smoothing the inner surface and polishing should be all that is needed.]

(c) Finish grinding with barrel-shaped mounted stones of medium grit. Use above precaution in grinding bars and clasps.

(d) Sandpaper the entire appliance using fine arbor bands, following the above precautions as to bars and clasps.

(e) . . . . rubber wheel the entire case carefully to remove all scratches. The better the case is rubber-wheeled, the easier the subsequent polishing steps become.

(f) The insides of the clasps and other inaccessible points may be polished readily and rapidly with [a pointed rubber cylinder. Retentive clasps should be shaped with a uniform taper in both width and thickness throughout their entire length.]

(g) The case is now ready for final polish. Use a B-20, 2-row brush wheel, with pumice or tripoli, or both, to remove all traces of rubber wheel marks.

(h) Finish this step with a tripoli-charged cloth buff or felt wheel and cones to get a velvety smooth finish.

(i) High gloss is imparted with a rouge-charged cloth or chamois buff.

(j) Boil case in a solution of [detergent] for several minutes and then with a hard brush remove all traces of polishing media. [This may also be accomplished by brushing with a solution of soap and household ammonia, or with commercial cleaning solutions.]*

4. Clean polishing wheels should be used. If contaminated wheels are used, foreign particles may become embedded in the surface which will lead to later discoloration.

5. Be sure each finishing operation completely removes all scratches left by the preceding one. Remember that each successive finishing step uses a finer abrasive and therefore cuts more slowly and requires more time to accomplish.

Heat Hardening. If the gold casting has been quenched in the investment, it is removed from the investment in its softest and most ductile condition. All grinding and finishing operations are performed while it is in this condition. After finishing, and just before final polishing, precious metal alloys should be heat hardened. While chrome-cobalt alloys cannot be heat hardened, they have satisfactory physical properties in their original state as cast, plus whatever work-hardening occurs from manipulation and use.

Hardening Gold Castings by Heat Soaking.† Dental gold castings, which are subject to heat hardening, may be effectively hardened as follows:

1. Quench the casting in the investment by shaking vigorously in an ample volume of water as soon as the sprue button has lost its heat color.

2. Remove the casting from the investment, thoroughly clean, and do all the finishing necessary.

3. When the casting is finished and ready for the final high polish, heat harden it as follows:

(a) Stabilize the furnace at the desired temperature by proper adjustment of the dial. See manufacturer's instructions for correct temperature for each alloy. (Yellow casting golds heat harden at temperatures between 600° and 700° F. White gold alloys heat harden more effectively at

---

*From Berger, H. R.: Finishing and Polishing Requires a Careful Technic, Jelenko Thermotrol Technician 1:7, Oct., 1947.

†From information taken from the physical properties chart of J. F. Jelenko & Co., Inc., New York, N. Y.

temperatures as high as 800° F., except Jelenko Palloro and alloys of its type which require somewhat different treatment. These should be quenched in the investment as soon as the casting machine stops, while the button is still red, and heat hardened by soaking for five minutes in a furnace stabilized at 600° F.)

(b) Place the casting on a metal tray in the furnace, close the door, and allow to heat soak for fifteen minutes.

(c) Remove the tray at the end of this period with the casting on it (do not touch the casting with cold tongs) and allow to bench cool.

This treatment will produce from 85 to 100 per cent of the strength given by the variable cooling-heat hardening process and avoids any possibility of warpage due to heat treatment.

Adapting Wrought-Wire Retentive Arms. Where wrought-wire retentive clasp arms are being used, these are adapted to the abutment tooth after the finished casting has been fitted back onto the master cast. With gold and Ticonium castings, the wrought wire will have been invested as part of the pattern and the metal cast around its base, thus securing it to the casting. With higher fusing chromium-cobalt alloys, the wrought wire must be soldered to the casting, usually after the fitting and finishing of the casting has been completed.

In either case, the retentive portion of the wrought-wire clasp must be adapted in relation to the survey line on the master cast. This line, representing the height of contour of the abutment tooth for a given path of insertion, should be crossed by the contoured wrought-wire at about one half of its length. (This differs from the cast clasp which, because of its lesser flexibility, should engage the tooth undercut with no more than one third of its length.)

The following technique is for the adaptation of that portion of the wrought-wire retentive arm that was originally adapted to the proximal-buccal or proximal-lingual aspect of the abutment tooth and then inclined downward toward the retentive area without engaging the undercut:

1. Resurvey the master cast (or the fitting cast) and delineate the height of contour on the abutment teeth in relation to the path of insertion.

2. Place a mark on this line at approximately the center of the retentive surface of the abutment tooth. Proximally, the clasp should be adapted to, or just above, this line. Distally (from its point of origin) the clasp should be adapted to lie in an infrabulge, or undercut, area. The terminus should engage the undercut to the degree previously determined by the survey. Remember that its length and diameter and the angle of cervical convergence must be taken into consideration when determining the location of the retentive terminal. The exact course of the wrought wire should be outlined in red pencil, in contrast to the lead pencil mark representing the height of contour.

3. Using Nos. 53 G (Dixon) and 200 (three-pronged) pliers, adapt the wire so as to conform to the contour of the tooth surface and follow the red pencil line. Take care not to nick the wire at any point. Any surface nick will be a potentially weak spot, because future flexures may be concentrated at this spot. Never use a plier beak that is not rounded. Work from the proximal end toward the terminus, cutting away any excess length as the required length

becomes known. As each portion is satisfactorily adapted, be careful not to alter it in adapting the remainder.

4. After the clasp arm is completely adapted, round the terminal end with a fine stone or rubber wheel. Then taper slightly the outer surface of the terminal one third and repolish, being careful not to alter its round form nor the uniformity of the taper. Thus tapered, not only is flexibility increased in the terminal one third but a smoother surface for the tongue and cheek to contact is provided as well. Also, when the clasp arm is properly tapered, there is less danger of it becoming distorted away from the tooth during insertion and removal.

THE MAKING OF IMPRESSION TRAYS AND DENTURE BASES

An individual impression tray may be made of self-curing resin, modeling plastic, or double-thickness baseplate.

The resin tray materials are packaged as a powder and liquid with activating chemicals added to induce polymerization when the two are mixed. They are mixed together in a jar in measured proportions and then adapted while in a doughy state to a moistened or lubricated cast. Polymerization is usually rapid with considerable exothermic reaction. They may be trimmed with scissors while soft and further trimmed after polymerizing. While considered "dead" materials (i.e., without elastic memory), they are not accurate enough to use as denture bases for jaw relation records or as trial bases where accuracy is essential.

Trial bases and bases for jaw relation records should either be made of materials possessing accuracy or be relined to provide such accuracy. Relining may be accomplished by seating the previously adapted base onto the tin-foiled or lubricated cast with an intervening mix of some zinc oxide-eugenol paste or with self-curing resin. Some use has been made of the mercaptan and silicone impression materials for this purpose, but the wisdom of using an elastic lining for jaw relation record bases is questionable. However, when rigid setting materials are used for this purpose, any undercuts on the cast must be blocked out with wax or clay to facilitate their removal without damage to the cast.

The ideal jaw relation record base and trial base is one that is processed (or cast) to the form of the master cast, becoming the permanent base of the completed prosthesis. Cast metal bases for either complete or partial dentures offer this advantage over resin-based dentures. Resin bases (either methyl methacrylate, vinyl combinations, or styrene) may likewise be processed directly to the master cast, thus becoming the permanent denture base. In either case, where undercuts are present, the master cast must be destroyed during removal of the base. Existing undercuts must then be blocked out inside the denture base before a cast is poured into it for the purpose of making an articulator mounting. A second cast, which includes the undercuts, must be poured against the entire base for the purpose of supporting it during the processing of the resin superstructure. Where both the base and the superstructure are of resin, some care must be taken to avoid visible junction lines between the original resin base and the resin which supports the teeth and establishes facial contours.

Some self-curing acrylic resin materials are sufficiently accurate for use as trial and jaw relation bases. These are used with a sprinkling technique, which, when properly done, permits a base to be made that compares favorably with a processed base. A material must be selected that will polymerize in a reasonable time (usually a twelve-minute monomer) and will retain its form during the sprinkling process. Since polymerization with typical shrinkage toward the cast begins immediately, alternate addition of monomer and polymer in small increments results in reduced over-all shrinkage and greater accuracy.

Technique for Making a Sprinkled Acrylic Resin Denture Base. The technique for sprinkling a denture base will be given here. However, the accuracy and stability obtainable by this method makes it equally applicable to the making of impression trays. I prefer to use sprinkled self-curing acrylic resin in every case where an impression tray or a trial denture base is needed.

Some blockout of the cast is necessary in all cases, depending upon the purpose for which the base is to be used. An individual impression tray requiring space for the impression material may be further relieved with sheet wax or wet asbestos. Sheet asbestos, such as is used to line inlay rings, may be dipped in water and adapted to the cast for this purpose. More than one thickness may be used, or wet asbestos may be added using the wet asbestos as one would modeling clay. By painting the asbestos relief with a tin-foil substitute, it may be easily stripped out of the impression tray, leaving no trace of the relief material on either the cast or the tray. This is a decided advantage over wax, which is sometimes removed with difficulty.

Relief of undercut areas on the cast is best accomplished with a water-soluble modeling clay. Modeling clay is easily formed and shaped on the cast and is easily removed from either the cast or the base with a natural bristle toothbrush under warm running water. Wax, on the other hand, must be flushed off the cast with boiling water. It must be removed from the inside of the base by scraping, as hot water would soften and distort the resin.

Impression trays to be used with an alginate hydrocolloid impression material must be perforated to assure retention of the impression material within the tray. Areas over soft tissue areas also require perforation to avoid displacement of those tissues by hydraulic pressure. Perforation is best accomplished by using a bi-beveled surgical drill, which fits the dental handpiece but will not become clogged when drilling holes in resin materials.

The amount of relief used for an impression tray will depend upon the type of impression material being used and the quality of the tissues being recorded. Trial bases and bases for jaw relation records, on the other hand, must have maximum contact with the supporting tissues. The accuracy of the base will be in proportion to the total area of intimate tissue contact provided. Those areas most frequently undercut and requiring blockout are the distolingual and retromylohyoid areas of the mandibular cast, the distobuccal and labial aspects of the maxillary cast, and, frequently, small multiple undercuts in the palatal rugae. These areas and any others are blocked out with a minimum of clay, so as to obliterate as little of the surface of the cast as possible. A close-fitting base may then be made that will have the necessary accuracy and stability and yet may be lifted from and returned to the master cast without abrading it.

Except for the presence of relief, the technique for sprinkling an impression tray is the same as that for a trial or jaw relation record base. The purpose for which it is to be used will influence the relief as follows: (1) An individual impression tray will have over-all relief sufficient to accommodate the impression material. (2) An impression tray for the purpose of making a fluid-wax functional impression prior to the making of the cast framework will have relief over the ridge areas to be recorded, with three or more tooth-bearing areas exposed and a clay matrix over the remainder of the cast. (3) An impression tray attached to the partial denture framework for the purpose of making a fluid-wax functional impression will have sufficient relief to accommodate the impression wax and permit its flow in the mouth. (4) A trial or jaw relation record base will have undercuts blocked out but no relief over the supporting areas of the ridge.

If the impression tray or base is to be attached to a partial denture framework, the framework is first seated on the cast in its terminal position and secured in that position with sticky wax. This is done after the necessary blockout and/or relief has been placed. The cast and the blockout and/or relief is then painted with a tin-foil substitute of a type that may be painted onto a cold surface without leaving a heavy or uneven film, such as Al-Cote. This is essential to the accuracy of a denture base, but not all tin-foil substitutes are suitable for this purpose.

As soon as the tin-foil substitute has dried, the cast is wet with the monomer from a dropper bottle. The ordinary medicine dropper is not suitable for this purpose because the lumen is too large, resulting in an uncontrollable excess of monomer. The glass may be drawn to a fine tip over a flame but is easily broken. Instead, the simple addition of a hypodermic needle of about 23 gauge to the glass lumen by flaming the glass tip around the needle provides a suitable syringe tip for the application of monomer in small quantities as needed (Fig. 235).

After wetting the surface with the monomer, the polymer is sprinkled or dusted onto the wet surface until all of the monomer has been absorbed. Sprinkling is best accomplished using a large-mouthed bottle with a single hole in the lid near the rim. The hole should be about the size of a No. 8 round bur. This facilitates the placement of the polymer without excess in any one area. A flexible bottle with suitable applicator tip may also be used for this purpose. However, it seems that better control over the application of the polymer is possible when a bottle with a hole in the cap is used. The objective should be the uniform application of polymer over the entire ridge rather than the allowing of excess to accumulate at the periphery to be trimmed later. A self-curing acrylic resin material must be used, such as Yates Flash Acrylic, that will retain its form during the sprinkling procedure without objectionable flow into low areas.

Once the polymer has been sprinkled in slight excess, the monomer is again added. Flooding must be avoided; therefore, the monomer must be directed

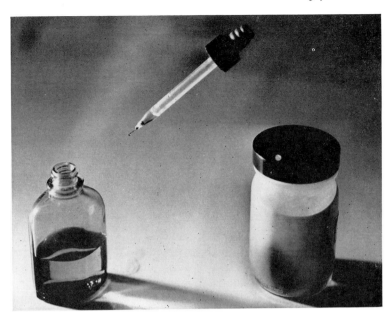

Fig. 235. Rapid self-curing acrylic resin in bottles used for sprinkling resin bases, etc. A 23-gauge hypodermic needle has been sealed into the tip of the dropper barrel to limit the size of the drop and facilitate wetting the monomer without flooding. The large-mouthed bottle is of a size that can easily be held in the hand, and it has in the rim a hole the size of a No. 8 or No. 10 round bur to allow the powder to be applied selectively to the area involved.

over the entire surface gradually until the polymer has just absorbed the monomer. *A few seconds' delay prior to the addition of excess monomer will allow the mass to reach a tacky consistency and prevent it from flowing when more monomer is added.* Then the monomer may be added in excess, which is immediately absorbed by the application of more polymer as before. This process is repeated selectively until a uniform layer has been built up, just thick enough so that none of the underlying cast or relief may be seen. Some areas will require further addition, particularly ridge crests and other prominent areas.

The final step in sprinkling is the addition of monomer sufficient to leave a wet surface. *Immediately,* the cast should be placed in a covered glass dish or covered with an inverted bowl. This permits final polymerization in a saturated atmosphere of monomer and prevents evaporation of surface monomer. The cast should not be placed in water or any attempt made to accelerate polymerization. Slow polymerization is necessary so that shrinkage *toward* the cast will occur, earlier layers polymerizing first. Only thus will over-all shrinkage be negligible and accuracy of fit be assured. While this is of little consequence in the making of an impression tray, it is most essential in the making of a sprinkled resin base.

Although polymerization will be about 90 per cent complete within an hour, and an impression tray may even be lifted within a half hour, a sprinkled denture base should be left *overnight* before being separated from the cast. It should then be lifted either dry or under lukewarm tap water. It should not be immersed in hot water or some warpage may occur.

A sprinkled acrylic base made with the precautions outlined above will retain its accuracy for days, or even for an indefinite period, comparable to that of a heat-cured resin base. Failure to do so can be attributed to faulty technique rather than to any inherent inaccuracy in the material itself, provided the proper material for this purpose has been used. As with any resin base, storing in air results in some distortion due to dehydration. However, since the stone cast itself may not be stored in water, possible distortion of the resin from being immersed off of the cast must be weighed against that occurring due to dehydration. Generally, the latter is not sufficient to warrent keeping the resin base in water.

OCCLUSION RIMS

It has been explained that jaw relation records for partial dentures should always be made upon accurate bases that are either part of the denture casting itself or attached to it in exactly the same relation as the final denture base will be. Further, it has been stated that, although the use of the final denture base is best for jaw relation records, a sprinkled or corrected acrylic base may be used satisfactorily. In any case, accuracy of the base supporting the occlusion record must be a foregone conclusion before considering the function of occlusion rims.

Occlusion rims may be made of several materials. The most commonly used material for the purpose of establishing static occlusal relationships is the baseplate wax rim. However, use of a wax occlusion rim is likely to be inaccurate, because of the fact that uniform softening cannot be assured. Also, some errors in repositioning wax occlusion rims for mounting on the articulator are likely to occur. When some soft material which sets to a rigid state, such as impression plaster or impression paste, is used in conjunction with wax rims to record static occlusal relations, many of the errors common to wax rims are eliminated. Vertical stops should first be established on chilled wax rims, which are then scored or serrated and the final record made in soft plaster or impression paste. As mentioned previously, an adjustable bite frame may be used to advantage with wax occlusion rims.

Modeling plastic may be used instead of wax for occlusion rims, with several advantages over the latter. It may be softened uniformly by flaming, yet becomes rigid and sufficiently accurate when chilled. It may be trimmed with a sharp knife to expose the tips of the opposing cusps for the purpose of rechecking or positioning an opposing cast into the record rim. Opposing occlusion rims of modeling plastic may be keyed with greater accuracy than opposing wax rims. Preferably, however, even those should be trimmed short except for vertical stops, and plaster or impression paste should be interposed for the final record. As with wax rims, an adjustable bite frame to support the final record may also be used.

Occlusion rims of either baseplate wax or modeling plastic may be used to support intraoral central bearing devices and/or intraoral tracing devices. However, because of its greater stability, modeling plastic is preferable for this purpose also, where the edentulous situation permits the use of flat plane tracings.

An example of such a situation is where an opposing complete denture is being made concurrently with the partial denture. In such case, modeling plastic occlusion rims provide greater stability than wax rims, with corresponding improvement in the predictable accuracy of such a jaw relation record. While the sealing of opposing occlusion rims or the use of clips for complete denture jaw relation records, particularly for an initial articulator mounting, may be acceptable, the existence of a partial denture framework makes this practice hazardous. Since it is necessary that the operator be able to see that the partial denture framework is in its original relation to the supporting teeth before the casts are articulated, the framework and attached base should be seated on its cast with accuracy before the opposing cast is repositioned in occlusion to it.

Occlusion rims for the purpose of recording functional, or dynamic, occlusion must be made of a hard wax that can be carved by the opposing dentition. This method, outlined previously in Chapter 16, Occlusal Relationships for Partial Dentures, presumes that the opposing arch is intact or has been restored. Functional occlusion records by this method cannot be made when both arches are being restored simultaneously.

Rather, an opposing arch must be as intact as the treatment plan calls for or must be restored by whatever prosthetic means the situation dictates. Opposing partial dentures or an opposing complete denture may be carried concurrently up to the final occlusal record. One denture is then completed and inserted and the functional record made in opposition to it. Frequently, this requires that all opposing teeth be articulated first in wax for the purpose of establishing optimal ridge relations and the correct occlusal plane. One denture is then carried to completion, and the teeth remaining in wax on the opposing denture are removed while the functional occlusal record is being made.

No single wax has been manufactured specifically for the purpose of establishing functional occlusal records. Some inlay waxes are used for this purpose because they can be carved by the opposing dentition and because most of them are hard enough to support occlusion over a period of hours or days. A wax for recording functional crown and bridge occlusion, since it is established entirely in the dental office, is selected on the basis of how well it may be carved by the opposing dentition in a relatively short period of time. Therefore, a softer wax may be used than is required for the recording of occlusal paths over a period of twenty-four hours or more. For this latter purpose, Peck's purple hard inlay wax seems to best satisfy the requirements for a wax that is durable yet capable of recording a functional occlusal pattern. This wax is packaged in the form of sticks. A layer of sticky wax is first flowed onto the surface of the denture base. Two sticks of the inlay wax are then laid parallel along the longitudinal center of the denture base and secured to it with a hot spatula. This is the only preparation prior to the dental appointment. Since neither the height nor the width of the occlusion rim can be known in advance, and since deep warming of a chilled wax rim is difficult, the rim is not completed prior to the appointment.

With the patient in the chair, a hot spatula is inserted into the crevice between the two sticks of wax, making the center portion fluid between two supporting walls. Some transfer of heat to the supporting walls occurs, resulting in the occlusion rim becoming uniformly softened. The patient is asked to close into this wax rim until the natural teeth are in contact, which establishes both the height and the width of the occlusion rim. Wax is then added or carved away as indicated and the patient asked to go into lateral excursions. Any excess wax is then removed, and any unsupported wax is supported by addition. Finally, wax is added to increase the vertical dimension sufficient to allow (1) for denture settling, (2) for changes in jaw relation brought about by the re-establishment of posterior support, and (3) for carving in all mandibular excursions. When sufficient height has been established, as well as sufficient width to accommodate all excursive movements, the patient is instructed and dismissed.

While the above has been included in this chapter on laboratory procedures, the entire procedure of establishing occlusion rims for recording functional occlusion should be considered a chairside procedure rather than a laboratory procedure. It is necessary, however, that the purpose of a functional occlusal record be clearly understood so that subsequent laboratory steps may be accomplished in a manner that the effect of such an occlusal record may be reproduced on the finished denture.

Making a Stone Occlusal Template From a Functional Occlusal Record. After final acceptance of the occlusal record as registered by the patient, the effectiveness of this method for establishing functional occlusion on the partial denture will depend upon how accurately the following procedures are carried out. For this reason it will be given as a step-by-step procedure, as follows:

1. If the base of the master cast (or processing cast) has not been keyed previously, do this before proceeding. First reduce the thickness of the base if it is so thick that difficulty will be encountered in flasking. The base may not be reduced on this account after removal from the articulator, since the mounting record would be lost.

The use of metal mounting plates is difficult if not impossible with partial denture casts because the impression is inverted rather than boxed, as for most complete denture impressions. The addition of mounting plates later is hazardous and unadvisable because of the danger of separation of the two layers of stone and the subsequent loss of the remounting record.

Keying may be done in several ways, but a method whereby the keyed portions are visible on the articulator mounting eliminates some possibility of remounting error. According to the preferred method, form a 45-degree bevel on the base of the cast by hand or with the model trimmer and then add three V-shaped grooves on each side and the dorsal aspect of the base of the cast at the bevel (Fig. 236). The bevel serves to facilitate reseating the cast on the articulator mounting, and the mounting surfaces are made still more definite by the triangular grooves. Being placed at the beveled margin, the triangular grooves are visible at all times and any discrepancy may be clearly seen.

2. Inspect the underside of the cast framework and any denture bases, removing any particles of wax or other debris. Similarly, inspect and clean the master cast of any particles of stone, wax, blockout material, or any other debris that might prevent the casting from being seated accurately upon it.

Now seat the denture framework on the cast in its original terminal position.

Fig. 236. The base of any cast should be beveled and keyed as shown before mounting on the articulator. Petroleum jelly is used as a separating medium to facilitate removal and re-mounting subsequent to processing. Keying should always be done prior to boxing and pouring an occlusal registration, because the cast and template must be mounted on the articulator before they are separated.

This is the position that was maintained by securing with sticky wax while the trial denture base was being made, with all of the occlusal rests seated. It is also the position that the casting assumed in the mouth while the occlusal record was being made and must be duplicated upon returning the denture framework to the master cast. Holding the framework in this terminal position, secure it again with sticky wax. (If a processing cast is being used in place of the master cast, the denture base will have been made upon that cast and the same precautions in returning the framework to its original position apply.)

3. With the denture framework and the occlusal record in position, form a matrix of clay around the occlusal record to confine the hard stone which will form the stone occlusal template. (Should electroforming have been done as mentioned in Chapter 16, the electroforming precedes Step 1. The clay matrix is the same for a metallized surface as for the wax record.)

The clay matrix should rise at a 45-degree angle from the buccal and lingual limits of the occlusal registration. Then arch either clay or a sheet of wax across from one side to the other, forming a vault which will permit lingual access when articulating the teeth.

Leave the occlusal surfaces of the adjacent abutment teeth or the corresponding surfaces of a processing cast, exposed so that they may act as vertical stops. This will serve to maintain the vertical relation on the articulator. Unless such stone-to-stone stops are used, the vertical relation on the articulator may be altered by the technician, either accidentally or otherwise. Any change in vertical relations is incompatible with a concept of dynamic occlusion, since the occlusal pattern is directly related to the degree of jaw separation. Although it may be true that vertical dimension may be changed when casts are mounted in relation to the opening axis of the mandible, *as long as natural cusps remain to influence mandibular movement, the vertical relation established with a functional occlusal record must not be changed on the articulator.*

Treat the surfaces of the adjacent abutment teeth left exposed with sodium silicate, Microfilm, or some other separating medium to ensure separation of the stone vertical stops.

4. If the wax record has not been metallized, use a very hard dental stone to form the opposing template. This may be an improved stone such as Duroc, but the use of a stone die material such as Vel-Mix is preferred. Only the occluding surface need be poured in the harder stone, a less costly laboratory stone being used to back it up. If this is done, add the second layer to the first before the former takes its initial set, to avoid any possibility of accidental separation between the two materials.

Vibrate the stone only into the wax registration and against the stone stops. Pile on the rest of the stone and leave uneven to facilitate firm attachment to the mounting plaster. Attach the occlusal template to the articulator without provision for remounting, since only the working cast need be keyed for remounting.

5. After the stone template has set, attach the occluded casts to both arms of the articulator before separating. The type of articulating instrument used is of little importance, since all eccentric positions are recorded on the template, and whatever instrument is used acts purely as a simple hinge or a tripod. Therefore, any laboratory articulator or tripod may be used. Because of the easy access afforded in setting teeth and adjusting occlusion, the Hagman Junior Balancer is preferred over most other instruments for this purpose.

Since both casts are not usually attached to the articulator with the same mix of material, the first mounting may be done with plaster without fear of error being introduced by the expansion of the plaster. Mounting to the opposing arm of the articulator, however, should be accomplished with stone to avoid such expansion. (When mounting complete denture casts, the upper cast, being mounted with the aid of a face-bow, may be attached to the upper arm of the articulator with plaster. The lower cast is then attached to the lower arm with stone to avoid error in jaw relations caused by the expansion of the plaster.) If preferred, both attachments may be accomplished with stone, but stone should always be used to attach the opposing arch.

It must be remembered which arch is represented by the working cast, and the articulator mounting should be made accordingly. For example, for a mandibular denture the template is attached to the upper arm of the articulator, whereas for a maxillary denture the template is mounted upside down on the lower arm. The keyed base of the working cast attached to the opposing arm must be coated with mineral oil or petroleum jelly to facilitate its separation from the mounting plaster.

6. After the mounting has been completed, separate the casts and remove the clay. The template with its mounting may be removed from the articulator if a mounting ring or mounting stud permits, otherwise trimming must be done on the articulator. With pencil, outline the limits of the occlusal registration and carefully knife-trim any excess stone around its borders. Trim the vertical stops to a sharp edge on the buccal surface where they contact the working

cast. Also remove any overhanging stone, leaving the occluding template and vertical stops clearly visible and accessible.

Remove the wax registration preparatory to setting denture teeth to the occluding template.

SETTING POSTERIOR TEETH TO AN OCCLUDING CAST OR TEMPLATE

Whether posterior teeth are to be set to occlude with an opposing cast or an occlusal template, unless metal bases are part of the denture framework, the denture base upon which jaw relation record has been made must first be removed and discarded. Since record bases that are entirely tissue supported have no place in recording occlusal relations for partial dentures, the bases must be attached to the denture framework. Metal bases, being part of the prosthesis, present no problem. The teeth may be set in wax or replaced on the metal base, depending on the type of posterior tooth being used, and these occluded directly to the opposing cast or template.

Unless occlusal relations are recorded on final resin bases, self-curing acrylic resin bases by the sprinkling method are the most accurate and stable bases that may be used for this purpose. (An alternate method is the relining of the original impression bases, thus accomplishing the same purpose.) While static relations may be recorded successfully on corrected bases, functional registrations are best accomplished on new resin bases made for that purpose. In either case, the denture cannot be completed on these bases, nor can the bases be removed conveniently from the retentive framework during the boilout after flasking. Therefore, the metal framework must be lifted from the cast and the original record base removed by flaming its underside. *Care must be taken not to allow the resin to catch on fire or the cast framework will become discolored with carbon.* The framework is then returned to its original position on the master cast and secured there with sticky wax before proceeding with the set-up.

Posterior Tooth Forms. Posterior tooth forms for partial dentures should not be selected arbitrarily in accordance with the personal preference of the dentist or the technician. One should bear in mind at all times that the objective in partial denture occlusion is harmony between natural and artificial dentition. Whether the teeth are set to occlude with an opposing cast or to an occlusal template, they should be modified to harmonize with the existing dentition. In this respect, both partial denture occlusion and occlusion on a single full denture differ from complete denture occlusion. In the latter, posterior teeth may be selected and articulated according to the dentist's own concept of what constitutes the most favorable complete denture occlusion, whereas partial denture occlusion must be made to harmonize with an existing occlusal pattern. Thus, the occlusal surfaces on the finished partial denture may bear little resemblence to the original occlusal surfaces of the teeth as manufactured.

Posterior teeth for partial dentures should be considered *material from which a suitable occlusal surface may be formed rather than teeth to be articulated as well as possible with opposing surfaces.* The original occlusal form, therefore, is of little importance in forming the posterior occlusion for the partial denture.

While the posterior teeth may be made of porcelain or resin, resin teeth are more easily modified and subsequently reshaped for masticating efficiency by adding grooves and spillways. Resin teeth are also more easily narrowed buccolingually to reduce the size of the occlusal table without sacrificing strength or esthetics. They may also be more easily ground to fit minor connectors and irregular spaces and to avoid retentive elements of the denture framework. Ordinarily, resin teeth are used in all situations, except where the opposing teeth are porcelain. Even then, there is reason to believe that resin teeth may be used successfully in opposition to porcelain teeth when the original surface glaze of the porcelain teeth has been left intact or when ground vacuum-fired porcelain surfaces have been repolished.

Setting Teeth to an Occluding Surface. The procedure for setting teeth to a static relationship with an opposing cast is essentially the same as for setting teeth to an occluding template. On the other hand, articulation of artificial teeth on an adjustable instrument, which presumably reproduces to some extent mandibular movement, will follow more closely the customary pattern for complete denture occlusion.

The step-by-step procedure for setting posterior teeth to an occluding template is as follows:

1. First raise the vertical adjustment of the articulator approximately 1 mm. If vertical stops are used, this will separate the stone stops by that amount.

2. With the aid of marking tape or articulating ribbon, mark the mesial and the ridge lap surfaces of the tooth to be set against the most anterior minor connector on either side. Continue to mark and relieve this tooth until it conforms to and fits around the minor connector, occluding with the opposing surface at the existing vertical dimension. Modify the cusps of this tooth as required to occlude with the opposing surface.

3. Set the remaining teeth on that side in order, progressing posteriorly. Relieve the ridge lap and modify the occlusal surfaces as required to occlude optimally with the opposing surfaces. One or more teeth may have to be narrowed mesiodistally to establish a satisfactory mesiodistal relation with the opposing teeth. In other instances, it may be necessary to leave a space between the first two teeth to accomplish this effect. While intercuspation is desirable in most instances, it is not absolutely necessary when setting to an occlusal template, since modified occlusal surfaces will function satisfactorily in any mesiodistal relation.

4. If a posterior abutment is present, the last tooth may have to be narrowed mesiodistally to fit the remaining space. This tooth also should be ground to conform to the contour of the minor connector, thereby effecting a more natural marginal contact relation with the abutment tooth.

5. Proceed to the opposite side of the arch and set the tooth or teeth in the same sequence, with each tooth lying adjacent to a minor connector being ground to fit that minor connector.

6. When all teeth have been set to the opposing surfaces, having been modified to occlude optimally at the existing vertical dimension, release the vertical element (pin or screw), leaving the occlusion uniformly high. When vertical stops of stone are used the vertical element on the articulator may be

removed entirely, since the absolute vertical dimension will be ultimately maintained by the stone stops. Otherwise, the pin or screw should be returned to its original position. (This is, of course, difficult to re-establish without a calibrated pin, hence the value of having definite stone stops.)

Using marking tape or articulating ribbon as an indicator, the occlusal surfaces are now further modified until an optimal occlusal relationship at the absolute vertical dimension has been established. At least three factors must be considered:

(a) The opposing surface may be easily abraded or otherwise damaged by repeated closure against the denture teeth. This does not apply when opposing artificial teeth are being set and modified concurrently. When setting teeth on a single denture, however, an opposing surface made of hard metal is the only way of eliminating this possibility; otherwise, violent tapping must be avoided.

(b) Unreliable markings usually result when articulating paper is used. Areas of heavy contact become perforated, leaving only a small mark, while areas of lesser contact may make a heavier mark. This may be avoided by using a marking tape or an inked ribbon, which better conforms to irregular occluding surfaces, does not tear or become perforated, and remains constant with repeated use. Markings are thus more reliably interpreted. A ribbon holder has been described in Chatper 16, under Setting Teeth to an Occluding Template.

(c) Wax from articulating paper eventually is deposited on opposing surfaces, having the effect of increasing the vertical dimension and leading to false interpretation of occlusal interference. This too is avoided by using a marking tape or an inked ribbon, since the ink or dye does not create a false surface.

Regardless of the type of indicator used, stone stops are best left unmarked for better interpretation of absolute contact. Wax from articulating paper may create a false surface here also, changing the vertical relation. While marking ink does not do this, it does make visualization of the vertical relation at the stops more difficult to interpret.

7. Except for the addition of spillways, perfect the occlusion while the teeth are still in wax. Only those errors occurring as a result of processing will then need to be corrected by remounting. Final waxing may be done off of the articulator, but the cast should be returned to it to correct for any tooth displacement resulting from waxing and carving.

TYPES OF ANTERIOR TEETH

Anterior teeth on partial dentures are concerned primarily with esthetics and the function of incising. These are best set in the mouth, since an added appointment for try-in would be necessary anyway. They may be set arbitrarily on the cast and then tried in, but in any case a stone index of their labial surfaces should be made on the master cast after the final arrangement has been established.

From a purely mechanical standpoint, all missing anterior teeth are best replaced with fixed restorations rather than with the partial denture. However, for economic or cosmetic reasons or in cases where a number of missing anterior teeth are involved, such as in a Class IV partially edentulous arch, their replacement with the partial denture may be unavoidable.

Some types of anterior teeth used on partial dentures are as follows:

1. Porcelain or resin denture teeth, attached to the framework with denture resin.

2. Ready-made resin denture teeth processed directly to retentions on the metal framework with a matching resin. This is called a "pressed-on" method and has the advantage of permitting prior selection and try-in of the anterior teeth, plus the advantage of using ready-made resin teeth for labial surfaces. These are then hollowed out on the lingual surface to facilitate their permanent attachment to the denture framework with resin of the same shade.

3. Resin teeth processed to a metal framework in the laboratory. Teeth may be carved on the denture framework and tried in the mouth, adjusted for esthetics and occlusion, and then processed in a resin of a suitable shade. There is some question as to whether or not the shade and durability of such teeth is comparable to manufactured plastic teeth, but improvements in materials has led to improved quality and appearance of laboratory-made teeth. Moreover, such teeth may frequently be shaped and characterized to better blend with the adjacent natural teeth.

4. Porcelain or resin facings cemented to the denture framework. These may be tried in the mouth on a baseplate wax base and adjusted for esthetics. Ready-made plastic backings may be used which become part of the pattern for the partial denture framework, and the teeth are then ultimately cemented to the denture framework. Esthetically, these are less satisfactory than other types of anterior teeth, but they have the advantage of greater strength and are easily replaced. A record of the mold and shade of each tooth should be kept, and only the ridge lap of the replacement teeth need to be ground to fit. When replaceability is the main reason for its use, the stock facing should not be beveled or difficulty will be encountered in replacing it. Replacement may also be accomplished by waxing and processing a resin facing directly to the metal backing. Stock tube or side-groove teeth are not ordinarily used for anterior teeth on partial dentures because of the horizontal forces that tend to dislodge them.

5. The denture pattern may include anterior teeth hollowed out to receive resin veneers, the same as for veneer crowns and veneer pontics on fixed bridges. This is most applicable where the denture framework is to be cast in gold. Labial surfaces may then be waxed and the final carving for esthetics done in the mouth. A modification of this method is the waxing of the veneer coping on a previously cast gold base. These are then cast separately and attached to the framework by soldering. Esthetically, the result is comparable to that obtained with resin veneer crowns. This method is particularly applicable where there is a desire to make the replaced teeth match adjacent veneered abutment crowns.

WAXING AND INVESTING THE PARTIAL DENTURE PRIOR TO PROCESSING RESIN BASES OR ATTACHMENTS

Waxing the Partial Denture Base. Waxing the partial denture base prior to investing differs little from the waxing of a complete denture; the only difference is the waxing to and around exposed parts of the metal framework. Here, undercut finishing lines should be provided whenever possible. Then the waxing is merely butted to the finishing line with a little excess to allow for finishing. Otherwise, small voids in the wax may become filled with investing plaster, or fine edges of the investment may break off during boilout and packing. In either case, small pieces of investment may become embedded in the resin at the finishing lines. This is avoided by slightly overwaxing and then finishing the resin back to the metal finishing line with finishing burs. Abrasive wheels and disks should not be used for this purpose, as they will cut into the metal and may burn the resin. Pumice on a rag wheel should not be used for polishing because it will cut the resin more rapidly than the metal and leave the finishing line elevated above the adjacent resin.

When waxing to polished metal parts not possessing a finishing line, it must be remembered that no attachment will exist and that over a period of time there will inevitably be some seepage, separation, and discoloration of the resin in this area. This may be avoided to some extent by roughening the metal whenever possible to effect some mechanical attachment. The wax should be left thick enough so that the resin will have some bulk at its junction with the polished metal. Thin films of resin over metal should be avoided, and, in finishing, these should be cut back to an area of bulk with finishing burs. Otherwise, any thin film of resin will eventually separate and become discolored and unclean due to marginal seepage.

Gingival form should be waxed in accordance with modern concepts of cosmetics and should be made as self-cleansing as possible. The dental student should familiarize himself with normal gingival architecture as found on study casts of natural dentition, beginning with the casts of each other's mouths usually made in basic technique exercises. In this manner he may have a better concept of gingival contours to be reproduced on prosthetic restorations.

In general, students and technicians alike seem to lack a clear concept of natural gingival architecture and are prone to leave too much tooth embedded in wax. Artificial teeth should ordinarily be fully uncovered to expose all of the anatomic crown and even beyond where gingival recession is to be simulated. Relatively few prosthetic patients are in an age bracket where some gingival recession and exposed cementum would not normally be present, and this should be reproduced on prosthetic restorations in proportion to the patient's age. With partial dentures, gingival contours around the remaining natural teeth should be used as a guide to the gingival contours to be reproduced on the prosthesis.

The denture should be waxed and carved as for a cast restoration, which it actually is, regardless of the material to be used or the method of processing. The fact that a split-mold technique is used for processing does not alter the fact that the form of the denture base is to be reproduced by a casting procedure. Therefore, the denture pattern should be waxed with care in the same form as that desired for the finished restoration rather than attempt to shape facial contours on the prosthesis during the polishing phase. Polishing should consist primarily of trimming away the flash, stippling polished surfaces where desired, and polishing lightly with brush wheels and pumice followed by final polishing with a brush wheel coated with wax or soap. Gross trimming and polishing with pumice should not be necessary if the denture has been properly waxed prior to investing.

Since the polished surfaces of any denture play an important part in both retention and in the control of the food bolus, buccal and lingual contours should generally be made concave. Peripheral thickness of the denture should be left as recorded in the impression. The only exceptions are the distolingual aspect of the lower denture base to avoid interference with the tongue, the distobuccal aspect of the upper denture base to avoid interference with the coronoid process of the mandible, and labial flanges which must be made thin for esthetic reasons. These are the only areas that cannot ordinarily be waxed to final contour before investing and may need to be thinned at the time of final polishing.

Investing the Partial Denture. In investing a partial denture for the purpose of processing a resin base, it must be kept in mind that the denture cast must be recovered from the flask intact for the purpose of remounting. The practice of cutting the teeth off of the cast to expose the connectors and retainers which are then embedded in the upper half of the flask is permissible only when an existing denture base is being relined and no provision has been made for re-mounting. (In such case, it seems that this practice has no advantage over in-vesting the denture being so relined upside-down in the lower half of the flask.) Since some increase in vertical dimension has, in the past, been inevitable in any split-mold processing technique, this method results in the denture frame-work being raised from the supporting teeth by the amount of increase. While occlusal adjustment in the mouth may temporarily re-establish a harmonious occlusal relation with the opposing teeth, the denture framework must then settle into supporting contact with the abutment teeth at the expense of the underlying ridge.

Changes in vertical dimension may be held to a minimum by using denture resins that can be placed in the mold in a fluid rather than a doughy state or those that may be injected in a fluid state into a closed mold. Dimensional changes occurring during relining may also be held to a minimum by using cold curing resins for this purpose, thus avoiding the thermal expansion of a mold subjected to elevated temperatures.

When two opposing partial dentures are being made concurrently, one is sometimes processed and inserted first and then the final occlusion established on the second denture to a fully restored arch. In such case, where there are no natural teeth in opposition, it is not necessary that the first denture be remounted after processing. In all other cases, remounting to correct for errors in occlusion is necessary. Flasking must be so accomplished that the cast may be recovered from the flask undamaged.

Since the partial denture impression may not be boxed prior to pouring the cast, metal mounting plates cannot be used as with complete denture impres-sions. Adding a mounting plate later with additional stone is not dependable, for should the cast separate between the two layers of stone, the mounting record is lost. The base of the stone cast must therefore be keyed by beveling and notch-ing on at least three sides.

Minute voids in the base of the cast will have been reproduced in the plaster mounting, and although the obvious larger blebs may be trimmed away, smaller blebs will remain. Should the voids in the cast become filled with investing material, the effect is two particles trying to occupy the same space. This may be prevented by covering the base with tin foil prior to investing. By coating the base and sides of the cast with petroleum jelly, tin foil may be easily adapted by burnishing it on with a towel. Not only does this keep the cast isolated from the investing material but the cast may also be more easily recovered from the surrounding investment.

After tin-foiling, the remainder of the cast should be coated with some reliable separator, such as mineral oil, petroleum jelly, sodium silicate, or tin-foil substitute. The entire cast, except for the wax and teeth, may then be invested in the lower half of the flask. As with a complete denture, only the supplied teeth and wax are left exposed to be invested in the upper half. Also, as with a complete denture, the investment in the lower half must be smooth and free of undercuts, and must be coated with a separator to facilitate separation of the two halves of the flask.

An alternate and preferred procedure is to invest the cast only to the top of the tin-foiled base, smoothing the investment and applying a reliable separator. Then, a second layer of investment is placed around the anatomic portion of the cast, covering the natural teeth and the exposed parts of the denture framework. This is likewise smoothed and made free of undercuts and coated with a separator prior to pouring the top half of the flask. Recovery of the cast is thus made easier by having a shell of investment over the anatomic portion of the cast which may be removed separately.

Where the denture base is to be characterized by applying tinted resins to the mold, care should be taken not to embed the wax periphery in the lower half of the flask. Bennett has pointed out the need for investing only to the periphery of the wax, leaving the entire surface to be tinted reproduced in the upper half of the flask. With this precaution, tinting may be carried all the way to the periphery and later removal of the flask will not mar the tinted surface. If tinting is not to be done or is to be done only at the necks of the teeth and the interdental papillae, the wax periphery should be embedded in the lower half where it may be faithfully reproduced and preserved during polishing.

The use of resin materials that require trial packing is complicated by the presence of the retentive framework of the partial denture. With their use, trial packing must be done with a sheet of cellophane between two layers of the resin dough; otherwise, the flask could not be opened without pulling the resin away from either the teeth in one half of the flask or the metal framework in the other. Resin dough is placed in each half of the flask, the sheet of cellophane placed between them, and the flask closed for trial packing. The flask is then opened, the cellophane removed, and the excess flash trimmed away. Final closure is then effected without the intervening sheet of cellophane.

More recently, resin materials have been developed which require no trial packing. These are mixed as usual but are either poured into the mold or placed in the mold in a very soft state. They offer little or no resistance to closure of the flask, yet the finished product is comparable if not superior to resin materials packed in a doughy state. They must be used in some excess, with the excess escaping between the halves of the flask. While they are soft enough to allow the escape of gross excess, the use of a land space is advisable to avoid a thin film on the land area. Any film existing on the land area after deflasking may be interpreted as an opening of the flask by that amount, hence the need for some provision for an intervening space to accommodate the excess and to facilitate its escape as the flask is closed.

To provide such a land space, the land area on the lower half of the flask may be painted with melted baseplate wax prior to pouring the top half. After wax elimination, a space then remains to accommodate any excess resin remaining after the flask is completely closed. It is necessary that no plaster or wax be allowed to remain on the rim of the flask and that the flask make metal-to-metal contact before pouring the second half. Only in this way is it possible to see that the flask is completely closed prior to placing it in the curing unit.

The pouring of the top half of the flask follows the same procedure as with a complete denture. While it is not absolutely necessary that the entire top half be poured in stone, it is necessary that a stone cap of some sort be used to prevent tooth movement in an occlusal direction. This is due to the inability of plaster to withstand closing pressures. All plaster remaining on the occlusal surfaces of the teeth should be removed and a separator added prior to pouring the stone cap to facilitate its removal during deflasking. Should the use of stone investment be preferred, a shell of improved stone or die stone may be painted or applied with the fingers onto the wax and teeth and this allowed to harden before filling the remainder of the flask with plaster. If a full stone investment is preferred (which is neither necessary nor advantageous), some provision should be made for easy separation during deflasking. Not only should a separate stone cap be used but metal separators or knife cuts radiating out to the walls of the flask should also be placed in the partially set stone. Deflasking is then easily accomplished by removing the stone cap and inserting a knife blade between the sections of stone.

Boilout should be deferred until the investing plaster has set for several hours or, preferably, overnight. Boilout must effectively eliminate all wax residue; therefore an adequate source of clean hot water must be available. After wax elimination with boiling water, it should be flushed with a solution of grease-dissolving detergent and again with clean boiling water.

Immediately following boilout, the hot mold should be painted with a very thin film of tin-foil substitute, being careful not to allow it to collect around the necks of the teeth. A second coat should never be applied, and packing of the mold should proceed immediately after the film has dried. Once the tin-foil substitute becomes completely dry it will wrinkle and lift away from the plaster, defeating the purpose for which it is used.

Where the master cast for a free-end partial denture has been repoured from a secondary impression, any supporting "foot" on the retention frame that the laboratory may have provided will no longer be in contact with the cast. Closing pressure within the flask may distort the unsupported extension of the metal framework, with subsequent rebound upon deflasking. The finished denture base will then lack contact with the supporting tissues, resulting in denture rotation about the fulcrum line similar to that occurring following tissue resorption. To provide support for the distal extension of the metal framework during flask closure, a self-curing resin should be sprinkled or painted around the distal end of the framework and allowed to harden before proceeding with packing the denture resin.

PROCESSING THE DENTURE

Processing follows the same procedure as that for a complete denture. Denture base characterization may be added just prior to packing. This is most desirable where denture base material will be visible. Posterior resin bases alone ordinarily do not require characterization, but the dentist should select a denture base material that closely resembles the color of the surrounding tissues. The ideal resin base material for partial dentures is therefore one that (1) may be used without trial packing, (2) possesses a shade that is compatable with surrounding tissues, and (3) is dimensionally stable and accurate.

Layered Silicone Rubber Flasking. There has never been any question as to the merits of tin-foiling the denture before investing, which results in a tin foil-lined matrix and eliminates the need for a separating film. The fact remains, however, that the use of a tin-foil substitute has become almost universal.

At best, any tin-foil substitute creates an undesirable film at the gingival margins of the teeth, resulting in microscopic separation between the teeth and the surrounding resin. This may be shown by sectioning a finished denture and by observing the marginal discoloration around the necks of the teeth after several months in the mouth. To some extent, injection molding obviates this objection to the use of a tin-foil substitute—which is one of the principal advantages of injection molding over compression molding.

Since the use of compression molding is widespread and is likely to continue, some method is needed which eliminates the use of a tin-foil substitute. The layered silicone rubber method results in more complete adaptation of the resin around the necks of porcelain teeth and more complete bonding to resin teeth. In addition, denture base tints may be applied directly to the mold without first applying a separating film.

A room-temperature-curing silicone rubber which has sufficient body and toughness for the purpose is applied to the wax surface of the denture and over the teeth just prior to pouring the upper half of the flask. The manufacturer's instructions must be followed as to mixing and time elapsed before adding the outer stone investment to ensure curing and bonding to the overlying investment. Boilout is then completed in the usual way.

A further advantage of the layered silicone rubber method is the ease with which deflasking is accomplished. If the wax carving of the denture has been completed with care prior to flasking, denture tints remain unaltered by unnecessary trimming and polishing of the processed denture.

All resin base materials available up to the present time exhibit some dimensional change, both during processing and in the mouth. The fit of the denture is therefore dependent, to a large extent, upon the accuracy, or lack of accuracy, of the denture base material, since impression and cast materials in use today are themselves reasonably accurate. In an attempt to minimize dimensional changes in the denture base, materials and techniques are constantly being improved. Some of these (such as Luxene, Jectron, and Tilon) use injection molding to provide a continuous source of material to the mold as curing shrinkage occurs. One technique (Hydro-cast denture processing) utilizes hydraulic pressure within the top half of the flask to limit the shrinkage toward the cast only. It is claimed, by the originator of this technique, that processing by any other means results in both a distorted mold and a distorted cast, due to collapse of the stone or plaster around the myriad of small air voids inevitably present. Evidence of this distortion can be seen when the cast is returned to the remounting surface on the articulator and seems to lend support to the claim that compression molding does result in a slightly distorted cast.

Compression molding resins in a doughy state are giving way to the use of materials such as Duraflow, Muco-Tone, and Pour-a-Densene that may be poured into the mold or placed into the mold in a very soft state, thus eliminating trial packing and excessive pressures which lead to open flasks and altered vertical dimension. Activated, or cold curing, resins are sometimes used to avoid mold expansion occurring at higher temperatures. Materials other than acrylic resins are used with various techniques, some of these being styrene, vinyl, and, experimentally, epoxy resins. The main objective behind the development of newer techniques and materials is greater dimensional accuracy and stability, combined with strength and better appearance.

The study of the history of denture base materials is a most interesting one that has been covered elsewhere in dental literature. The future of denture base materials promises to be just as fascinating a study, but such a discussion cannot be included within the scope of this book. With newer materials, the future of methyl methacrylate as a denture base material is uncertain despite its acceptance as the best material available for this purpose since its introduction in 1937. While it has made possible the simulation of natural tissue color and contours combined with ease of manipulation, the fact remains that it leaves much to be desired so far as accuracy and dimensional stability are concerned. Whether or not other and newer materials will eventually supplant methyl methacrylate as a denture base material remains to be seen. The fact is that the denture base of the future (1) must be capable of accurately reproducing natural tissue tones faithfully through the use of characterizing stains and customizing procedures and (2) must not require elaborate processing procedures and equipment which would make the cost prohibitive for general usage.

REMOUNTING AND OCCLUSAL CORRECTION

As long as dimensional changes continue to occur during the processing of resin denture bases or the resin attachment of denture teeth to metal bases, the processed denture will need to be remounted on the articulating instrument for the purpose of correcting the altered occlusion. Even with improved denture base materials and processing techniques, some errors will still occur due to the dimensional instability of the set-up wax. So until both sources of error can be eliminated, remounting will continue to be necessary.

The only alternate to remounting is the correction of the occlusion in the mouth. As has been discussed previously, the limitations to doing so successfully depends upon the number of teeth involved, the stability of the denture bases, the accessibility of the occlusion, and the ability of the dentist to interpret and correct occlusal discrepancies.

How well the occlusion may be perfected by remounting will depend upon the manner in which jaw relations were transferred to an instrument and how closely the instrument is capable of reproducing functional occlusion. But even though the articulator is capable of reproducing only a static, centric relation, that relation at least should be re-established prior to delivery of the denture.

While it is admitted that there are limitations to the perfection of eccentric occlusion in the mouth, there are some who believe that it can be done with more accuracy than on an instrument that is incapable of reproducing eccentric positions. Correction for errors in centric occlusion, however, should not be included in this philosophy, for such is based upon a premise that centric occlusion may be satisfactorily established by intraoral adjustment, followed then by a perfecting of eccentric occlusion. Because of denture instability and the inaccessibility of the occlusion for analysis, this is presuming more than anyone can justify. Even occlusal adjustment of natural dentition, where each tooth has its own support, can best be done when preceded by an analysis of articulated study casts.

One cardinal premise must be accepted if prosthetic dentistry is to be anything more than a haphazard procedure. This is *that it is possible to transfer centric jaw relations to an instrument with accuracy and maintain this relation throughout the fabrication of the prosthesis.* If this is true, then centric occlusion, coinciding either with centric jaw relation or with centric occlusion of the remaining natural teeth, or both, must have been established prior to delivery of the prosthesis. This means that occlusal correction by remounting after final processing is an absolute necessity to the success of the restoration. The term *remounting* is also applied to the mounting of a completed prosthetic restoration back onto an instrument using some kind of intraoral interocclusal record. This should not be confused with remounting for the purpose of perfecting occlusion *prior* to delivery of the denture. The latter is for the purpose of correcting for processing errors, whereas the former is for the purpose of adjusting to denture settling and to denture movement caused by tissue instability. Remounting after delivery is not ordinarily done with partial dentures because of the presence of some remaining natural teeth which are capable of supporting and stabilizing the prosthesis during post-insertion adjustments. With complete dentures, on the other hand, remounting from an intraoral interocclusal record permits occlusal adjustment with a degree of accuracy not possible intraorally. There are those who believe strongly that all complete dentures should be so remounted and that occlusal adjustment should be done on an instrument at some reasonable interval after delivery of the dentures. In this way, occlusal discrepancies arising from denture settling may be interpreted and the necessary adjustments therefor made.

Remounting after processing is accomplished by returning the cast to a keyed relationship with the articulator mounting. While the use of metal mounting plates attached to both surfaces may be desirable, it is not practical to do so with a partial denture cast. Stone to stone or stone to plaster, properly keyed and free of debris, provides a sufficiently accurate surface for remounting.

A simple procedure which greatly enhances the accuracy of the remounting surfaces is the making of a stone split cast. After beveling and keying the base of the master cast, a separating film is applied and the inverted cast is encircled with a strip of lead boxing material. A thin layer of hard stone of a different color is then vibrated onto the base of the cast, and the exposed surface is left purposely uneven. Paper clips or washers may be partially embedded for added retention. After this thin layer of stone has hardened, it is attached to the articulator with mounting plaster. Separation of the cast from the articulator and any subsequent remounting are then accomplished with opposing stone surfaces, resulting in greater accuracy than is possible with a stone cast against mounting plaster alone.

It is most important that the mounting surfaces be free of particles that would prevent re-establishment of their original relationship. Therefore, tin foil of about .002 inch thickness should be applied to the base of the cast prior to investing. This is easily accomplished by coating the surface of the cast with petrolatum and then applying the tin foil smoothly with the aid of a cloth towel. The original mounting surface of the cast is thus protected from contamination, and, on stripping away the tin foil after deflasking, the original surface may be returned to its original position. The opposing mounting surface on the articulator should be brushed and blown free of particles and then the base of the cast secured to it with sticky wax or modeling plastic. Plaster may then be used for additional security, but only after the cast has first been secured with some reliable thermoplastic material. *A layer of cement, such as Duco cement, should never be used as it introduces an intervening film that interferes with the accuracy of the remounting.*

Precautions to Be Taken in Remounting. The following precautions should be taken to assure the accuracy of remounting for the purpose of making final occlusal adjustment prior to the polishing and delivery of the denture. These apply to all types of occlusal relationship records but are directed particularly to remounting to an occlusal template, where stone vertical stops are used.

1. Make sure that the base of the cast has been reduced before keying and mounting, so that it will not have to be altered later to get it into the flask.

2. Bevel the margins of the base of the cast so that it will seat in a definite boxlike manner in the articulator mounting.

3. Notch the two sides and the dorsal aspect of the base to further assure its return to its original position. Notches at the margins are preferable to depressions within the base, as the former permits a visual check of the accuracy of the remounting.

4. Lubricate lightly the base and sides of the cast before mounting to facilitate easy removal from the mounting plaster.

5. Tin-foil the base and sides of the cast prior to flasking, so that traces of investment will not be present to interfere with remounting.

6. When remounting, secure the cast to the articulator with sticky wax or modeling plastic, followed by plaster over both the mounting and the sides of the cast.

7. Before adjusting the occlusion, make certain that no traces of investment remain on the vertical stops.

8. Take care not to abrade the opposing occlusal surface during occlusal adjustment. The use of marking tape or inked ribbon is preferable to articulating paper. The denture tooth is less likely to cut through and mar the opposing surface, and ink or dye will not build up a false opposing surface as will the wax from articulating paper.

9. Occlusal readjustment to an occlusal template is complete when the stone vertical stops are again in contact. With other types of articulator mountings, readjustment is complete when the vertical pin is again in contact and any valid horizontal excursions are freed of interference.

Occlusal readjustment, as was the original articulation, is at the expense of the original tooth anatomy. Occlusal surfaces should be reshaped by adding grooves and spillways and by reducing the area of the occlusal table, thus improving the masticating efficiency of the denture tooth. While this may be done immediately following occlusal readjustment and prior to delivery of the denture, it may be deferred until final adjustment in the mouth has been completed. In any case, it is a necessary step in the completion of any removable prosthesis.

Porcelain teeth may be reshaped with abrasive or diamond mounted points. Plastic teeth lend themselves better to reshaping since inverted cone and fissure burs may be used to restore functional anatomy. Either should be repolished judiciously to avoid reduction of cusp contacts. While cusps may be narrowed, spillways added, and the total area of contact reduced to improve masticating efficiency, critical areas of contact, both vertical and horizontal, must always be preserved.

POLISHING THE DENTURE

The areas to be considered in the polishing of a partial denture are (1) the peripheries of the denture bases, (2) the facial surfaces, and (3) the teeth and adjacent areas.

The peripheries on full metal bases will have been established previously. On partial metal bases and full resin bases, the accuracy with which the periphery may be finished will depend upon the accuracy of the impression record and how well this was preserved on the stone cast. Edentulous areas recorded from impressions in stock trays generally lack the accuracy at the peripheries that is found on casts made from impressions in individual trays and by secondary impression methods. Peripheral accuracy is determined also by whether or not the impression recorded a functional or a static relationship of the bordering tissue attachments.

Denture Peripheries. The principal objectives to be considered in making an impression of edentulous areas of a partially edentulous arch are (1) maximum support for the partial denture base and (2) extension of the peripheries to obtain maximum coverage compatible with moving tissues. While this second objective may be obtained with an adequate individual impression tray, it is best accomplished with a secondary impression method such as a correctable fluid-wax impression. Not only should the *extent* of the periphery be recorded accurately but also its *width*. Both extent and width as recorded should be preserved on the stone cast. With the exception of certain areas which are arbitrarily thinned in polishing (mentioned previously in this chapter), finishing and polishing the denture peripheries should consist only of removing any flash and artifactual blebs. Otherwise the periphery should be left as recorded in the impression.

When the impression is made in a stock tray, both the extent and the width of the periphery will have been influenced by the tray itself. Some areas will be left short of the total area available for denture support, while others will be extended beyond functional limits by the overextension of the tray. In such areas the technician must interpret the anatomy of the mouth as best he can and arbitrarily trim the denture borders just short of obvious overextension. This presumes an intimate knowledge of the anatomy of the mouth which the technician may or may not possess. Any overextension remaining after arbitrarily trimming the periphery may then be corrected in the mouth.

Facial Surfaces. The facial surfaces of the denture base are those polished surfaces lying between the peripheries and the supplied teeth. Methods have been proposed for making sectional impression records of buccal contours, thereby permitting the denture base to be made to conform to facial musculature. These have never received wide acceptance and may be considered impractical.

Facial surfaces may be established in wax or may be carved into the denture base after processing. Generally, it is desirable that it be done in wax as part of the wax pattern, both because it is easier to do so and because contours can best be established at a time when additions can be made if desired. Buccal surfaces should be made concave to aid in the retention of the denture by muscle molding, to preserve the peripheral roll and thereby prevent food impaction, and to facilitate return of the food bolus back onto the masticating table. Lingual surfaces should be made concave to provide tongue room and to aid in the retention of the denture. If such contours are established previously in wax, finishing is not only more easily accomplished but peripheral and gingival areas are also less likely to be inadvertently altered. Polishing of concave surfaces is always more difficult than flat and convex surfaces, and this can largely be avoided by taking care to contour and polish the wax pattern prior to investing.

Finishing Gingival and Interproximal Areas. The contouring of gingival and interproximal areas in the cured resin is difficult and generally unsatisfactory. The practice of doing so dates back to the days when vulcanite rubber was trimmed and shaped with Pearson-type chisels and a trimming block was a necessary piece of equipment in any dental laboratory. Finishing was done with vulcanite burs and with brush wheels and pumice, creating the vertical interproximal grooves that for many years were typical of the "denture look." Not only is this contrary to modern concepts of denture esthetics but also gingival and interproximal carving of the denture resin around plastic teeth may not be done without some damage to the teeth themselves.

Modern cosmetic considerations demand that gingival carving be done around each tooth individually, with variations in the height of the gingival curve and in the length of the interdental papillae. Interproximally, the papillae should be convex rather than concave. The gingival attachment should be free of grooves and ditches that would accumulate debris and stain and should be as free-cleansing as possible. All of this precludes gross shaping and trimming of gingival areas *after* processing. Gingival carving should be done in wax, and investing should be done with care to avoid blebs and artifacts. Finishing should consist only of trimming around the teeth and the interdental papillae with small round burs to create a more natural simulation of living tissue, plus light stippling with an off-center round bur for the same reason. Polishing should consist only of light buffing with brush wheels and pumice and finally with a brush wheel coated with wax or soap.

Pumicing of gingival areas can only serve to polish the high spots, and although it may be done lightly, its use should be limited to light buffing of areas already made as smooth as possible by other means. Not only does heavy pumicing of the denture resin create a typical "denture look" but it also alters the surface of any plastic teeth present. If pumicing must be done, plastic teeth should be protected with adhesive tape during the process.

Any polishing operation on a partial denture done on a lathe is made hazardous by the presence of clasp retainers, which can easily become caught in the polishing wheel. While the least damage that might occur is the distortion of a clasp arm, there is a greater possibility that the denture may be thrown forceably into the lathe pan with serious damage to the framework or other parts of the denture. The operator must be ever conscious of this possibility and always cover any projecting clasp with the finger while it is near the polishing wheel. In addition, it is wise to keep a pumice pan well filled with wet pumice to cushion the shock should an accident occur. Any other lathe pan used in polishing should be lined with a towel or with a resilient material such as automotive undercoating material for the same reason.

Frush has listed the following rules for varying the height of the gum line at the necks of the teeth:

(a) Slightly below the high lip line at the central incisors.
(b) Lower than the central incisor gum line at the lateral incisors.
(c) Higher than the central or lateral incisor gum line at the cuspid.
(d) Slightly lower than the cuspid at the bicuspid and variable for both bicuspids and molars.*

The correctly formed interdental papilla should be so formed that it will be self-cleansing. It should be so carved that it is in harmony with the interpretation of age and will be the deciding factor in the visible outline form of the tooth. As Frush has pointed out, even a drop of wax properly placed can change the appearance of a square tooth to one of tapering or ovoid appearance. A properly formed interdental papilla further enhances the natural appearance by increasing the color in this area.

---

*From Frush, J. P.: Dentogenic Restorations and Dynesthetics, Los Angeles, 1957, Swissedent Foundation.

The rules for forming the interdental papilla are given by Frush as follows:

(a) The papilla must extend to the point of tooth contact for cleanliness.
(b) The papillae must be of various lengths.
(c) The interdental papilla must be convex in all directions.
(d) The papillae must be shaped according to the age of the patient.
(e) The papilla must end near the labial face of the tooth and never slope inward to terminate towards the lingual portion of the interproximal surface.*

Frush's instructions for finishing a denture that has been carefully waxed prior to investing are as follows:

(1) Trim excess flash from the periphery and, if any, from around the necks of the teeth.
(2) Trim the lingual of the teeth and establish lingual "cutaways" or valleys behind any anterior interdental spaces.
(3) Stipple the labial-buccal surfaces with a No. 5 round bur (eccentric).
(4) Refine the papillae with first a No. 1 round and finally with a No. ½ round (eccentric) bur.
(5) Polish the periphery and the palatal or lingual surfaces. Then lightly polish the stippled surface (labial-buccal) with a No. B-12 brush wheel and pumice.
(6) High shine the periphery and palate (and lingual), but not the labial-buccal surface.*

The instruments for finishing the denture* are as follows:

CC trimmers	2B and 5A	Periphery and palate
Fissure bur	No. 562	Frenum
No. 2 bur	Straight	For cleaning the necks of the teeth and interdental spaces
No. 8 bur	Eccentric	Rough carving of the labial face of the denture
S. S. White	Points No. 12, B2, and B28	Lingual cutaway on the palate of the denture behind the anterior teeth
Torit wet or dry fine water-proof discs ⅞″		Outline the necks and the papillae
No. 5 bur	Eccentric	Carve the papillae, the labial face of the denture, the necks of the teeth and finer stippling
Nos. 1 and ½ burs	Eccentric	Refine the carving and facial shape of the papillae

*From Frush, J. P.: Dentogenic Restorations and Dynesthetics, Los Angeles, 1957, Swissdent Foundation.

Chapter 18

Delivery, adjustment, and servicing of the partial denture

Delivery of the completed partial denture should never be sandwiched in between other scheduled appointments. Too often this is done in the delivery and insertion of both complete and partial denture restorations. Both, being removable restorations not requiring the elaborate preparations common to the cementation of fixed restorations, can be quickly inserted and the patient dismissed with instructions to return when soreness or discomfort develops. Perhaps this is where the word "patient" originated, because of the patience and fortitude required in accommodating to a new denture.

While it is true that this is a necessary part of adjusting to new dentures, many other factors are also pertinent. Among these are how well the patient has been informed as to the mechanical and biologic problems involved in the fabrication and wearing of a removable prosthetic restoration and how much confidence he has acquired in the excellence of the finished product through his own observation of the various steps in its construction. Knowing in advance that every step has been carefully planned and executed with skill, and having acquired confidence both in the dentist and in the excellence of the restoration, the patient is better able to accept the adjustment period as a necessary, but transient, step in learning to wear the prosthesis. Much of this confidence can be dissipated when the dentist inserts the prosthesis with an air of finality as though to imply that "my part in the fabrication of this restoration is now completed. The rest is up to you, including payment of the fee on your way out of the office."

The term "adjustment" has two connotations, each of which must be considered separately. First is the adjustments to the bearing surfaces of the denture and the occlusion made by the dentist at the time of delivery and thereafter. Second is the adjustment or accommodation by the patient, psychologically and biologically, to the presence of a foreign body which is to serve as a prosthetic res-

437

toration of some missing part or parts of the body, in this particular case, an oral prosthesis.

It must be presumed that the partial denture has been fabricated with care and that the prosthesis is representative of the best that the dentist and technician are capable of producing. Certainly it is not within the scope of this book to suggest ways and means of adjusting a faultily designed or poorly fabricated prosthesis to fit the patient's mouth. But, as in industry, a casting is rarely, if ever, considered a precision product. Certain machining operations are necessary before the casting is considered finished and acceptable. So it is with a partial denture restoration. First, the rough metal alloy casting must be ground, adjusted, and polished by the technician to fit an accurate stone cast of the patient's mouth. Following the processing of resin bases, the occluding teeth must be ground so as to perfect the occlusal relationship between opposing artificial dentition or between artificial dentition and an opposing cast or template. Denture bases then must be ground to eliminate excess and to perfect the contours of polished surfaces for the best functional and esthetic result. All of these are machining operations made necessary by the inadequacies of casting procedures, for actually both the metal and resin parts of a prosthetic restoration are produced by casting methods. Unfortunately, such machining operations in the laboratory do not eliminate entirely the need for final adjustment in the mouth, which is also, in effect, a machining process to perfect the fit of the restoration to the oral tissues.

Included in this final step in a long sequence of machining procedures necessary to produce a biologically acceptable prosthetic restoration are the adjustment of the occlusion to accommodate the occlusal rests and other metal parts of the denture, the adjustment of the bearing surfaces of the denture bases in harmony with the supporting soft tissues, and the final adjustment of occlusion on the artificial dentition to harmonize with natural occlusion in all mandibular positions.

Occlusal Interference From the Denture Framework. Any occlusal interference from occlusal rests and other parts of the denture framework will usually have been eliminated prior to or during the establishment of occlusal relations. Assuming that the denture framework will have been tried in the mouth before establishing a final jaw relation, any such interference should have been detected and eliminated. Much of this need not exist at all if mouth preparations and the design of the denture framework are carried out with a specific treatment plan in mind. In any case, occlusal interference from the framework itself should not ordinarily require further adjustment at the time the finished denture is inserted. For the dentist to have sent an impression or casts of the patient's mouth to the laboratory and receive back a finished partial denture prosthesis without having once tried the cast framework in the mouth is not only a dereliction of his responsibility to the patient but is also, in effect, handing the practice of prosthetic dentistry over to the dental laboratory technician. However, where such is done, it is obvious that occlusal interference from the casting itself must be first detected and eliminated before proceeding with other adjustments to the denture.

Adjustments to the Bearing Surfaces of the Denture Bases. The machining of bearing surfaces to perfect the fit of the denture to the supporting tissues should be accomplished by the use of some indicator paste. The paste must be one that will be readily displaced by positive tissue contact and will not adhere to the tissues of the mouth. An area of the denture base showing through the film of indicator paste may be erroneously interpreted as a pressure spot, when actually the paste had adhered to the tissues in that area. Therefore, only those areas showing through an intact film of indicator paste should be interpreted as pressure areas and be relieved accordingly.

Rather than dismiss the patient with instructions to return when soreness develops and then over-relieve the denture over a traumatized area to restore patient comfort, the use of pressure indicator paste should be routine with any tissue-bearing prosthetic restoration. The paste should be applied in a thin layer over the bearing surfaces and then both occlusal and digital pressure applied to the denture. The patient cannot be expected to apply a heavy enough force to the new denture to register all of the pressure areas present. Therefore, the dentist should apply both vertical and horizontal forces with his fingers in excess of that which might be expected of the patient. The denture is then removed and inspected. Any areas heavy enough to displace a thin film of indicator paste should be relieved and the procedure repeated with a new film of indicator until pressure areas have been eliminated.

Pressure areas most frequently encountered are as follows: in the mandibular arch—the lingual slope of the mandibular ridge in the premolar area, the mylohyoid ridge, the peripheral extension into the retromylohyoid space, and the distobuccal periphery in the vicinity of the ascending ramus and the external oblique ridge; in the maxillary arch—the inside of the buccal flange of the denture over the tuberosities, the periphery of the denture lying at the malar prominence, and the pterygomaxillary notch where the denture may impinge on the pterygoid bursa. In addition, in either arch there may be bony spicules or spicules of the denture base itself which will require specific relief.

The amount of relief by machining that will be necessary will depend upon the accuracy of the impression registration, the accuracy of the master cast, and the accuracy of the denture base. Despite the accuracy of modern impression and cast materials many denture base materials leave much to be desired in this regard, and the element of technical errors is also always present. It is therefore essential that discrepancies in the denture base be detected and corrected before the tissues of the mouth are subjected to the stress of supporting a prosthetic restoration. This is one of our major responsibilities to the patient, that trauma be always held to a minimum. Therefore, the appointment time for the delivery of the denture must be adequate to permit such adjustment at the time of initial insertion.

Adjustment of Occlusion in Harmony With Natural and Artificial Dentition. The final step in the adjustment of the partial denture at the time of insertion is the adjustment of the occlusion to harmonize with the natural occlusion in all mandibular excursions. Where opposing partial dentures are inserted concurrently, the adjustment of the occlusion will parallel, to some extent, the adjustment of occlusion on complete dentures. This is particularly true where the few remaining natural teeth are out of occlusion. But where *one or more* natural teeth may occlude in any mandibular position, those teeth will influence mandibular movement to some extent. It is necessary, therefore, that artificial dentition on the partial denture be made to harmonize with whatever natural occlusion remains.

The methods by which occlusal relations may be established and recorded have been discussed in Chapter 16, Occlusal Relationships for Partial Dentures. In this chapter the advantages of establishing a functional occlusal relationship with an intact opposing arch have been discussed and also the limitations which exist to the perfecting of harmonious occlusion on the finished prosthesis by intraoral adjustment alone. Even when the occlusion on two opposing partial dentures is being adjusted entirely in the mouth, it is best that one arch be considered an intact arch and the other one adjusted to it. This is accomplished by first eliminating any occlusal interference to mandibular movement imposed by one denture and adjusting any opposing natural dentition to accommodate to the denture teeth. Then the opposing partial denture is inserted, and occlusal adjustments are made to harmonize with both the natural dentition and the opposing denture which is now considered part of an intact dental arch. Which denture is adjusted first and which one made to occlude with it is somewhat arbitrary, with the following exceptions: If one partial denture is entirely tooth supported and the other has a tissue-supported base, the tooth-supported denture is adjusted to final occlusion with any opposing natural teeth and then that arch is treated as an intact arch and the opposing denture adjusted to occlude with it. If both partial dentures are entirely tooth borne, the one occluding with the most natural teeth is adjusted first and the second denture then adjusted to occlude with an intact arch. Tooth-borne segments of a composite (tooth- and tissue-supported) partial denture are likewise adjusted first to harmonize with any opposing natural dentition. The final adjustment of occlusion on opposing tissue-supported bases is usually done on the mandibular denture since this is the moving member, and the occlusion is made to harmonize with the maxillary denture which is treated as part of an intact arch.

Intraoral occlusal adjustment is accomplished by using some kind of indicator and suitable mounted points and burs. Diamond or other abrasive points must be used to reduce enamel and metal contacts. These may also be used to reduce plastic tooth surfaces, but burs may be used for this purpose with greater effectiveness. Articulation paper may be used as an indicator if one recognizes that heavy interocclusal contacts may become perforated, leaving only a light mark, while secondary contacts, being lighter and frequently sliding, may make a heavier mark. Although articulation ribbon does not become perforated, it is not easy to use in the mouth, and the differentiation between primary and secondary contacts is difficult to ascertain.

In general, occlusal adjustment of multiple contacts between natural and/or artificial dentition where partial dentures are involved follows the same principles as those for natural dentition alone. This is because the partial dentures are retained by devices attached to the abutment teeth, whereas with complete dentures no mechanical retainers are present. The use of more than one color of articulation paper or ribbon to record and differentiate between centric and eccentric contacts is just as helpful in adjusting partial denture occlusion as natural occlusion, and for the initial adjustment this method may be used.

For final adjustment, however, since one denture will be adjusted to occlude with an intact arch, the use of an occlusal wax is necessary to establish points of excessive contact and interference. This cannot be done by articulation paper alone. An occlusal wax, such as Kerr occlusal indicator, which is adhesive on one side, or strips of 28-gauge Kerr green casting wax or other similar soft wax, may be used. It should always be used bilaterally, with two strips folded together at the midline. Thus the patient is not as likely to deviate to one side as he is when wax is introduced unilaterally. (Fig. 237.)

For centric contacts, the patient is asked to tap into the wax and then the wax is removed and inspected under transillumination for perforations. All perforated areas are either premature contacts or excessive contacts and must be removed. One of two methods may be used to locate specific areas to be relieved. Articulation paper may be used to mark the occlusion, and then those marks representing areas of excessive contact are identified by referring to the wax bite and are relieved accordingly. A second method is to introduce the wax strips a second time, this time adapting them to the buccal and lingual surfaces for

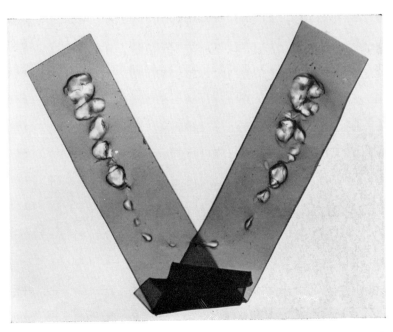

Fig. 237. Two strips of 28-gauge soft green (casting) wax are inserted in the mouth between opposing dentition. These are first folded over anteriorly to unite the two halves, and then the patient is asked to tap in centric occlusion two or three times. Viewed out of the mouth, against a source of light, uniform contacts free of perforations may be considered to be simultaneous contacts. Perforations in the wax represena occlusal prematurities which should be relieved.

retention. After having the patient tap into the wax, perforated areas are marked with waterproof pencil. The wax is then stripped off and the penciled areas are relieved. This procedure has been outlined in some detail by Jankelson.

Whichever method is used it must be repeated until occlusal balance in centric occlusion has been established and more uniform contacts without perforations are evident from a final interocclusal wax record. After centric adjustment has been completed, Jankelson suggests that the patient should be asked to "open and eat the wax lightly" several times. Any remaining areas of interference are then reduced, thus assuring that there is no interference during the chewing stroke. Adjustments to relieve interference during the chewing stroke should be confined to buccal surfaces of mandibular teeth and lingual surfaces of maxillary teeth. This serves to narrow the cusps so that they will go all the way into the opposing sulci without wedging as they travel into centric contact. Skinner proposed that the patient be given a small bite of soft banana to chew rather than to expect him to chew without food actually being present. The small bolus of banana promotes normal functional activity of the chewing mechanism, yet by its soft consistency does not itself cause indentations in the soft wax. Any interfering contacts encountered during the chewing stroke are thus detected as perforations in the wax, which are marked with pencil and relieved accordingly.

Kyes has described some of the advantages to be had with an alginate interocclusal record, supplementing or replacing the use of soft wax strips for this purpose (Fig. 238). An alginate hydrocolloid impression material is applied to the occlusal surfaces of the mandibular teeth, and the patient is asked to bring the teeth together as previously rehearsed until the first point of contact is made. This occlusion is then held until the material has set. The gelled hydrocolloid is carefully removed from the open mouth and the excess carefully trimmed away with scissors; it is then dropped into a plaster bowl of water until it has become firmer and easier to handle without tearing. This record of occlusion may be observed in water with a dark bowl as a background, or it

Fig. 238. An alginate hydrocolloid interocclusal record. Perforations in the alginate are interpreted as areas of hyperocclusion. These are then located on the teeth with articulating ribbon and relieved accordingly.

may be observed by transillumination. In any case, areas of prematurity may be seen as perforations in the alginate and the over-all areas of occlusal contact interpreted for evidence of hyperocclusion. Occlusal adjustment may then proceed, using either articulating ribbon or perforations in suitable wax strips as a specific indication of areas to be relieved.

This method is primarily diagnostic and is usually supplemented by the use of articulating ribbon or occlusal wax. However, it has definite advantages over the latter two as a diagnostic aid because the impression materials offer no resistance to closure. Further, because of its soft consistency and because it is applied over all occluding surfaces simultaneously, a natural stimulus to closure is effected. This method may be used effectively between natural, artificial, or mixed dentition.

Adjustments to occlusion should again be repeated at a reasonable interval after the dentures have settled to a point of equilibrium and the musculature has become adjusted to the changes brought about by restoration of occlusal contacts. This second occlusal adjustment may usually be considered sufficient until such time as tissue-supported denture bases no longer support the occlusion and corrective measures, either by reoccluding the teeth or relining the denture, must be employed. However, a periodic recheck of occlusion at intervals of six months or annually is advisable to avoid traumatic interference resulting from changes in denture support or tooth migration.

Following the adjustment of occlusion, the anatomy of the artificial teeth should be restored to maximum efficiency by restoring grooves and spillways (food escapeways) and by narrowing the teeth buccolingually to increase the sharpness of the cusps and reduce the width of the food table. Mandibular buccal and maxillary lingual surfaces in particular should be narrowed to assure that these areas will not interfere with closure into the opposing sulci. Since artificial teeth used on partial dentures opposing natural or restored dentition should always be considered *material* out of which a harmonious occlusal surface is created, final adjustment of the occlusion should always be followed by the meticulous restoration of the most functional occlusal anatomy possible. While this may be done following a subsequent occlusal adjustment at a later date, there is always the possibility that the patient may fail to return on schedule and, in the meantime, broad and inefficient occlusal surfaces may cause an overloading of the supporting structures, which would be traumatogenic. Therefore, the restoration of an efficient occlusal anatomy is an essential part of the denture adjustment at time of insertion. Again, this requires that sufficient time be allotted for the insertion of the partial denture to permit all of the necessary occlusal corrections to be accomplished.

Instructions to the Patient. Finally, before dismissing the partial denture patient, he should be advised of the difficulties that may be encountered and of the care that must be given the prosthesis and the abutment teeth.

The patient should be advised that he will experience some discomfort initially and that in the beginning the body will reject the prosthesis as an unwanted foreign object. While this is to some extent due to the presence of bulk which the tongue in particular must become accustomed to, any strange object, however comfortable, must be accepted biologically and psychologically before it can become an integral part of the oral mechanism.

The patient must be advised also of the possibility of soreness developing despite every attempt on the part of the dentist to prevent its occurrence. Since patients vary widely in their ability to tolerate discomfort, it is perhaps best to advise every patient as though soreness is inevitable, with every assurance that any needed adjustments will be made. On the other hand, the dentist himself should be aware of the fact that some patients are unable to ever accommodate to the presence of a removable prosthesis. Fortunately, these are few in any practice. But the dentist must avoid any positive statements which might be interpreted or construed by the patient to be positive assurance tantamount to a guarantee that he will be able to wear the prosthesis with comfort and acceptance. Too much depends upon the patient's ability to accept a foreign object and to tolerate reasonable pressures to make such assurance possible.

Perhaps the less said to the patient the better regarding the influence of a prosthesis on normal speech. Demosthenes long ago demonstrated the ability of the human organ to adapt to hindrances to clear speech. Most people who are otherwise free of oral or pharyngeal abnormalities that interfere with the control of air fail to enunciate clearly only because of a lazy or sluggish tongue. Any normal person who is desirous of enunciating clearly may do so if he will make a conscientious effort to form each syllable clearly and distinctly. Furthermore, anyone who has been able to speak clearly before receiving a denture has already demonstrated that he has the necessary anatomic and physiologic equipment for doing so. While new kinesthetic senses must be acquired in order to speak clearly with a prosthesis in the mouth, the adaptiblity of the human speech mechanism is more than adequate to cope with the changes in contours caused by the partial denture.

The hazard of discussing phonetics with the patient in regard to his new dentures is to imply that this is a unique problem to be overcome because of the influence of the prosthesis on speech. With few exceptions, and these are usually due to excessive and avoidable bulk in the denture design or to improper placement of teeth and the contour of denture bases, the average patient will experience little difficulty in wearing the partial denture. Most of the hindrances to normal speech will disappear in a few days.

Similarly, perhaps little or nothing should be said to the patient about the possibility of gagging or the tongue's reaction to a foreign object. Most patients will experience little or no difficulty in this regard, and the tongue will normally accept smooth, nonbulky contours without objection. Contours that are too thick, too bulky, or improperly placed should be avoided in the construction of the denture, but, if present, these should be detected and eliminated at the time of insertion of the denture. The dentist should palpate the prosthesis in the mouth and reduce excessive bulk accordingly before the patient has an opportunity to object to it. The area most frequently needing thinning is the distolingual flange of the mandibular denture. Here the denture flange should always be trimmed during the finishing and polishing of the denture base. Sublingually, the denture flange should be reproduced as recorded in the impression, but distal to the second molar the flange should be arbitrarily trimmed to almost a knife edge. Then, upon inserting the denture, the dentist should palpate this area to ascertain that a minimum of bulk exists which might be encountered by the side and base of the tongue. Should this need further reduction, it should be done and the denture repolished before dismissing the patient.

The patient should be advised of the need for keeping the dentures and the abutment teeth meticulously clean. If cariogenic processes are to be prevented, the accumulation of debris should be avoided as much as possible, particularly around abutment teeth and beneath minor connectors. Furthermore, inflammation of gingival tissues is prevented by removing acccumulated debris and by substituting toothbrush massage for the normal stimulation of tongue and food contact with areas that will be covered by the denture framework.

The mouth and partial denture should be cleaned after eating and before retiring. Brushing before breakfast may also be effective in reducing the bacterial count, which may help to lessen acid formation in the caries-susceptible individual after eating. A partial denture may be effectively cleaned by the use of a small, stiff-bristle brush. Debris may be effectively removed through the use of dentifrices, since they contain the essential elements for cleaning. Household cleaners should not be used as they are too abrasive for use on resin surfaces. The patient, and the elderly or handicapped patient in particular, should be advised to clean the denture over a basin partially filled with water so that the fall will be broken should the denture be accidentally dropped during cleaning.

In addition to brushing with a dentifrice, additional cleaning may be accomplished by the use of a solvent cleaning solution such as D.O.C. (denture oxygen cleanser) or a solution made of one part Clorox to two parts Calgon. The patient should be advised to soak the dentures in the solution for fifteen minutes once daily, followed by a thorough brushing with a dentifrice.

In some mouths, the precipitation of salivary calculus on the partial denture necessitates the taking of extra measures for its removal. Such patients may need to be provided with a small bottle of Taxi liquid stain detergent, with instructions to apply the solution to the denture at weekly intervals to dissolve the accumulated calculus. The Taxi should be used on the denture only when it is out of the mouth and then the denture should be rinsed thoroughly before returning it to the mouth.

Since many patients will dine away from home, the informed patient should provide some means of carrying out a midday oral hygiene. Simply rinsing the partial denture and the mouth with water after eating is beneficial if brushing is not possible.

Opinion is divided on the question of whether or not a partial denture should be worn during sleep. Conditions should determine the advice given the patient, although generally the tissues should be allowed to rest by removing the denture at night. In such case, the denture should be placed in a container and covered with water to prevent its dehydration, with subsequent dimensional change. About the only situation that justifies the wearing of partial dentures at night is where stresses generated by bruxism would be more destructive since they would then be concentrated on fewer teeth. Broader distribution of the stress load, plus the splinting effect of the partial denture, may make the wearing of the denture at night advisable in such cases.

There occurs frequently the question of whether an opposing complete denture should be worn when a partial denture in the other arch is out of the mouth. The answer is that if the partial denture is to be removed at night, the opposing complete denture should not be left in the mouth. There is no more certain way of destroying the alveolar ridge which supports a maxillary complete denture than to have it occlude with a few remaining anterior mandibular teeth.

After all of the necessary adjustments to the partial denture have been made and the patient has been advised as to the proper care of the denture, he must also be advised as to the future care of the mouth to ensure health and longevity of the remaining structures. How often the mouth and denture should be examined by the dentist depends upon the oral and physical condition of the patient. If the patient is caries-susceptible or has tendencies toward periodontal disease or alveolar atrophy, his mouth should be examined more frequently. Every six months should be the rule if conditions are normal. At least once a year a roentgenographic examination should supplement clinical examination and oral prophylaxis.

The need for increasing retention on clasp arms to make the denture more secure will depend upon the type of clasp that has been used. Increasing retention should be accomplished by adjusting the clasp arm to engage a deeper part of the retention undercut rather than by bending the clasp in toward the tooth. The latter creates only frictional retention which violates the principle of of clasp retention. Being an active force, such retention contributes to tooth and/or appliance movement in a horizontal direction, disappearing only when either the tooth has been moved or the clasp arm returns to a passive relationship with the abutment tooth. Unfortunately, this is almost the only adjustment that can be made to a half-round cast clasp arm. On the other hand, the round wrought-wire clasp arm may be adjusted cervically and brought into a deep part of the retentive undercut. Thus the passivity of the clasp arm in its terminal position is maintained, but retention is increased by its being forced to flex more in order to withdraw from the deeper undercut. The patient should be advised that the abutment tooth and the clasp will serve longer if the retention is held to a minimum, which is only that amount necessary to resist reasonable dislodging forces.

Denture rocking or looseness developing in the future may be due to a change in the form of the supporting ridges instead of to a lack of retention. This should be detected as early as possible after it occurs and corrected by relining or rebasing. The loss of tissue support is usually so gradual that the patient may be unable to detect the need for relining. This must usually be determined by the dentist at subsequent examinations as evidenced by rotation of the free-end denture about the fulcrum line. If the partial denture is opposed by natural dentition, the loss of base support causes a loss of occlusal contact which may be detected by having the patient close upon wax strips placed bilaterally. If, however, a complete denture or free-end partial denture opposes the partial denture, the interocclusal wax test is not dependable since occlusal contact may have been maintained by posterior closure, changes in the temporomandibular joint, and/or migration of the opposing denture. In such case, evidence of loss of ridge support is determined solely by the indirect retainer leaving its seat as the free-end denture rotates about the fulcrum line.

There can be no assurance given to the patient that uncrowned abutment teeth will not decay at some future time. Even with full cast crowns, there can be no positive assurance that the tooth will not ever decay gingival to the crown, as a result of gingival recession and caries attack of exposed cementum. The patient can be assured, however, that prophylactic measures in the form of meticulous oral hygiene and the avoidance of carbohydrates, coupled with routine prophylactic care by the dentist, will be rewarded by greater health and longevity of the remaining teeth.

The patient should be advised that maximum service may be expected from the partial denture if he observes the following rules:

1. Avoid careless handling of the denture which may lead to distortion or breakage. Damage to the partial denture occurs while it is out of the mouth, as a result of dropping it during cleaning or an accident occurring when the denture is not being worn. Fractured teeth and denture bases can be repaired, as can broken clasp arms, but a distorted framework can rarely, if ever, be satisfactorily readapted or repaired.

2. Teeth should be protected from caries by proper oral hygiene, proper diet, and frequent dental care. The teeth will be no less susceptible to caries where a partial denture is being worn but may be more so due to the retention of debris. At the same time, the remaining teeth have become all the more important as a result of oral rehabilitation, and abutment teeth have become even more valuable because of their importance to the success of the partial denture. Therefore, the need for a rigid regime of oral hygiene, diet control, and periodic clinical observation and treatment is essential to the future health of the entire mouth. Also the patient must be more conscientious about responding to being recalled at stated intervals by the dentist for examination and necessary treatment.

3. Periodontal damage to the abutment teeth can be avoided by maintaining tissue support of any free-end bases. As a result of periodic examination this can be detected and corrected by relining or whatever procedure is indicated.

4. Partial denture service must be accepted as something that cannot be considered permanent but must receive regular and continuous care by both the patient and the dentist. The obligations for maintaining caries control and for returning at stated intervals for servicing must be clearly understood, as well as the fact that regular charges will be made by the dentist for whatever service is rendered.

The partial denture patient should not be dismissed as completed without at least one subsequent appointment for observation and minor adjustment if needed. This should be made at an interval of two to four days after delivery of the denture. It need not be a lengthy appointment but should be made as a definite rather than a drop-in appointment. Not only does this give the patient assurance that any necessary adjustments will be made and provide the dentist with an opportunity to check on the patient's acceptance of the prosthesis but it also avoids giving the patient any idea that he may break into the dentist's schedule at will and serves to give notice that an appointment is necessary for future adjustments.

Chapter **19**

Miscellaneous partial prosthodontics

*John J. Sharry, B.S., D.M.D.**

The prosthetic replacement of tissue defects, which were either surgically or developmentally acquired, depends very often upon removable appliances that are retained by clasps on the teeth.

We shall discuss certain considerations which do not supplant but rather supplement those general principles of design that apply in the usual partial denture. Such things as the pharyngeal portion of a cleft palate appliance and the obturator that closes the defect resulting from a hemisection of the maxilla impose further burdens on the usual designs. These dislodging forces must be considered and included in that design which will be used for any particular case.

There are several types of prostheses which depend for their retention on a partial denture framework. We shall attempt to describe a representative few because the variations are myriad and do not lend themselves to classification.

CLEFT PALATE PROSTHESES

The cleft palate obturator is one of the most common and is the obturator concerning which most has been written. (Various other appliances often referred to as maxillofacial prostheses will be discussed in more general than specific terms later.)

Classification. Cleft palates lend themselves to morphologic classifications. The simplest and perhaps the most easily remembered is that of Veau. He proposed four classes: Class I, where the cleft involves only the soft palate; Class

___
*Professor and Chairman, Department of Prosthetic Dentistry, University of Alabama School of Dentistry, Birmingham, Ala.

Fig. 239. Veau's classification of cleft palates.

II, which involves the soft and hard palates but not the alveolus; Class III, which involves the soft and hard palates, continuing through the alveolus on one side of the premaxillary area; and Class IV, which involves the soft and hard palates, the cleft continuing through the alveolus on both sides, leaving a free premaxilla (Fig. 239). The latter two classes are usually, though not always, associated with a cleft lip.

Etiology. The etiology of cleft palate is not clear but seems at the present time to have some basis in heredity, although many other factors have been mentioned, such as infectious diseases of the mouth, mechanical interferences in the fetus, nutritional inadequacies, and various changes in the intrauterine environment.

Personality Evaluation. The personality range of individuals with a cleft palate is not much different from that of the general population. Perhaps more of them fall into the quiet, unresponsive, withdrawn category and a few exhibit a brashness or bravado (which disappears with continued association). We find, however, that a large share are well-adjusted, pleasant people. Sometimes we wonder how so many can be happy when the attitude of the parents and the public is often such that a considerable degree of overprotection or rejection is the fare of these cleft palate individuals when they are children.

There are a few areas in which certain differences of approach are necessary in treating such persons. For example, we find so often that their speaking habits are so poor that we cannot understand them. This difficulty will usually disappear with continued association, but initially a relative can interpret for them. If they are alone, then a paper and pencil will solve the problem.

Anatomy. During the examination of clefts that have not been operated upon, the practitioner should examine the nasal and pharyngeal cavities and their component structures and, by using a blunt instrument, ascertain the tissue consistency of various areas. It should be noted here that the gag reflex of the person with a cleft palate is markedly diminished and does not usually hinder palpatory examination.

The knowledge of the anatomic structure of these cavities serves not merely to satisfy our intellectual curiosity but, more important, it also places us on familiar ground when and if we should have to remove impression materials that may inadvertently be forced through the cleft or perforation while obtaining impressions of the dental arches.

The normal soft palate either closes the nasal cavity from the pharynx or the oral cavity from the pharynx, or it just relaxes as the occasion demands (Fig. 240). If this "valve" is not whole, then, of course, it cannot effectively perform these closing functions but rather allows food to enter the nasopharynx during deglutition and air to enter the nasal cavity during the production of those speech sounds wherein the air should be directed into the oral cavity. Further, it makes the production of such sounds as "puh" and "kuk" practically impossible.

There is a group of muscles attached to the soft palate which are responsible for the closure of the nasal cavity. This total action (closing off the nasal cavity) is called the velopharyngeal closure. To accomplish this the following, more or less simultaneous, muscular contractions take place.

The levator veli palatini muscle, which originates on the petrous portion of the temporal bone and the cartilage of the eustachian tube and runs downward and forward to insert into the palatine aponeurosis, contracts, pulling the soft palate upward and backward (Fig. 241). This is a paired muscle, and upon entering the soft palate it merges with its fellow of the opposite side, form-

Fig. 240. The three positions of the soft palate during normal activity.

MED. PTERYGOID PLATE

EUSTACHIAN TUBE

SALPINGOPHARYNGEUS

LEVATOR PALATINI

TENSOR PALATINI

HAMULAR PROCESS

PALATOPHARYNGEUS

SUPERIOR CONSTRICTOR

VERTEBRA

Fig. 241. Dissection of the velopharyngeal area as seen from the side.

A

B

TENSOR VELI PALATINI

LEVATOR VELI PALATINI

SALPINGOPHARYNGEUS

AZYGOS UVULAE

SUPERIOR CONSTRICTOR

C

Fig. 242. Musculature of the soft palate as seen from above. **A,** The area of section **B,** The portion of section used. **C,** Detail of section.

Fig. 243. Passavant's cushion in the posterior pharyngeal wall.

ing a sling. At the same time, the tensor veli palatini, which arises from the
scaphoid fossa, the sphenoid spine, and eustachian cartilage, travels downward
and forward to the lateral aspect of the hamulus (which is used as a pulley),
swings medially to enter the soft palate, contracts, and effects tension on the
soft palate. Now the soft palate has been pulled backward and upward.

But the pull is not sufficient to close the gap between the distal limits of the
soft palate and the pharynx, so the pharynx accommodates by moving forward
and medially. This is accomplished by the joint action of three muscles. The
pterygopharyngeal portion of the superior constrictor, which originates usually
on the medial pterygoid plate, travels backward fanwise to terminate in a
median raphe in the posterior pharynx. It contracts and pulls the posterior
pharyngeal wall forward to meet the soft palate. (Fig. 242, *A*, *B*, and *C*.) Meanwhile, since this action may not be quite enough in certain instances, the palatopharyngeus muscle, which we can see in the throat as the posterior pillars of
the tonsil and which has two parts, the thyropalatal and pharyngopalatal portions, comes into play. The latter part, which arises in the palatal aponeurosis
and travels backward and downward to insert in a fanwise fashion in the posterior pharynx anterior to, but interlaced with the superior constrictor fibers, contracts strongly. It is more or less circular and it further attempts to approximate
the soft palate and pharynx and, in doing so, produces a ridge or "bunching up"
of the posterior pharyngeal musculature, called Passavant's cushion (Fig. 243).
This is usually, though not always, visible in the patient with a cleft palate. It it
located at levels varying from as high as the region of the atlas to as low as the
level of the distally projected mandibular occlusal plane. Now the soft palate
is touching the posterior pharyngeal wall, but there is a leak where the lateral
aspect of the soft palate does not meet the lateral aspect of the pharynx. This
will be closed by the salpingopharyngeus muscle. This muscle arises from the
cartilage of the eustachian tube and travels downward and laterally to fan out

and insert in the lateral pharyngeal wall. When it contracts it pulls the lateral wall medially, thus closing the last gap in velopharyngeal closure. All these muscle contractions take place almost simultaneously. The velopharyngeal mechanism has now closed the nasal cavity from the oral cavity and pharynx. This movement is used in deglutition to prevent food from entering the nose and in speech when pronouncing the so-called plosive sounds, puh, buh, tuh, duh, kuh, guh. These sounds are produced by closing off the nose and building up pressure in the mouth and suddenly releasing it. Thus the name "plosive."

The second position, the closure of the oral cavity, is a result of the contraction of the following. The thyropalatal portion of the palatopharyngeus muscle arises from the posterolateral rim of the thyroid cartilage and courses upward through the posterior pillar to insert into the palatine aponeurosis, where it merges with its fellow of the opposite side, forming an inverted U. When it contracts it pulls the soft palate down toward the tongue. Meanwhile, the tensor is flattening the dome of the soft palate to bring down that portion of the structure which may not come down with the action of the thyropalatal muscle. Concurrently, the tongue is forced upward and backward. To finally eliminate the possibility of a leak, the palatoglossus muscle, which is attached superiorly to the palate and inferiorly to the tongue, forming more or less a sphincteric structure in this motion, contracts and completes the approximation. Therefore, it can now be seen that velopharyngeal closure *is not* a simple sphincteric action of the superior constrictor and palatopharyngeus muscles (which run in a nearly horizontal direction) but is instead the resultant contraction of these and others running in a vertical direction, such as the levator, tensor, and the salpingopharyngeus muscles. This second position is used in sucking and in the pronunciation of sounds such as "ng" in the word sing. The third position finds the palate relaxed as in normal breathing.

Pathology. The patient with a cleft palate, because of his inability to close off the nose, is constantly the victim of nasal infections and middle ear infections sometimes resulting in deafness. He cannot correctly pronounce the plosive sounds and tries to overcompensate with his tongue. He tries to make the latter obturate the cleft and articulate at the same time. These habits are an obstacle to the speech correctionist who must attempt to train the patient to forget these habits and learn a new set of movements.

Despite some of these difficulties, the patient can be nourished adequately, and aside from the possibility of constant nasal and pharyngeal infections, he may be generally quite healthy. Nevertheless, the inability to speak properly constitutes his greatest problem.

Physiology of Speech. Speech is a function of respiration, phonation, resonation, articulation, and integration. Respiration is, of course, concerned with the exchange of air by the lungs; phonation is accomplished by the abduction and adduction of the vocal cords which change the pitch of the voice; resonation is realized in the nasal, oral, and pharyngeal cavities, which are the prime resonation chambers. The teeth, tongue, lips, and palate serve as articulatory mechanisms, and all, of course, would be nothing without the integrating facilities of the human brain. (Fig. 244.)

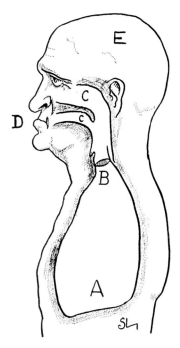

Fig. 244. The mechanisms of speech. **A,** Respiratory organ (lungs). **B,** Phonating organ (vocal cords). **C,** Resonating chambers (oral and nasal cavities). **D,** Articulating organs (lips, tongue, and teeth). **E,** Integrating center (brain).

The soft palate performs any one of the following basic functions in speech. It closes off the nasal cavity, as in producing "k" and hard "g"; it closes off the oral cavity for production of the sounds "m," "n," and "ng" (as in "ring"), or it may close neither cavity completely but allow varying portions of the air stream to enter the appropriate resonating chambers.

Although the soft palate is but one part of the velopharyngeal mechanism (the other part being the pharyngeal muscles), it is of such importance that when cleft, the individual cannot effect velopharyngeal closure.

Surgical Treatment. Two general types of physical treatment can restore partially or completely the function of the soft palate. The first concerns surgical procedures to close the soft palate (and the hard palate when involved). The other utilizes an artificial appliance, called an obturator, which serves not to close the soft palate but rather to fill the space between the two halves of the palate. (Both the surgical and prosthetic approaches are usually of little avail without speech therapy, given previously, conjointly, or subsequently.) The surgical approach is generally concerned with the closure and, in many cases, the lengthening of the palate. Closure is achieved by denuding the opposing edges of the two halves of the cleft palate and suturing them together. This may necessitate lateral relaxing incisions parallel to the long axis of the cleft which will allow it to be apposed and sutured together (Fig. 245, *A* and *B*). Lengthening of the palate may be accomplished by an anterior incision of the palatine mucosa which

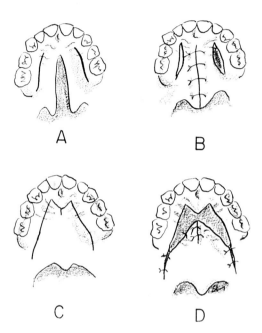

A   B

C   D

Fig. 245. Surgical procedures in cleft palate therapy. A, Relaxing incisions in the palatal mucosa. B, Mucosa elevated and displaced medially where freshened edges of the cleft are sutured together. C, Incision for push-back operation. D, Push-back completed and sutured.

Fig. 246. The pharyngeal flap operation viewed from the side. The flap is based below.

may run from the area of the molars on one side around back of the anterior teeth (avoiding the anterior palatine foramen) to the molars on the opposite side (Fig. 245, *C* and *D*). The palatine mucosa posteriorly and medially to this incision is dissected from the palatine bone and displaced backward, thus lengthening the soft palate. The denuded palatine bone anteriorly becomes epithelized via granulation tissue.

In those cases where the general types of operation are not feasible, the surgeon may perform a pharyngeal flap operation, wherein a longitudinal flap is dissected from the posterior pharyngeal wall (its attachment being located either below or above) and is brought forward and sutured to the denuded posterior edge of the soft palate (Fig. 246). This then forms a continuous tissue bridge between the soft palate and the pharynx, which functions well as part of the velopharyngeal mechanism. The flap, as dissected, tends to curl medially, leaving lateral space for air transmission through the nasal cavity. Since a great deal of the pharyngeal closing movement is in a medial direction, one can see that this action can aid in velopharyngeal closure because the lateral walls converge medially toward the flap. There are more definitive surgical approaches to the cleft palate, but they are generally concerned with either of these two aims.

Prosthetic Treatment. The prosthetic approach utilizes a metal framework on the order of a partial denture framework in which is included a posterior latticework extension into the area of the cleft (Fig. 247). This extension supports an acrylic resin bulb, which is the obturator.

Fig. 247

Fig. 248

Fig. 247. The ladderlike extension of the framework into the area of the cleft.
Fig. 248. The use of utility wax to confine impression material to the tissues.

The preservation of the patient's teeth is of prime importance, for although obturators have been made for edentulous cases, they can never be as efficient as those that utilize the teeth for stabilization. Therefore, we must immediately do all of the restorative dentistry necessary. In a large percentage of cases we are faced with the problem of restoring occlusal harmony, and therefore our patient may first require orthodontic treatment. When we see a patient with good occlusion, no active caries, and no periodontal disease or other oral lesions, we may start construction of the prosthetic appliance.

Impressions With Alginate Hydrocolloid Impression Materials. The examination will reveal the nature of the unrepaired cleft or, if repaired, those perforations which sometimes result from tissue breakdown. One should look particularly in the anterior mucobuccal fold for minute oronasal perforations following the repair of Classes III and IV clefts.

A resilient impression material must be used because of the many tissue undercuts. The alginate hydrocolloid impression materials serve this purpose adequately.

The problems incident to impressions are divided into two groups; the unrepaired cleft presenting one situation, the repaired cleft, another. We shall consider first the unrepaired cleft palate, Classes II, III, and IV. (The method of obtaining impressions of the teeth are not modified by Class I clefts.) When using a hydrocolloid impression material, we should dam the posterior of the tray with boxing or utility wax to prevent material from flowing down the throat. In addition, the use of this wax adjacent to the cleft or perforation will more accurately record the mucosal detail by confining the impression material to those areas. (Fig. 248).

The material should be prevented from entering the nasal cavity in such a large quantity that it may fracture from the main body of material. Such an accident requires a tedious process of fragmentation and removal. To prevent this, we simply underload the tray in the area of cleft. The tooth-bearing section of the tray is completely filled with the alginate, but the area corresponding to the cleft is loaded to a height of only 2 to 3 mm. Thus, when the tray is seated, the material is not likely to be forced upward into the cleft in sufficient quantity to "lock."

Cleft palates previously repaired present slightly different problems. The palatal repair itself may look adequate, and yet we find that there may be an oronasal perforation in the labial mucobuccal fold as previously mentioned. If it is present, we must either pack this perforation with wet gauze (in many cases the perforations are too small for this approach) or else we must "underload" the tray in this area so that great amounts of the impression material will not be forced into the nasal cavity.

Amounts small enough to be dislodged by blowing the nose should not concern us. Larger amounts, however, require a considerable degree of skill in their fragmentation and removal as *they cannot be pushed into the mouth as in unrepaired cases and must be manipulated within the nasal cavity.*

Those perforations which may exist on the palate itself should be approached in a similar manner. If the area is large enough to pack off with wet gauze, then

Fig. 249. Arrow shows buccal bar which may occasionally be used.

this is the method of choice. If the diameter is a half inch or more, then perhaps it is better to handle it like an open cleft, using utility wax damming and under-loading the tray in that area.

Framework. The design of the so-called framework is of primary importance, as it must be so balanced as to eliminate, as much as possible, harmful torque effects on the teeth. The essential requirements for the casting consist of the following: (1) The metal to be used should be as thin as possible commensurate with strength so that metal bulk does not cause an added obstacle to speech. (2) The tip of the clasp should engage a distal undercut on the most posterior abutments because the displacing force downward is usually concentrated in the pharyngeal area. The type of clasp will vary with the case and will follow the precepts of good partial denture design. The patient with a full complement of teeth presents us with some little difficulty in clasping. This may be solved by the use of a buccal bar, making possible the crossing of only one embrasure on each side (Fig. 249). However, if adequate undercuts are not present or if the caries index is very high and the patient must have full crowns, this is not neces-sary, as embrasure space may be included in the crowns. One disadvantage to the buccal bar is the imperfect esthetic effect on those patients who show their molars when smiling. However, this is a question of values, and thus it may be that the bar is preferable to cutting healthy teeth. Generally, we prefer to use full crown coverage and thus eliminate the buccal bar while at the same time pro-tecting the teeth.

Of course, as in any partial denture case, there should be adequate bracing for each retaining arm of the clasp, as well as proper occlusal rests.

The pharyngeal portion is usually attached to the framework by a distal loop or "ladder" from the casting. The superoinferior position of the loop will vary according to the type of prosthesis.

Obturator Design. There are three main types of obturators: the so-called hinge or movable type, the fixed type, and the meatus type (Fig. 250, *A, B,* and *C*). The hinged type is connected to the main framework by means of a

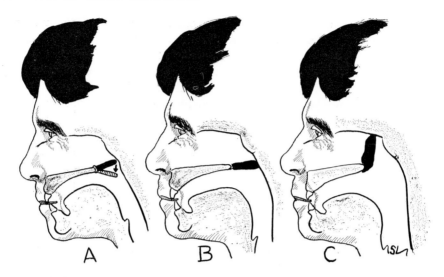

Fig. 250. The location of the pharyngeal portion of the several obturators. **A,** The hinge type. **B,** The fixed type. **C,** The meatus type.

hinge. Its bulk is located above the cleft edges and supposedly serves an anatomic purpose in that it moves up and back, supported by the soft palate edges, as does the normal soft palate to effect velopharyngeal closure. Theoretically, this is workable, but in practice it is not quite true because many cleft palates have limited motion and many authors feel that this type of obturator is limited in use to a very few cases. The fixed type is stationary and is directed toward Passavant's pad. It depends on the forward movement of the pad and lateral movement of the pharynx to effect closure. This is the obturator in most general use today and, if made well, is relatively efficient. The meatus obturator we shall speak of later because of the difference in construction.

PHARYNGEAL IMPRESSIONS. The method of obtaining impressions for the hinge type or the fixed type is essentially the same. It involves the following steps: A mound of modeling plastic approximating the pharyngeal defect in shape and size is placed on the distal extension and warmed. This bulk is directed as high above the area of Passavant's pad as feasible and is placed into the patient's mouth while still warm. When the framework is seated properly on the teeth, the patient is instructed to swallow, tilt the head back, and then place the chin on the chest. Keeping it there, he should turn the head from left shoulder to right shoulder. (Fig. 251). This total routine should be accomplished quickly in order to mold the modeling plastic while it is still warm. The resultant impression is then removed from the mouth and compared with the defect. Gross inadequacies are noted and, if necessary, more material is added. The modeling plastic impression is then removed and all excess trimmed. It should have a superoinferior thickness of not more than 5 to 6 mm. in order to keep it as lightweight as possible.

Experience in making impressions for a fixed type of appliance (and occasionally the hinge type) has taught us that attempts to obtain accurate detail in impressions by means of the "wash" materials may be abandoned. There is a certain amount of leakage that will occur around any obturator, and this leakage does not affect the efficiency of the appliance. When the patient swallows, there is a vigorous excursion of the pharyngeal musculature; when he talks, there is less movement of it. Because the appliance must be made comfortable enough to enable the patient to swallow, an air leak will occur during ordinary speech. Furthermore, the musculature changes its shape, and the detail obtained from a wash impression will not be maintained on tissue topography for any length of time.

The procedures used for making impressions for cleft palate prostheses may well be due for re-evaluation. Recently, several children for whom orthodontic appliances were to be constructed were examined jointly by an orthodontist and a prosthodontist. It was decided that removable appliances which combined orthodontic and prosthodontic treatment should be constructed. However, it was believed that it would be wise to provide the prosthodontic treatment in several progressing steps in order to avoid any antagonism on the part of the child toward the obturating section.

Accordingly, impressions of the pharyngeal area were avoided, and some firm wax was attached to the palatal portion of the acrylic resin appliance which had been finished. The wax extension was constructed initially to such a dimen-

Fig. 251. Positions of the head for muscle-trimming the pharyngeal impression.

sion that it would not contact the pharyngeal tissues at any time. Acrylic resin was then substituted for the wax and the patient wore this "bulb" for one week. The next week the "bulb" was enlarged to contact one or two small areas during swallowing. We were planning to accustom the child gradually to a mass of material in the nasopharynx and then to obtain an impression of the tissues in that region. However, it was noted that when the "bulb" was enlarged (by means of hand molding), there was a marked improvement in the nasal quality of the voice.

Further empirical enlargement of the "bulb" was made at the next appointment. There was some further improvement of the voice, but it was not as dramatic as that of the second appointment. Finally, the pharyngeal impression was made, and the finished appliance was placed. The voice quality was not improved over that of the previous week. The results in several succeeding patients treated in this same manner suggested that it may not be necessary to obtain detailed impressions for pharyngeal obturators.

It has been interesting to note again and again the secondary role that surgical and prosthetic procedures play in the correction of cleft palate speech. We may work hard and provide our patients with an excellent technical result, but even with our understandable enthusiasm, we are not entirely satisfied with the vocal results. Conversely, we often see patients for whom relatively little has been done, and yet with all their lack of physical equipment, they speak reasonably well. We are convinced that the procedures per se do not always make the correction. They merely provide the equipment, and personality, either the patient's or the therapist's, or both, heals. Nevertheless, we need to provide the best equipment possible.

MEATUS OBTURATOR. We shall consider the pharyngeal impression for a meatus obturator as a separate section here. The meatus obturator is formulated on the presumption that complete occlusion of the oropharynx from the nasopharynx is not necessary for good cleft palate speech. It is believed, rather, that the partial occlusion of the nasal cavity will result in a marked diminution and, in many cases, complete elimination of the nasal sound that is so apparent and so objectionable in the patient with a cleft palate. If the appliance fulfills this objective, the logopedist, who, when using other appliances, has to train certain muscles to reduce the hypernasality and others to conquer the articulative defects, need direct his efforts only toward correcting the latter. He need not concern himself with the muscle-training incident to reducing nasality. This in turn should reduce the number of training sessions necessary to improve speech for any particular patient.

This type of obturator ignores Passavant's pad and the posterior pharyngeal wall. Instead it makes contact with the superior aspect of the nasal cavity at the junction of nasal and pharyngeal cavities.

In other words, whereas the usual fixed type of obturator is directed in a line more or less parallel to and continuous with the palate, this type is inclined perpendicularly to the palate (Fig. 252).

The construction is not complicated. The upper casting is finished with the usual loop projecting into the cleft and is checked in the mouth for accuracy.

Fig. 252. Side view of a meatus obturator showing its relation to the framework.

Fig. 253. Frontal view of the meatus obturator showing the vents.

Using this framework as a vehicle, softened modeling plastic is molded around the distal loop with its greatest bulk directly above the loop. When the modeling plastic is hard, it is removed. More softened material is added and the denture framework is reinserted. Then an attempt by the patient is made to blow air through the nose. If air escapes, then small amounts of modeling plastic are added in likely areas until no air escapes through the nose and the patient talks as though he had a bad cold (the so-called rhinolalia clausa). The impression is removed from the mouth, and at this time any projection of material into the eustachian tubes should be cut from the impression to allow free interchange of air.

The completed impression is invested, boiled out, and processed in acrylic resin. After polishing, it is placed in the patient's mouth to check for gross errors in processing. When it is satisfactory, a vent about 3 mm. in diameter is cut in an anteroposterior direction, approximately in the center and free of the turbinates and vomer. If the latter is very large, it may be necessary to make two smaller holes on either side. (Fig. 253.)

This opening serves as a means of breathing through the nose. The appliance is put back into the mouth and the patient is instructed to speak. If the voice sounds "closed," the aperture is enlarged until a balance between the closed and open "nose" is reached. Immediately upon inserting the prosthesis and balancing

Fig. 254. Model of repaired cleft palate with its appliance. Four remaining maxillary teeth, which do not occlude with mandibular teeth, are crowned and act as retentive mechanism for a façade prosthesis. The occlusion is established entirely on the denture.

the size of the hole, the resultant nasality should improve. Only the articulative defects remain and these are not as unpleasant because of the normal nasal quality. There is usually no gagging tendency and no irritation of the mucous membrane. When the physical situation permits the use of any type of obturator, the decision as to which should be used must be determined by individual preference rather than by intrinsic value.

We prefer to use the meatus type whenever possible because it generally brings the fastest and most dramatic results. It can be used whenever the opening is almost as large as the nasopharynx or when the palatal sides are soft and pliable enough to admit the bulk of impression material to that area. The fixed obturator can be used in any case suitable for a palatal prosthesis and is used probably most often. Its results are not consistently as dramatic as the meatus obturator or it would be preferred in all cases. The hinge type has been used successfully by many workers and has much merit, although we have made only infrequent use of it because of personal preference for the other two types.

Psychologic Aspects. The psychologic aspects of cleft palate prostheses cannot be overemphasized. We often see maxillary dental arches which are underdeveloped in those patients who have had early surgical closure. If the orthodontist is unable for any reason to correct these malocclusions, the patient is left with an underdeveloped middle third of the face. This pseudo-Class III appearance can be somewhat diminished by a façade prosthesis. In these instances, all teeth have to be crowned and the prosthesis is fashioned anterior to these teeth for proper appearance. Fig. 254 shows an extreme case where only four teeth remained and these were not occluding with any of the mandibular teeth. The façade prosthesis was fashioned to improve the appearance and also to provide a masticating unit.

MAXILLOFACIAL PROSTHESES

There are many oral defects that are the results of corrective surgery or of accidental trauma. The prosthetic replacement of lost oral structure has to be approached with some caution since the remaining tissues are very often scarred and more reactive to pressures. The presence of teeth is a great boon to the prosthodontist who may treat such persons. It is well known that attempts to replace the tissue lost in a hemisection of the palate is extremely difficult *in the edentulous patient*. If worn at all, such prostheses are maintained largely by the active will of the patient and to a lesser degree by the usual biophysical factors.

When teeth are present in the mouth, the construction of the prosthesis is divided into three phases: (1) the complete and perfect restoration of all the remaining teeth and periodontal tissues; (2) the design and construction of the metal framework; and (3) the construction of the tissue replacement section. The first phase should include full crown coverage whenever necessary for restoration of carious areas, for protection from carious processes, and whenever necessary to provide retentive areas for clasp arms.

As in cleft palate therapy, the loss of any of the teeth places a burden on remaining teeth, and the loss of all teeth is catastrophic. We must resort to any measures that will preserve the integrity of the remaining teeth, including the splinting together of several teeth.

Although the detailed design of the metal framework will vary with each case, two general principles must be considered. First, the bracing aspects of the design must be emphasized. For example, every molar and premolar tooth remaining after a hemisection of the maxilla should have a bracing arm, in order to distribute torque forces adequately (Fig. 255). Second, retentive clasp arms should be so designed that they resist the displacement forces of the finished appliance. It must be remembered that weight alone is often an important displacement force in these appliances. We shall further consider weight in a subsequent paragraph.

Fig. 255. Prosthetic treatment of maxillary hemisection. **A,** All of the posterior teeth remaining after a hemisection of the maxilla should have reciprocal arms in order to distribute widely the downward dislodging force of the unsupported side. **B,** When the corrected impression is obtained, all of the original cast except the teeth and adjacent gingival tissues is cut away, and a new cast is poured into the corrected impression. The dotted line separates the new section from the original section of the cast.

The tissue replacement section of the prosthesis is very important because, of course, it serves the primary function of this type of appliance. When the framework has been checked in the mouth for accurate fit, an acrylic resin impression tray is fashioned as part of the framework. This impression tray is underextended at least 1 mm. in all directions. The periphery is now accurately recorded in low-fusing stick compound. When this is done, all compound areas which contact tissue are scraped 0.5 mm. and the final impression is obtained in polysulfide rubber material.

The original cast is now sawed so as to remove all the tissue-borne section and leave only the teeth and adjacent gingival portion. The impression and framework is replaced accurately on the remainder of the cast, and a new tissue section is poured into the final impression. Thus a corrected cast is available for processing.

The utmost care must be exercised to avoid even the slightest compression in the area of remaining tissue. This is extremely important in patients whose defects are due to cancer surgery, because any tissue irritation in these areas is potentially dangerous. This is especially true if irradiation therapy followed surgery. Mechanical attempts to lock appliances into tissue undercuts by ingenious sectional devices are hazardous.

As we mentioned previously, weight is a considerable displacing factor, and when prostheses demand thickness and bulk, they should be constructed in such a way that they are hollow. This is an easy process today with the autopolymerizing resins which are available. These enable us to process a hollow appliance and cap it with a lid sealed with autopolymerizing resin.

When constructing prostheses after radical surgery of the face or neck, one must be prepared to alter them to accommodate for changes in tissue topography. The latter result from altered physiology in connection with lymph drainage and fluid drainage in general. Sometimes these patients will have a very marked difference in the tissue fluid content of their facial tissues from morning to night. This may prove very difficult to the prosthodontist because if the prosthesis fits in the morning, it will be loose in the afternoon, and if it fits in the afternoon, it may cause sore spots in the morning. In general, the former situation is to be preferred. Accordingly, it may be better to take all impressions in the morning.

Furthermore, the process of scar contraction may continue for several weeks or months, which will demand continual revision of the prosthesis.

One final word about scarring. We should never attempt to restore facial contour when considerable pressure against scar tissue is required to do so. This again may cause ulcers, displacement of the appliance, movement of the teeth, or all three.

When setting teeth in an appliance such as that which replaces a hemisection of the maxilla, it should be remembered that the tissue which bears the force of occlusion is of poor quality. Therefore, the occlusion should be set to just lightly contact on the affected side. In some instances, it may be preferable to eliminate occlusal contact entirely, in order to avoid any pressure. The patient should be instructed to avoid chewing on the affected side. He now has a difficult situation, but it is better for him to eat only on one side without soreness than to eat on both and develop constantly irritated tissue areas.

This brings us to the psychologic aspects of such prostheses. We realize that these particular patients have been through a difficult period. The thoughts of losing large tissue blocks are matters of concern to the most callous. The realization that the resultant defects in speech or appearance may be permanent does not encourage him. The patient should therefore be informed that the prostheses are available, and a clear assessment of their role should be offered to him.

The practitioner should never dispel this hope with talks of failure. Nor should he build false hopes with talk of great success. Indeed, he should consider his own chances of creating a successful prosthesis. Then the patient should be encouraged to cooperate in the building of the appliance and be encouraged to wear it. Negative approaches are poor. If you dwell unduly on the chance of failure, you are making a bad mistake. Instead, tell the truthful story of the happy people who wear these types of appliances successfully.

It occurs to me that there is a great deal of difference between the following statements:

1. There are 40 per cent of people who wear these appliances happily and successfully.
2. There are 60 per cent of people who cannot wear these appliances.

The former is encouraging, the latter deadening. Use a positive bright approach, being careful not to build up false hopes. Building a very bleak picture can seriously affect the patient's attitude toward the prosthesis.

Years of constructing these cleft palate and surgical prostheses have convinced us that it is perhaps the most rewarding branch of prosthetic dentistry. These patients are not petty, arrogant people; they are indeed appreciative and cooperative and a pleasure to know.

Temporary and treatment
partial dentures

Temporary dentures may be classified according to the purpose for which they are used.

Temporary Partial Dentures. Temporary partial dentures are made for economic or other reasons where the use of such an appliance is justified. For example, a patient may be preparing to make a trip and time does not permit the making of adequate mouth preparations and a more complete partial denture service. Or the patient may be in poor health or be facing some medical or surgical emergency. Or a very young person may have lost teeth prematurely through accident or is missing teeth for other reasons. Either for the sake of appearance or for the purpose of maintaining a space, or both, a temporary partial denture must be made until such time as fixed restorations can be made or more definitive partial denture service is possible.

Where recent extractions must be replaced temporarily while tissues heal or, in younger patients, until the adjacent teeth have reached sufficient maturity to be used as abutments for fixed restorations, the use of a temporary partial denture maintains mesiodistal and occlusal relations until other restorative treatment can be done, and a very acceptable esthetic result can usually be obtained. It is important, however, that the patient or the parents of the younger patient be made aware that any such removable restoration is temporary and may jeopardize the integrity of the adjacent teeth and the health of the supporting soft tissues if worn for a period of years without supportive care. The need for strict oral hygiene and diet control must also be clearly understood and provisions made therefor while a temporary partial denture is being worn. Generally, the younger patient is even more susceptible to caries when wearing a removable temporary appliance, and adequate prophylactic measures must be taken to prevent decalcification and caries in the teeth contacted.

A temporary partial denture may replace only one or more missing anterior teeth or it may replace a number of teeth, both anterior and posterior, in a partially edentulous dental arch. Such an appliance is usually made of acrylic resin, either by a sprinkling method or by waxing, flasking, and processing with either self-curing or thermal-curing resin. It may be retained by wrap-around wrought-wire clasps, Crozat-type clasps, interproximal spurs, or wire loops. In rare instances, separate cast circumferential type clasps may be used, attached to the resin base by a retaining lug.

Whatever the materials and methods of retention used, such partial dentures are *temporary dentures* and a destinction must be made between this type of appliance and a partial denture prosthesis with prepared abutments and rigid all-cast framework construction. *Too frequently a partial denture is constructed by dental laboratories on orders from the dentist, who then delivers it to the patient as a "partial denture," with a fee that is a multiple of the laboratory cost, when it should be considered nothing more than a temporary partial denture.* The patient is being misled (perhaps the word "fleeced" is more appropriate) when such an appliance is purported to be representative of modern restorative dentistry.

Interim Partial Dentures. Interim partial dentures are made for one or more of the following reasons: (1) to maintain a space, (2) to re-establish occlusion, (3) to replace visible missing teeth while definitive restorative procedures are being accomplished, or (4) while the patient is undergoing periodontal or other treatment. Such an appliance serves much the same purpose as a temporary crown or bridge during oral rehabilitation. It may be fabricated the same as a temporary partial denture and may serve for a rather prolonged period of time as mouth preparations proceed toward the time when more permanent partial denture(s) can be constructed.

In some instances, an existing partial denture can be used with modifications as an interim partial denture. Such modifications may include relining and the adding of the teeth and clasps to an existing denture. In other instances, an existing partial denture may be converted to a temporary complete denture for immediate insertion while tissues heal and an opposing arch is prepared to receive a partial denture. In still other instances, a new temporary partial denture must be made to replace missing anterior teeth in a partially edentulous arch which are ultimately to be replaced with fixed restorations. In some instances, the anterior portion of the appliance is then cut away when the fixed restorations are inserted, leaving the remainder of the temporary denture to be worn while posterior abutment teeth are being prepared.

Still another type of interim denture is one where missing posterior teeth are replaced temporarily with a resin occlusion rim rather than with denture teeth. In dental school clinics, it is sometimes impossible to complete treatment in a school year and the continuing student may desire to resume treatment following the summer recess. In such case, occlusion may be maintained, and as in the case of treatment dentures, the tissues may be conditioned by having the patient wear a temporary appliance with posterior occlusion rims that have been adjusted to occlusal harmony.

In the category of interim appliances must also be placed the partial denture that is made to aid the patient in making the transition to complete dentures where total loss of teeth is inevitable. Such a partial denture may also be considered a treatment appliance, since the patient is at the same time being conditioned to the wearing of a removable prosthesis. It should be considered strictly a temporary appliance that provides the patient with an interim restoration for the remaining life of the natural teeth when further restorative treatment of those teeth is impractical or economically or technically impossible.

Such a partial denture may be worn for several years, in the meantime undergoing revision, modification to include additional teeth lost, and/or relining when such becomes necessary or advisable. The dentist should agree to provide such a partial denture only under certain conditions. These are (1) that a definite fee for the service is impossible to predict and that the cost will depend upon the servicing necessary and (2) that when, in his opinion, further wearing of the interim appliance is unwise and jeopardizes the health of the remaining tissues, the transition to complete dentures will proceed.

Treatment Partial Dentures. Treatment partial dentures are used for the following reasons: (1) to establish a new occlusal relationship or vertical dimension, (2) to condition teeth and ridge tissues to better support the partial denture to follow, and (3) to condition the patient to the wearing of a removable prosthesis. In the latter case, the patient's response to wearing a more costly restoration may be evaluated and, in some rare instances, further treatment may be interrupted while the patient becomes conditioned to the wearing of a removable restoration.

Treatment partial dentures may be used as occlusal splints in much the same manner as cast or resin occlusal splints on natural teeth (Figs. 256 and 257). Where total tooth support is available there is little difference between a fixed and a removable occlusal splint except that a removable splint is too likely to be left out of the mouth unless the patient is actually made more comfortable by its presence. This is usually true where temporomandibular joint pathology is alleviated by the wearing of an occlusal splint. In other cases, it may be advisable to cement the removable appliance to the teeth until such time as the patient has become accustomed and dependent upon the jaw relationship provided by the splint.

Both fixed and removable tooth-supported occlusal splints have much in common. Either of them may be eliminated sectionally as restorative treatment is being done, thus maintaining the established jaw relation until all restorative treatment has been completed. It is usually up to the operator whether these be fixed or removable and whether they are made of a cast (silver or gold) alloy or of a resin material.

Where one or more free-end bases exist on an occlusal splint a different situation exists. The establishment of a new occlusal or vertical relation depends too much upon the quality of support the splint receives to ignore the need for the best possible support for any existing free-end base. Both broad coverage and functional basing of tissue-supported bases are desirable, as well as some sort of occlusal rest on the nearest abutments. Any tissue-supported occlusal splint should at least be relined in the mouth with a self-curing reline resin to afford optimal coverage and support for the free-end base.

Fig. 256. Four views showing the use of a removable occlusal splint. **A,** Evidence of over-closure to be corrected by occlusal reconstruction. **B,** A removable occlusal splint for the lower arch using tooth-colored acrylic resin for occlusal surfaces. **C,** The removable splint in the mouth. The occlusal anatomy is the result of an occlusal registration done in wax on the resin base, which is then invested and to which tooth-colored resin is added to reproduce the functional occlusal surfaces that were recorded in wax. **D,** The resulting occlusion with removable splint. This may be adjusted until satisfactory, and then it becomes the vertical dimension, to be maintained by oral rehabilitation.

O. C. Applegate in an article on the choice of partial or complete denture service has emphasized the advantages of conditioning edentulous areas to provide stable support for free-end partial dentures. This is accomplished by having the patient wear a treatment partial denture for a period of time prior to construction of the final base. In the absence of opposing occlusion, stimulation of the underlying tissues by applying intermittent finger pressure to the denture base is advised. Whether the stimulation is from occlusal or finger pressure, there seems to be little doubt that the tissues of the residual ridge become more capable of supporting a free-end partial denture when they have been conditioned by the wearing of a previous appliance.

Abutment teeth also benefit from the wearing of a treatment appliance where such an appliance applies an occlusal load to those teeth, either through occlusal coverage or through occlusal rests. Frequently a tooth that is to be used as an abutment for a partial denture has been out of occlusion for some time. Immediately upon applying an occlusal load to that tooth sufficient to support any

Fig. 257. Cast gold occlusal splints. Following occlusal adjustment, the splints are cemented to the teeth. Since these are made to fit the unprepared natural teeth, they cannot extend beyond the height of contour of each tooth. Surveying is therefore necessary prior to their construction. The splints may be eliminated tooth by tooth as subsequent restorations are being done, thus maintaining the established vertical relationship.

type of removable prosthesis, some intrusion of the tooth will occur. If such intrusion is allowed to occur following the delivery of the final prosthesis, the occlusal relationship of the prosthesis and its relation to the adjacent gingival tissues will be altered. Perhaps this is one reason for gingival impingement which occurs after the denture has been worn for some time, even though seemingly adequate relief had been provided initially. Where a treatment partial denture is worn, such abutment teeth have an opportunity to become stabilized under the loading of the treatment appliance, and intrusion will have occurred prior to making the impression for the master cast. There is sufficient reason to believe that both abutment teeth and supporting ridge tissues are better capable of providing continuing support for the partial denture when they have been previously conditioned by the wearing of a treatment appliance.

Another example of the use of a treatment partial denture is to facilitate the eruption of posterior teeth through the use of an acrylic resin bite plane. Particularly in the younger patient, early loss of some posterior teeth results in either depression or incomplete eruption of the remaining teeth. The most frequently seen example of this is where the molar teeth in one arch are missing and the premolar teeth remain in occlusion. These are then either depressed or were never able to erupt fully because of excessive occlusal loading. Overclosure results, with anterior teeth likewise in excessive contact, leading to orthodontic movement of those teeth and/or excessive vertical overlap. Prosthetic replacement of missing teeth with a partial denture can thus only perpetuate an overclosed relationship unless one of two things is done first. One is to increase the occlusal height of the remaining teeth arbitrarily with restorations. The other is to permit the remaining posterior teeth to attain full eruption by opening the bite anteriorly. Usually the latter method is preferable.

For such treatment, an acrylic resin appliance is made which causes the lower anterior teeth to close against a bite plane while the posterior teeth remain out of occlusion. Some depression of the lower anterior teeth may occur but without ill effect. More important, posterior teeth which have become depressed or were not fully erupted may migrate into a new vertical occlusion as dictated by the amount of opening anteriorly. Once this has occurred, prosthetic replacement of the missing teeth may proceed and the established vertical dimension be maintained with fixed or removable restorations or a combination of both.

• • •

These are the various types of prosthetic appliances for the partially edentulous mouth which are, or should be, considered temporary partial dentures. It is imperative that a distinction be made between these and a true partial denture service and that the patient be advised of the purposes and limitations of such a restoration. In no instance should the patient be misled into believing that an inadequate temporary partial denture is representative of modern prosthetic dentistry.

Relining and rebasing the partial denture

Differentiation between relining and rebasing has been discussed previously in Chapter 1, Terminology. Briefly, *relining* is the resurfacing of a denture base with new material to make it fit the underlying tissues more accurately, whereas *rebasing* is the replacement of a denture base with new material without changing the occlusal relations of the teeth.

In either case, a new impression registration is necessary, using the existing denture base as an impression base for either a closed-mouth or an open-mouth impression. One of several types of impression materials may be used. The impression may be made with a metallic oxide impression paste, with one of the rubber-base or silicone impression materials, with an activated resin used as an impression material, or with a mouth-temperature wax.

In making the decision between a closed-mouth and an open-mouth impression method for relining, one must first consider the reasons for doing so and the objectives to be obtained. Again, it is necessary to differentiate between the two basic types of partial dentures, one being the all-tooth-borne restoration and the other being the tooth-and-tissue-supported restoration or the true partial denture.

RELINING TOOTH-BORNE DENTURE AREAS

When total abutment support is available, but for one reason or another a removable bridge has been the restoration of choice, support for that restoration is derived entirely from the abutment teeth lying at each end of each edentulous span. This support is effective through the use of occlusal rests, boxlike precision rests, internal attachments, and/or supporting ledges on abutment restorations. Except for intrusion of abutment teeth under functional stress, settling of the restoration toward the tissues of the residual ridge is prevented by the supporting abutments. Tissue changes occurring beneath tooth-borne denture bases does not affect the support of the denture and therefore relining or rebasing is usually done for other reasons. These are (1) unhygienic conditions and the trapping of debris between the denture and the residual ridge, (2) an unsightly condition due to the space which has developed, and/or (3) patient discomfort associated with lack of tissue contact arising from open spaces between the denture base and the tissues. Anteriorly, some loss of support beneath a denture base may lead to some denture movement, despite occlusal support and direct retainers located posteriorly. Rebasing might be the treatment of choice if the denture teeth are to be replaced or rearranged, or if the denture base needs to be replaced for esthetic reasons or because it has become defective.

For either relining or rebasing to be accomplished, the original denture base must have been made of a resin material that can be relined or replaced. Frequently, tooth-borne partial denture bases are made of metal as part of the cast framework. These cannot be satisfactorily relined, although they may sometimes be altered by drastic grinding to provide mechanical retention for the attachment of an entirely new resin base. Ordinarily, a metal base, with its several advantages, is not used in a tooth-borne area where early tissue changes are anticipated. A metal base should not be used following recent extractions or other surgery, nor for a long span where relining to provide secondary tissue support may become necessary. (A free-end metal base is ordinarily used only where a partial denture is being made over tissues that have become conditioned to supporting a previous denture base.)

Since the tooth-borne denture base cannot be depressed beyond its terminal position with the occlusal rests seated and the teeth in occlusion, and since it cannot rotate about a fulcrum, a closed-mouth impression method is used. Virtually any impression material may be used, provided sufficient space is allowed beneath the denture base to permit the excess material to flow to the peripheries, where it is either turned by the bordering tissues or, as in the palate, allowed to escape without unduly compressing the underlying tissues. The qualities of each type of impression material must be kept in mind when selecting the material to be used for this purpose. Ordinarily, for short spans a mucostatic type of impression material is used, whereas for longer spans the displacing quality of mouth-temperature wax may be utilized to advantage.

A word should be said in favor of relining a tooth-borne resin base with one of the immediate reline materials, such as Durbase or Self-Set. Where one or more relatively short spans are to be relined, the making of an impression for that purpose requires that the denture be flasked and processed. The possibilities of increased vertical dimension resulting and the denture becoming distorted during laboratory procedures must be weighed against the disadvantages of using a direct reline material. Fortunately these materials are constantly being improved with greater predictability and color stability. The possibility that the original denture base will become crazed or distorted by the action of the activated monomer is nonexistent when the base is made of modern cross-linked resin. However, for this reason earlier resin bases should not be subjected to relining with direct reline resins.

When relining in the mouth with a resin reline material is done with a definite technique, the results can be quite satisfactory, with complete bonding to the existing denture base, good color stability, and with permanence and accuracy. The procedure for applying a direct reline of an existing resin base is as follows.

1. Relieve generously the tissue side of the denture base and just over the peripheries. This not only provides space for an adequate thickness of new material but also eliminates the possibility of tissue impingement due to confinement of the material.

2. Apply masking or adhesive tape over the polished surfaces from the relieved border to the occlusal surfaces of the teeth.

3. Mix the powder and liquid in a glass jar according to the proportions recommended by the manufacturer. First stir red fibers into the monomer, if not already incorporated into the powder, according to the color characteristics of the base being relined.

4. While the material is reaching the desired consistency, have the patient rinse the mouth with cold water. At the same time, wipe the fresh surfaces of the dried denture base with a cotton pellet saturated with some of the monomer. This facilitates bonding and makes sure that the surface is free of any contamination.

5. When the material has first begun to take on some body, but while still quite fluid, apply it to the tissue side of the denture base and over the peripheries. Immediately place the denture in the mouth in its terminal position and have the patient close into occlusion. Then, with the mouth open, manipulate the cheeks to turn the excess at the periphery and establish harmony with bordering attachments. If a mandibular denture is being relined, have the patient move the tongue into each cheek and then against the anterior teeth to establish a functional lingual periphery. It is necessary that the direct retainers be effective to prevent displacement of the denture while molding of the borders is accomplished. Otherwise the denture must be held in its terminal position with finger pressure on the occlusal surfaces.

6. Immediately, remove the denture from the mouth and with fine curved iris scissors trim away gross excess material and any material that has flowed onto proximal tooth surfaces and other components of the denture framework. While this is being done, have the patient again rinse the mouth with cold water. Then reinsert the denture to its terminal position, bringing the teeth into occlusion. Then repeat the border movements with the mouth open. By this time or soon thereafter the material will have become firm enough to maintain its form out of the mouth.

7. Remove the denture, rinse quickly in water, and dry the relined surface with compressed air. Apply a generous coating of glycerine or Tect-ol with a brush or cotton pellet to prevent frosting of the surface due to evaporation of monomer. The material is then allowed to bench cure, thus eliminating patient discomfort and tissue damage from exothermic heat or prolonged contact with raw monomer. While it is preferable that twenty to thirty minutes elapse before trimming and polishing, it may be done as soon as the material hardens. The masking tape must be removed before trimming but should be replaced over the teeth and polished surfaces below the junction of the new and old materials to protect those surfaces during final polishing.

Properly done, a direct reline is entirely acceptable for most all tooth-borne partial denture bases made of a resin material except where some tissue support is desired for long spans between abutment teeth. In the latter case, a reline impression in wax should be accomplished, the denture then flasked, and a processed reline added for optimal tissue contact and support.

RELINING FREE-END PARTIAL DENTURE BASES

A free-end partial denture, deriving its major support from the tissues of the residual ridge, requires relining much more frequently than tooth-supported denture areas. Because of this, free-end bases are usually made of a resin material that can be relined to compensate for loss of support due to tissue changes. While tooth-supported areas are relined for other reasons, the sole reason for relining a free-end base is to re-establish tissue support for that base.

The need for relining a free-end base is determined by evaluating the stability and occlusion at reasonable intervals following delivery of the denture. At the time of delivery, the patient must be advised that periodic examination is imperative and relining also when it becomes necessary and that the success of the partial denture and the health of the remaining tissues and abutment teeth depends upon periodic examination and servicing of both the denture and the abutment teeth. The patient should also be told that a charge will be made in proportion to the service required.

There are two indications of the need for relining a free-end partial denture base. First, a loss of occlusal contact between opposing dentures or between the denture and opposing natural dentition may be evident. This is determined by having the patient close on two strips of 28-gauge soft green or blue (casting) wax. If occlusal contact between artificial dentition is weak or lacking, while the remaining natural teeth in opposition are making firm contact, the free-end denture needs to have occlusion re-established on the present base either by altering the occlusion or by re-establishing the original position of the denture framework and base and sometimes both. In most cases, re-establishing the original relationship of the denture is necessary and the occlusion will automatically be re-established.

Second, a loss of tissue support causing rotation and settling of the free-end base or bases is obvious when alternate finger pressure is applied on either side of the fulcrum line. Although checking for occlusal contact alone may be misleading, such rotation is positive proof that relining is necessary. If occlusal inadequacy is detected without any evidence of denture rotation toward the residual ridge, all that needs be done is to re-establish occlusal contact by resetting the teeth or by adding to the occlusal surfaces with resin or cast gold onlays. On the other hand, if occlusal contact is adequate but denture rotation can be demonstrated, it is usually due to migration or extrusion of opposing teeth or to a shift in position of an opposing maxillary denture, thus maintaining occlusal contact at the expense of the stability and tissue support of that denture. This is frequently the case where a partial denture is opposed by a maxillary complete denture. It is not unusual for a patient to complain of looseness of the maxillary complete denture and request relining of that denture when actually it is the partial denture which needs relining. In most every cast, relining and thus repositioning the partial denture results in repositioning of the maxillary complete denture with a return of stability and retention in that denture. Therefore, evidence of rotation of a free-end partial denture about he fulcrum line must be the deciding factor as to whether or not relining needs to be done.

Rotation about the fulcrum line always results in a lifting of the indirect retainers(s). The framework of any free-end partial denture must be in its original terminal position with indirect retainers fully seated during and at the end of any relining procedure. Any possibility of rotation about the fulcrum line due to occlusal influence must be prevented, and therefore the framework must be held in its original terminal position during the time the impression is being made. This all but eliminates the practicability of using a closed-mouth impression procedure effectively when relining unilateral or bilateral free-end bases. Although Steffel has outlined in detail the procedures for a functional reline impression (see Chapter 15, Support for the Free-End Denture Base), the use of posterior stops of modeling plastic does not eliminate the possibility of tissue displacement and denture rotation occurring when the mouth is closed and the teeth are in occlusion. Although adjusting the occlusion helps to prevent such rotation when the final impression is being made, one cannot always be sure that some rotation and lifting of the indirect retainers does not occur.

The only sure method, therefore, of making a reline impression for a free-end partial denture is with an open-mouth procedure done in exactly the same manner as the original functional impression. The denture to be relined is first relieved generously on the tissue side and then is treated the same as the original impression base for a functional impression. The step-by-step procedure is the same, with the operator's three fingers placed on the two principal occlusal rests and at a third point between, preferably at an indirect retainer farthest from the axis of rotation. The framework is thus returned to its original terminal position, with all tooth-supported components fully seated. The tissues beneath the free-end base are then registered in a relationship to the original position of the denture that will assure (1) the denture framework being returned to its intended relationship with the supporting teeth, (2) the re-establishment of optimal tissue support for the free-end base, and (3) the restoration of the original occlusal relationship with the opposing teeth.

While it is true that the teeth are not allowed to come into occlusion during an open-mouth impression procedure, the original position of the denture is positively determined by its relationship with the supporting abutment teeth. Since this is the relationship upon which the original occlusion was established, returning the denture to that position should bring about a return to the original occlusal relationship if two conditions are satisfied. First of these is that the laboratory procedures during relining must be done accurately without any increase in vertical dimension. This is essential with any reline procedure, but particularly with a partial denture because any change in vertical dimension will prevent occlusal rests from seating and will result in overloading and trauma to the underlying tissues. The second condition is that the opposing teeth have not extruded or migrated or that the position of an opposing denture has not become irreversibly altered. In the latter situation some adjustment of the occlusion will be necessary, but this should be deferred until the opposing teeth or denture and the structures associated with the temporomandibular joint have had a chance to return to their original position before denture settling occurred. Frequently, only minor occlusal adjustment or none at all will be necessary after the relined denture has been worn for a period of two or three days. One of the greatest satisfactions of a job well done is to be found in the execution of an open-mouth reline procedure as described above, which results in the restoration not only of the original denture relationship and tissue support but the original occlusal relationship as well.

In rare instances, following the relining of a free-end partial denture by this method, the occlusion is found to be negative rather than positive or the same as originally. This may be due to wear of occlusal surfaces over a period of time, to the original occlusion being high with resulting depression of opposing teeth, or to other reasons. In such case, occlusion on the denture must be restored to re-establish an even distribution of occlusal loading over both natural and artificial dentition. Otherwise, the natural dentition must carry the burden of mastication unaided and the denture becomes only a space-filling or cosmetic device.

METHODS OF RE-ESTABLISHING OCCLUSION ON A RELINED PARTIAL DENTURE

Occlusion on a relined partial denture may be re-established by one of several methods.

The best method is to remove the original teeth and replace them with a hard inlay wax occlusion rim upon which a functional registration of occlusal pathways is then established (see Chapter 16, Occlusal Relationships). Either the original teeth or new teeth may then be set to occlude with the template thus obtained and subsequently attached to the denture base with processed or self-curing resin. If the latter, the need for flasking may be eliminated by securing the teeth to a stone matrix while the resin attachment is applied with a brush technique. Regardless of the method used for reattaching the teeth, the occlusion thus established should require little adjustment in the mouth and should be typical of the occlusal harmony that is possible by this method.

Another method is also a functional method obtained by establishing occlusal pathways in wax, but it results in cast gold onlays being cemented to the original denture teeth. Recesses must be ground into the occlusal surfaces that are to be restored, and some lubricant must be used to ensure removal of the wax patterns. A hard inlay wax is used to record functional occlusion in all excursions, preferably over a period of twenty-four hours or more. The wax record is then carved as for full coverage inlay patterns, except that they are left in one piece for all adjacent teeth. Some occlusal anatomy should be carved into the patterns to provide escapeways and promote greater efficiency and less occlusal loading than the broad occlusal contacts registered in wax. The inlays are then cast in a B-type gold and cemented to the denture teeth.

While this method does not permit remounting to correct for technical errors, minor occlusal adjustment may be accomplished by leaving the occlusal surfaces unpolished, preferably with a sandblasted surface, and relieving obvious areas of interference after one or two days' wear. Occlusal adjustment should always be deferred until the denture and opposing teeth have returned to the relationship existing when the wax registration was completed.

The re-establishment of occlusion on a partial denture may be done by the simpler method of interposing wax or some other recording medium between the teeth for the purpose of recording a new occlusal relationship. Teeth may then be reset to an opposing cast. However, despite the fact that this method is by far the most commonly used, the advantages of a functional method over this one have been given in Chapter 16, under Establishing Occlusion by the Recording of Occlusal Pathways.

Tissue Conditioning Prior to Relining a Partial Denture Base. Free-end partial denture bases frequently need relining within a few months because of initial tissue changes following the insertion of a first partial denture. This is not observed where the patient has been wearing a previous partial denture. Applegate has shown the beneficial effects of a treatment base prior to completion of the final base. Whether as a result of wearing a treatment base or a previous partial denture, tissue changes are not as likely to occur once the tissues have become conditioned to supporting a denture base.

There has been much interest in the use of soft resins for tissue-conditioning purposes prior to relining a complete denture. This is due to the beneficial massage of a soft resin reline rather than to any medicinal action of the treatment material. It has been clearly shown that tissues which are unhealthy and edematous and even those which are hyperplastic and papillomatous due to an ill-fitting denture base are returned to a normal, healthy state by repeated applications of a soft relining material.

Tissues under a partial denture base generally remain healthy due to the supporting and stabilizing effect of the denture framework. Therefore, tissue treatment prior to relining is not usually necessary or indicated. On the other hand, there is no harm in utilizing one of the tissue treatment materials for this purpose where its use is indicated—but only for treatment purposes. These are not meant to be impression materials, nor can they provide the support necessary to restore the proper relationship of the denture framework to the supporting teeth. An open-mouth relining procedure as outlined previously in the chapter should follow any tissue treatment procedures.

Repairs and additions to
partial dentures

Inevitably, the need for repairing or adding to a partial denture will occasionally arise. However, the frequency of this occurring should be held to a minimum by careful diagnosis, intelligent treatment planning, adequate mouth preparations, and carrying out an effective partial denture design with all component parts properly constructed. Any need for repairs or additions will then be due to unforeseen complications arising in abutment or other teeth in the arch or to breakage or distortion of the denture through accident or careless handling by the patient rather than to faulty design or construction.

It is important that the patient be instructed in the proper insertion and removal of the restoration so that undue strain is not placed upon clasp arms or other parts of the denture nor upon the abutment teeth contacted. The patient should also be advised that care must be given the restoration when it is out of the mouth and that distortion occurring due to careless handling may be irreparable. It should be made clear that there can be no guarantee against breakage or distortion occurring from causes other than obvious structural defects.

CLASSIFICATION OF REPAIRS AND ADDITIONS

Repairs and additions to partial dentures may be classified according to the cause of occurrence—broken clasp arms, broken occlusal rests, distortion or breakage of other components, loss of an additional tooth, and miscellaneous causes.

Broken Clasp Arms. There are several reasons for breakage.

1. Breakage may result from repeated flexure into and out of too severe an undercut. If the periodontal support is greater than the fatigue limit of the clasp arm, failure of the metal occurs first; otherwise, the abutment tooth is loosened and eventually lost due to the persistent strain placed upon it. This type of breakage can be avoided by locating clasp arms only where an acceptable minimum of retention exists, as determined by an accurate survey of the master cast. The amount

of retention is predictable only by the proper utilization of guiding planes during insertion and removal.

2. Breakage may occur due to structural failure of the clasp arm itself. A cast clasp arm which is not uniformly tapered because the pattern was not properly formed or because of careless finishing and polishing will eventually break at its weakest point due to repeated flexure at that point. This can be avoided by providing a uniform taper to flexible retentive clasp arms and uniform bulk to all rigid nonretentive clasp arms.

Wrought-wire clasp arms may eventually fail because of repeated flexure at the point where a nick or constriction occurred due to careless use of the contouring pliers. They may also break at the point of origin from the casting due to excessive manipulation during initial adaptation to the tooth or subsequent re-adaptation. The latter can best be avoided by cautioning the patient against repeatedly lifting the clasp arm away from the tooth by application of the fingernail during removal of the denture. A wrought-wire clasp arm can normally be adjusted a number of times over a period of years without failure. It is only when the number of adjustments are excessive that breakage is likely to occur.

Wrought-wire clasp arms may also break at the point of origin due to crystallization of the metal. This usually occurs during initial adaptation or soon after completion of the restoration. It can be prevented by proper selection of the wrought wire used and by avoiding too high burnout and casting temperatures where a cast-to method is used. Where the wrought wire is attached to the framework by soldering, as must be done with all but one of the chromium-cobalt alloys, the soldering technique must avoid crystallization of the wire. For this reason, it is best that soldering be done electrically to prevent overheating the wrought wire.

3. Breakage may occur due to careless handling by the patient. Any clasp arm will become distorted or will break if subjected to excessive abuse by the patient. The most common cause of failure of a cast clasp arm is distortion caused by accidentally dropping the denture into the lavatory basin or onto other hard surfaces. The most common cause of failure of a wrought-wire clasp is due to repeated readjustment made necessary by the patient lifting improperly against the wrought wire during removal of the denture. This is avoided by instructing the patient before a mirror in how to remove the denture without distorting the wrought-wire clasp arms. Removal should be accomplished by lifting against some other part of the framework or at the point of origin of the wrought-wire clasp arm rather than along its course. It is also avoided by placing wrought-wire clasp arms on the lingual surface of abutment teeth whenever possible, where they are inaccessible to the fingernail during removal.

Broken Occlusal Rests. Breakage of an occlusal rest almost always occurs at the point where it crosses the marginal ridge, due to weakness at this point. Improperly prepared occlusal rest seats are usually the cause of such weakness, because an occlusal rest crossing a marginal ridge that was not lowered sufficiently during mouth preparations is either made too thin or is thinned by adjustment in the mouth to avoid occlusal interference. Failure of an occlusal rest is rarely due to a structural defect in the metal and rarely if ever due to accidental distortion. Therefore, the blame for such failure must frequently be assumed by the dentist for not having provided sufficient space during mouth preparations for the placement of an occlusal rest of adequate bulk.

Distortion or Breakage of Other Components, Such as Major and Minor Connectors. Assuming that these were made with adequate bulk originally, distortion can occur only from abuse by the patient. All such components should be designed and fabricated with sufficient bulk to assure their rigidity and permanence of form under normal circumstances. In such case, any distortion or breakage occurring when the restoration is out of the mouth is then the fault and obligation of the patient, the dentist's responsibility being limited to its repair or replacement at a reasonable fee.

Major and minor connectors occasionally become weakened by adjustment to avoid or eliminate tissue impingement. Such adjustment at the time of delivery is due to inadequate survey of the master cast or to faulty design or fabrication of the casting. This is inexcusable and reflects upon the dentist or his laboratory, and such a restoration should be remade rather than weaken the restoration by attempting to compensate for its inadequacies by relieving the metal. Similarly, tissue impingement arising from inadequately relieved components is due to faulty construction, and the casting should be remade with enough relief to avoid impingement. Failure of any component that was weakened by adjustment at the time of delivery is the responsibility of the dentist. However, adjustment made necessary by settling of the restoration due to abutment teeth becoming intruded under functional loading may be unavoidable, and subsequent failure due to the weakening effect of such adjustment may necessitate the making of a new restoration as a consequence of tissue changes. Frequently, repeated adjustment to a major or minor connector to relieve tissue impingement may not result in actual breakage but results in a loss of rigidity to the point that the connector can no longer function effectively. In such case, either a new restoration must be made or that part replaced by casting a new section and then reassembling the denture by soldering. This occasionally requires disassembly of denture base areas and replaced teeth, and the cost and probable success must then we weighed against the cost of an entirely new restoration. Frequently, the latter course is advisable.

Loss of an Additional Tooth or Teeth Not Involved in the Support or Retention of the Restoration. Such additions to a partial denture are usually simply made where the bases are made of resin. The addition of teeth to metal bases is more complex and necessitates either casting a new component, and attaching it by soldering, or creating retentive elements for the attachment of a resin extension. In most instances, where a free-end denture base is extended, the need for subsequently relining the entire base should be considered. Following the extension of the denture base, a relining procedure of both the new and old base should then be carried out to provide optimal tissue support for the restoration.

Loss of an Abutment Tooth Necessitating Not Only Its Replacement But Also the Substitution of a New Clasp Assembly on Another Abutment. This is usually the next adjacent tooth, which may or may not have to undergo restorative treatment. In the latter case, any new restoration should be done so as to conform to the original path of insertion, with proximal guiding plane, occlusal rest seat, and suitable retentive areas. Otherwise, modifications to the existing tooth should be done the same as would be done during any other mouth preparations, with proximal disking, preparation of an adequate occlusal rest seat, and any reduction in tooth contours necessary to accommodate retentive and stabilizing components. A new clasp assembly may then be cast for this tooth and the denture reassembled with the new replacement tooth added.

The most frequent cause of the loss of an abutment tooth is periodontal involvement. If an abutment tooth becomes carious or fractures, it can frequently be restored with a crown made to fit the existing denture clasp. Early pulpal involvement is usually amenable to endodontic treatment, by gaining access through the existing restoration. But an abutment tooth that becomes periodontally involved is too often lost. In many instances this could have been avoided initially by more careful evaluation of the periodontal support of a tooth which is to serve as an abutment and by the use of multiple abutments by splinting whenever advisable. When an adjacent tooth must be substituted as the new abutment, it must be considered as potentially a periodontally weakened tooth and treated accordingly. Occasionally, splinting of two teeth with double restorations is necessary before the denture is extended to include the new abutment. This is often made more necessary by the fact that the edentulous area is increased by one tooth and, in a free-end situation, the leverage on the abutment is increased correspondingly.

Other Types of Repairs and Replacements. Included in this category is the replacement of a broken or lost denture tooth, the repair of a broken resin base, or the reattachment of a loosened resin base to the metal framework. Breakage is sometimes due to poor design, faulty construction, or the use of the wrong material for a given situation. Other times it is due to an accident which will not necessarily repeat itself. If the latter, repair or replacement usually suffices. On the other hand, if fracture has occurred due to structural causes or if it occurs a second time after having been repaired once before, then some change in the design, either by modification of the original denture or with a new denture, may be necessary. Usually the share of responsibility by dentist and patient will depend upon the length of service given by the denture before breakage occurred and upon other contributing factors, such as the existence of an abnormal occlusion. Such matters are best approached by a frank and honest appraisal of all the factors involved, based on the patient's understanding that the permanence or longevity of any prosthetic restoration, since it is dependent upon the changing characteristics of living tissues, can never be assured.

PROCEDURES FOR MAKING REPAIRS AND ADDITIONS

Although most repairs or additions to partial dentures will be done by the laboratory, impressions and other chairside procedures must be done in accordance with the laboratory procedures to follow.

If a new clasp assembly is to be made, an impression is made for a new master cast. This is poured, surveyed, and the design of the new clasp outlined.

The same applies to the making of any new component part to be cast and subsequently attached to the original framework. Frequently the patient can continue to wear the denture while the new part is being made and must be without it only for the brief period of time it takes to reassemble the parts. Jaw relations are usually made with the original denture in the mouth, and at the same time an impression is made for an occluding cast.

For more simple repairs and additions, the laboratory technician usually prefers that the impression be made with the denture in place, the denture being removed in the impression. An alginate hydrocolloid impression material should be used which has sufficient toughness upon setting to permit withdrawal of the denture in the impression. To facilitate easy withdrawal, retentive clasp arms should be opened up slightly. They can then be readapted to the abutment teeth after the repair or addition has been made.

The impression should be poured immediately, either in stone or in a mixture of stone and plaster to facilitate later removal without difficulty. If a resin repair or addition is to be done, the stone and plaster mixture will be sufficiently strong. But if a new clasp arm is to be adapted, the cast should be made of the harder stone for obvious reasons. If an occlusal rest or some soldered clasp assembly is to be made, the soldering will be done on a refractory duplicate of the stone cast and the original stone cast will be used for the final fitting and finishing.

Replacing a Broken Clasp Arm With a Wrought-Wire Retentive Arm

A broken retentive clasp arm, regardless of its type, may be replaced with a wrought-wire retentive arm embedded in a resin base or attached to a metal base by electric soldering. Frequently this avoids the necessity of constructing an entirely new clasp assembly. Eighteen-gauge wrought wire is used to replace the original clasp arm.

Where a resin base is present the wire may be embedded into it with repair resin, thus eliminating the need for soldering (Fig. 258). The method for replacing a clasp in this manner is as follows:

The remains of the original clasp arm is first cut off flush with its point of origin. A hole is then drilled just below the adjacent denture tooth as close as possible to the minor connector from which it originated. This hole must be angled downward toward the opposite side, emerging approximately midway on the opposite side of the resin base. From this hole a groove is cut in the resin base long enough to accommodate a sufficient length of the wrought wire for adequate retention. At the opposite end of this groove, a hole is made which will accommodate a right-angle turn in the wire. A piece of 18-gauge wrought wire to be used as a clasp arm is shaped with a right-angle bend at one end, adapted to fit the lingual groove, and then bent to fit the hole passing through to the opposite side. A straight portion sufficient to be adapted later as a clasp arm is left emerging from the resin base at the point of origin of the new clasp arm.

After securing the projecting wrought wire with sticky wax, self-curing repair resin is painted into the resin base until the defect is overfilled. After polymerizing, this is trimmed and polished. The projecting wrought wire is then cut off

Fig. 258. Lingual view of the technique for replacing a broken retentive clasp arm with an 18-gauge wrought wire. The wrought wire is embedded securely with self-curing repair resin in a groove cut in the resin base.

to the required length and adapted to serve as a new retentive clasp arm. The abutment tooth must be surveyed to determine the location of the desired under-cut. The terminal portion of the adapted clasp arm is then rounded and tapered slightly.

This method is suitable any time a retentive clasp arm must be replaced and avoids any disassembly of the original denture. Because of the flexibility of wrought wire, it cannot be used to replace a stabilizing arm where rigidity is needed. In such case, where a rigid clasp arm has been lost, it is best that an entirely new clasp assembly be cast and attached to the framework by soldering.

Repairing by Soldering

It has been said that 80 per cent of all soldering in dentistry can be done electrically. Electric soldering units are available for this purpose, and most dental laboratories are so equipped. Electric soldering permits soldering close to a resin base without removing that base, due to the rapid localization of heat at the electrode. The resin base needs only to be protected with wet asbestos during soldering.

Gold solder is used for soldering both gold and chromium-cobalt alloys. For electric soldering, triple-thick solder should be used so that the additional bulk of the solder will retard melting momentarily while the carbon electrode conducts heat to the area being soldered. For chromium-cobalt alloys a color-matching white 19K gold solder is used which melts at about 1675° F. A liberal application of flux in a watery consistency is essential to the success of any soldering operation.

Following is a procedure* for electric soldering:

1. Roughen both sections to be joined.

---

*Adapted from Ticonium Technique Manual, Ticonium Division, Consolidated Metal Products Corp., Albany, N. Y.

2. Adapt platinum foil to the master cast to serve as a backing upon which the solder will flow. Lift the edges of the foil to form a trough to confine the flow of the solder.

3. Seat the pieces to be soldered onto the master cast and secure them temporarily with sticky wax. Over each piece add enough soldering investment or plaster to secure them after the sticky wax is eliminated, but leave as much metal exposed as possible.

4. After flushing off the sticky wax with hot water, secure the cast to the soldering stand. Cut sufficient solder and place conveniently nearby. Insert tweezers into the grounding terminal and the size carbon into the electrode holder which is best suited to the size and bulk of the sections to be joined (the smaller the piece of carbon used, the less power output needed).

5. Place the points of the tweezers so that both sections are grounded. Flux both sections liberally. Put sufficient triple-thick solder on or in the joint to complete the soldering in one operation, always starting with enough solder to complete the job.

6. Wet the carbon tip with water to aid conduction of the current and then touch the carbon to the solder. Press the foot pedal, allowing time for the solder to flow freely, and then let up on the foot pedal. Do not push the solder with the carbon tip, but let the heat alone make the solder flow. Do not remove the carbon from the solder while the soldering operation is in progress, as this will cause surface pitting due to arcing as the carbon is removed. After the solder has flowed and the foot pedal is released, remove the carbon and grounding tweezers and proceed to remove the work from the cast for finishing.

Torch soldering requires an entirely different approach. It is used when the solder joint is long or unusually bulky, and when a larger quantity of solder has to be used. The procedure* for torch soldering is as follows:

1. Roughen both sections to be joined.

2. Adapt platinum foil to the master cast so that it extends under both sections.

3. Seat the sections on the master cast in the correct relationship and secure them temporarily with sticky wax. Flow sticky wax also into the joint to be soldered.

4. Attach a dental bur or nail over the two sections with a liberal amount of sticky wax. Attach a second and even a third nail or bur across other areas to lend additional support. Never use pieces of wood for this purpose, because the wood will swell if it gets wet, thus distorting the relationship of the two sections.

5. Remove the assembled casting from the master cast carefully. Adapt a stock of utility wax directly under each section, on either side of the platinum foil. After boilout, investment will remain in the center to support the platinum foil.

6. Invest the casting in sufficient soldering investment to secure it, leaving as much of the area to be soldered exposed as possible. When the investment

---

*Adapted from Ticonium Technique Manual, Ticonium Division, Consolidated Metal Products Corp., Albany, N. Y.

has set, boil out the sticky and utility waxes. Then place the investment in a drying oven at a temperature not exceeding 200° F. until the contained moisture has been eliminated. Do not preheat the investment with a torch or oxides will be formed which will interfere with the flow of the solder.

7. Use the reducing part of the flame, which is that feathery part just outside the blue inner cone. Flux the joint thoroughly and dry out the flux with the outer part of the flame until it has a powdery appearance. Heat the casting until it is dull red and then, holding a strip of solder in the soldering tweezers, dip it into the flux and feed it into the joint while the casting is being held at a dull red heat with the torch. Once the soldering operation has begun do not remove the flame, as any cooling will cause oxides to be formed. The heat from the casting should be sufficient to melt the solder, so do not put the flame directly on the solder or it will become overheated, resulting in pitting.

8. After the soldering has been completed, allow the investment to cool slowly before quenching and proceeding with finishing. Remember that any soldering operation that heats the entire casting is in effect a heat-treating operation, and heat-hardening of a repaired gold alloy casting is desirable to restore its optimal physical properties.

Selected references

TEXTBOOKS

Applegate, O. C.: Essentials of Removable Partial Denture Prosthesis, Philadephia, 1954, W. B. Saunders Co.

Austin, K. P., and Lidge, E. F., Jr.: Partial Dentures, St. Louis, 1957, The C. V. Mosby Co.

Boucher, C. O.: Dental Prosthetic Laboratory Manual, St. Louis, 1950, The C. V. Mosby Co.

Brecker, S. C.: Clinical Procedures in Occlusal Rehabilitation, Philadelphia, 1958, W. B. Saunders Co.

Brecker, S. C.: Crowns, Philadelphia, 1961, W. B. Saunders Co.

Brumfield, R. C.: Dental Gold Structures, New York, 1949, J. F. Jelenko & Co., Inc.

Bulbulian, A. H.: Facial Prosthesis, Philadelphia, 1945, W. B. Saunders Co.

Clarke, C. D.: Facial and Body Prosthesis, St. Louis, 1945, The C. V. Mosby Co.

Craddock, F. W.: Prosthetic Dentistry, St. Louis, 1951, The C. V. Mosby Co.

Cummer, W. E.: Partial Denture Service. In Anthony, L. P. (editor): American Textbook of Prosthetic Dentistry, ed. 7, Philadelphia, 1942, Lea & Febiger, pp. 753-756.

Dental Laboratory Technician's Manual AFM 160-29, Department of the Air Force, Washington, 1959, U. S. Government Printing Office.

Dental Technician, Prosthetic, NAVPERS 10685B, Washington, 1962, U. S. Government Printing Office.

Denton, G. B.: The Vocabulary of Dentistry and Oral Science, Chicago, 1958, American Dental Association.

Ewing, J. E.: Fixed Partial Prosthesis, Philadelphia, 1954, Lea & Febiger.

Fenn, H. R. B., Liddelow, K. P., and Gimson, A. P.: Clinical Dental Prosthetics, London, 1953, Staples Press, Ltd.

Fish, E. W.: Principles of Full Denture Prosthesis, New York, 1948, Staples Press, Ltd.

Gehl, D. H., and Dresen, O. M.: Complete Denture Prosthesis, Philadelphia, 1958, W. B. Saunders Co.

Godfrey, R. J.: Manual of Removable Partial Denture Design, Toronto, 1948, University of Toronto Press.

Goldman, H. M., Schluger, S., and Fox, L.: Periodontal Therapy, St. Louis, 1956, The C. V. Mosby Co.

Granger, E. R.: Practical Procedures in Oral Rehabilitation, Philadelphia, 1962, J. B. Lippincott Co.

Johnston, J. F., Phillips, R. W., and Dykema, R. W.: Modern Practice in Crown and Bridge Prosthodontics, Philadelphia, 1960, W. B. Saunders Co.

Kazis, H., and Kazis, A. J.: Complete Mouth Rehabilitation Through Crown and Bridge Prosthodontics, Philadelphia, 1956, Lea & Febiger.

Kennedy, E.: Partial Denture Construction, Brooklyn, 1942, Dental Items of Interest Publishing Co.

Klatsky, M., and Fisher, R. L.: The Human Masticatory Apparatus, Brooklyn, 1953, Dental Items of Interest Publishing Co., Inc.

Langley, L. L., and Cheraskin, E.: The Physiological Foundation of Dental Practice, St. Louis, 1956, The C. V. Mosby Co.

Lucia, V. O.: Modern Gnathological Concepts, St. Louis, 1961, The C. V. Mosby Co.

McNeil, C. K.: Oral and Facial Deformity, New York, 1954, Pitman Publishing Corp.

Morley, M. E.: Cleft Palate and Speech, Edinburgh, 1954, E. & S. Livingstone, Ltd.

489

Nagle, R. J., Sears, V. H., and Silverman, S. I.: Dental Prosthetics, St. Louis, 1958, The C. V. Mosby Co.

Neurohr, F. G.: Partial Dentures, Philadelphia, 1939, Lea & Febiger.

Osborne, J., and Lammie, G. A.: Partial Dentures, Oxford, 1952, Blackwell Scientific Publications.

Peyton, F. A., et al.: Restorative Materials, St. Louis, 1960, The C. V. Mosby Co.

Prothero, J. H.: Prosthetic Dentistry, ed. 2, Chicago, 1916, Medico-Dental Publishing Co., p. 250.

Rebassio, A. D.: Protesis Parcial Removable, Buenos Aires, 1960, Editorial Mundi Republica Argentina.

Sarnat, B. F. (editor): The Temporomandibular Joint, Springfield, 1951, Charles C Thomas, Publisher.

Schlosser, R. O., and Gehl, D. H.: Complete Denture Prosthesis, Philadelphia, 1953, W. B. Saunders Co.

Schmidt, A. H.: Periodic Reviews and Demonstrations of Prosthetic Dentistry, San Antonio, 1955, Lackland Air Force Base.

Schwartz, L.: Disorders of the Temporomandibular Joint, Philadelphia, 1959, W. B. Saunders Co.

Schweitzer, J. M.: Oral Rehabilitation, St. Louis, 1951, The C. V. Mosby Co.

Schweitzer, J. M.: Restorative Dentistry, St. Louis, 1947, The C. V. Mosby Co.

Sharry, J. J. (editor): Complete Denture Prosthodontics, New York, 1962, The Blakiston Division, McGraw-Hill Book Co., Inc.

Sicher, H.: Oral Anatomy, St. Louis, 1949, The C. V. Mosby Co.

Silverman, M. M.: Occlusion in Prosthodontics and in the Natural Dentition, Washington, D. C., 1963, Mutual Publishing Co.

Skinner, E. W.: The Science of Dental Materials, Philadelphia, 1954, W. B. Saunders Co.

Steiger, A. A., and Boitel, R. H.: Precision Work for Partial Dentures, Zurich, 1959, Buchdruckerei Berichthaus.

Swenson, M. G.: Complete Dentures, St. Louis, 1953, The C. V. Mosby Co.

Swenson, M. G., and Terkla, L. G.: Partial Dentures, St. Louis, 1951, The C. V. Mosby Co.

Tylman, S. D.: Theory and Practice of Crown and Bridge Prosthesis, St. Louis, 1947, The C. V. Mosby Co.

Tylman, S. D., and Peyton, F. A.: Acrylics and Other Synthetic Resins Used in Dentistry, Philadelphia, 1946, J. B. Lippincott Co.

Wilson, J. H.: Partial Dentures, Philadelphia, 1957, Lea & Febiger.

ABUTMENT RETAINERS: EXTERNAL AND INTERNAL ATTACHMENTS

Adisman, I. K.: The Internal Clip Attachment in Fixed-Removable Partial Denture Prosthesis, New York J. Den. **32**:125-129, 1962.

Beder, O. E.: Evaluation of Conventional Circumferential Clasps, J. Pros. Den. **3**:88-95, 1953.

Blatterfein, L.: Study of Partial Denture Clasping, J.A.D.A. **43**:169-185, 1951.

Blatterfein, L.: Design and Positional Arrangement of Clasps for Partial Dentures, New York J. Den. **22**:305-306, 1952.

Caldarone, C. V.: Attachments for Partial Dentures Without Clasps, J. Pros. Den. **7**:206-208, 1957.

Cohn, L. A.: The Physiologic Basis for Tooth Fixation in Precision-Attached Partial Dentures, J. Pros. Den. **6**:220-244, 1956.

Conacher, F.: Stainless-Steel Finger Springs in Partial Denture Retention, Brit. D. J. **83**:147-148, 1947.

DeVan, M. M.: Preserving Natural Teeth Through the Use of Clasps, J. Pros. Den. **5**:208-214, 1955; Fort. Rev. Chicago D. Soc. **27**:7-12 (portrait), 1954.

Dietz, W. H.: Modified Abutments for Removable and Fixed Prosthodontics, J. Pros. Den. **11**:1112-1116, 1961.

Dolder, E. J.: The Bar Joint Mandibular Denture, J. Pros. Den. **11**:689-707, 1961.

Gilson, T. D.: A Fixable-Removable Prosthetic Attachment, J. Pros. Den. **9**:247-255, 1959.

Goncalves, A.: System of Modified Attachments for Removable Partial Dentures, J. Pros. Den. **5**:649-657, 1955.

Green, J. H.: The Hinge-Lock Abutment Attachment, J.A.D.A. **47**:175-180, 1953.

Grosser, D.: The Dynamics of Internal Precision Attachments, J. Pros. Den. **3**:393-401, 1953; Harvard D. Alum. Bul. **14**:7-9, 1954.

Grubb, H. D.: Partial Dentures With Precision Attachments, J.A.D.A. **42**:154-162, 1951.

Handlers, M., Lenchner, N. H., and Weissman, B.: A Retaining Device for Partial Dentures, J. Pros. Den. **7**:483-488, 1957.

Harris, F. N.: The Precision Dowel Rest Attachment, J. Pros. Den. **5**:43-48, 1955.

Hekneby, M.: The Spring-Slide Joint for Lower Free End Removable Partial Dentures, J. Pros. Den. **11**:256-263, 1961.

Hollenback, G. M., and Oaks, S.: Role of the Precision Attachment in Partial Denture Prosthesis, J.A.D.A. **41**:173-182, 1950.

Isaacson, D.: Cast Gold Crowns as Retainers for Clasp Partial Dentures, D. Digest **58**:213-217, 1952.

James, A. G.: Self-Locking Posterior Attachment for Removable Tooth-Supported Partial Dentures, J. Pros. Den. **5**:200-205, 1955.

Johnston, J. F.: The Application and Construction of the Pinledge Retainer, J. Pros. Den. **3**:559-567, 1953.

Jones, R. R.: Attachments for Partial Dentures and Abutments, J.A.D.A. **28**:410-420, 1941.

Knowles, L. E.: A Dowel Attachment Removable Partial Denture, J. Pros. Den. **13**:679-687, 1963.

Leff, A.: Precision Attachment Dentures, J. Pros. Den. **2**:84-91, 1952.

Mann, A. W.: The Lower Distal Extension Partial Denture Using the Hart-Dunn Attachment, J. Pros. Den. **8**:282-288, 1958.

Morrison, M. L.: Internal Precision Attachment Retainers for Partial Dentures, J.A.D.A. **64**:209-215, 1962.

Myers, G. E., Wepfer, G. G., and Peyton, F. A.: The Thiokol Rubber Base Impression Materials, J. Pros. Den. **8**:330-339, 1958.

Nelson, E. A., and Hinds, F. W.: Abutments as Applied to Fixed as Well as Removable Partial Denture Prosthesis, J.A.D.A. **29**:534-542, 1942.

Phillips, R. N.: A Problem of Retention in a Lower Partial Denture, J. Pros. Den. **6**:213-219, 1956.

Plotnick, I. J.: Internal Attachment for Fixed Removable Partial Dentures, J. Pros. Den. **8**:85-93, 1958.

Rispler, C. J.: Evaluation of Precision Attachments in Partial Denture Construction, J. Soc. D. Res. **1**:8-12, 1952; Bul. San Diego Co. D. Soc. **25**:8-9, 15, 1955.

Roach, F. E.: Roach Bar Clasp, D. Survey **21**:249, 1945.

Rosen, M. H.: Fixed-Movable Partial Dentures With Interlocking Onlay Attachments: Review of a Practical Case, J.A.D.A. **41**:306-307, 1950.

Rubin, J. G.: Precision Attachment Partial Dentures With Hydrocolloid Impressions: An Accurate, Rapid Precedure, D. Digest **60**:504-508, 1954.

Rybeck, S. A.: Simplicity in a Distal Extension Partial Denture, J. Pros. Den. **4**:87-92, 1954.

Scherrer, H.: Screw Clasps and Springs: Their Utilization for Partial Dentures and Removable Bridges, D. Abs. **1**:633-634, 1956.

Schuyler, C. H.: Analysis of the Use and Relative Value of the Precision Attachment and the Clasp in Partial Denture Planning, J. Pros. Den. **3**:711-714, 1953.

Smith, G. P.: Cast Clasps: Their Uses, Advantages and Disadvantages, Am. J. Orthodont. & Oral Surg. (Oral Surg. Sect.) **33**:479-483, 1947.

Swepston, O. L.: Some of the Fundamental Principles of Movable Removable Precision Partial Dentures, Texas D. J. **58**:389-391, 1940.

Terrell, W. H.: Specialized Frictional Attachments and Their Role in Partial Denture Construction, Australian J. Den. **55**:119-128, 1951; D. J. Australia **22**:471-483, 1950; J. Pros. Den. **1**:337-350, 1951.

Turkheim, H. J.: Modified Retaining Device for Upper Dentures, D. Practitioner & D. Record **2**:203-205, 1952.

Vig, R. G.: Splinting Bars and Maxillary Indirect Retainers for Removable Partial Dentures, J. Pros. Den. **13**:125-129, 1963.

ANATOMY

Bennett, N. G.: A Contribution to the Study of the Movements of the Mandible, J. Pros. Den. **8**:41-54, 1958.

Boucher, C. O.: Anatomy of the Mouth in Relation to Complete Dentures, J. Wisconsin D. Soc. **19**:161-166, 1943.

Boucher, C. O.: Complete Denture Impressions Based Upon the Anatomy of the Mouth, J.A.D.A. **31**:1174-1181, 1944.

Brodie, A. G.: Anatomy and Physiology of Head and Neck Musculature, Am. J. Orthodont. **36**:831-844, 1950.

Craddock, F. W.: Retromolar Region of the Mandible, J.A.D.A. **47**:453-455, 1953.

Haines, R. W., and Barnett, S. G.: The Structure of the Mouth in the Mandibular Molar Region, J. Pros. Den. **9**:962-974, 1959.

Harris, H. L.: Anatomic Landmarks of Value in Full Denture Construction, J.A.D.A. **28**:1765-1779, 1941.

Last, R. J.: The Muscles of the Mandible, D. Digest **61**:165-169, 1955.

Martone, A. L., et al.: Anatomy of the Mouth and Related Structures. Part I, J. Pros. Den. **11**:1009-1018, 1961; Part II, J. Pros. Den. **12**:4-27, 1962; Part III, J. Pros. Den. **12**:206-219, 1962; Part IV, J. Pros. Den. **12**:409-419, 1962; Part V, J. Pros. Den. **12**:629-636, 1962; Part VI, J. Pros. Den. **12**:817-834, 1962; Part VII, J. Pros. Den. **13**:4-33, 1963; Part VIII, J. Pros. Den. **13**:204-228, 1963.

Merkeley, H. J.: The Labial and Buccal Accessory Muscles of Mastication, J. Pros. Den. **4**:327-334, 1954.

Merkeley, H. J.: Mandibular Rearmament. Part I. Anatomic Considerations, J. Pros. Den. **9**:559-566, 1959.

Pendleton, E. C.: Anatomy of the Face and Mouth From the Standpoint of the Denture Prosthetist, J.A.D.A. **33**:219-234, 1946.

Pendleton, E. C.: Changes in the Denture Supporting Tissues, J.A.D.A. **42**:1-15, 1951.

Roche, A. F.: Functional Anatomy of the Muscles of Mastication, J. Pros. Den. **13**:548-570, 1963.

Silverman, S. I.: Denture Prosthesis and the Functional Anatomy of the Maxillofacial Structures, J. Pros. Den. **6**:305-331, 1956.

BIOMECHANICS

Abel, L. F., and Manly, R. S.: Masticatory Function of Partial Denture Patients Among Navy Personnel, J. Pros. Den. **3**:382-392, 1953.

Applegate, O. C.: Use of the Paralleling Surveyor in Modern Partial Denture Construction, J.A.D.A. **27**:1397-1407, 1940.

Brudevold, F.: Basic Study of the Chewing Forces of a Denture Wearer, J.A.D.A. **43**:45-51, 1951.

Brumfield, R. C.: Load Capacities of Posterior Dental Bridges, J. Pros. Den. **4**:530-547, 1954.

DeVan, M. M.: The Nature of the Partial Denture Foundation: Suggestions for Its Preservation, J. Pros. Den. **2**:210-218, 1952.

Frechette, A. R.: The Influence of Partial Denture Design on Distribution of Force to Abutment Teeth, J. Pros. Den. **6**:195-212, 1956.

Goodman J. J., and Goodman, H. W.: Balance of Force in Precision Free-End Restorations, J. Pros. Den. **13**:302-308, 1963.

Granger, E. R.: Mechanical Principles Applied to Partial Denture Construction, J.A.D.A. **28**:1943-1951, 1941.

Hindels, G. W.: Stress Analysis in Distal Extension Partial Dentures, J. Pros. Den. **7**:197-205, 1957.

Howell, A. H., and Brudevold, F.: Vertical Forces Used During Chewing of Food, J. D. Res. **29**:133, 1950.

Howell, A. H., and Manly, R. S.: An Electronic Strain Gauge for Measuring Oral Forces, J. D. Res. **27**:705-712, 1948.

Kaires, A. K.: Effect of Partial Denture Design on Bilateral Force Distribution, J. Pros. Den. **6**:373-385, 1956.

Kaires, A. K.: Effect of Partial Denture Design on Unilateral Force Distribution, J. Pros. Den. **6**:526-533, 1956.

Kaires, A. K.: Partial Denture Design and Its Relation to Force Distribution and Masticatory Performance, J. Pros. Den. **6**:672-683, 1956.

Knowles, L. E.: The Biomechanics of Removable Partial Dentures and Its Relationship to Fixed Prosthesis, J. Pros. Den. **8**:426-430, 1958.

Kratochvil, F. J.: Influence of Occlusal Rest Position and Clasp Design on Movement of Abutment Teeth, J. Pros. Den. **13**:114-124, 1963.

Moses, C. H.: Biomechanics and Artificial Posterior Teeth, J. Pros. Den. **4**:782-802, 1954.

Skinner, E. W., and Chung, P.: The Effect of Surface Contact in the Retention of a Denture, J. Pros. Den. **1**:229-235, 1951.

Smyd, E. S.: Dental Engineering Applied to Inlay and Fixed Bridge Fabrication, J. Missouri D. A. **32**:310-312, 347-349, 1952; J. Pros. Den. **2**:536-542, 1952.

Smyd, E. S.: Mechanics of Dental Structures: Guide to Teaching Dental Engineering at Undergraduate Level, J. Pros. Den. **2**:668-692, 1952.

Smyd, E. S.: Bio-Mechanics of Prosthetic Dentistry, J. Pros. Den. **4**:368-383, 1954.

Smyd, E. S.: Dentistry Is Biophysics. Part 2, D. Digest **61**:482-490, 517, 1955.

Smyd, E. S.: Role of Mechanical Stress in Dentistry, New York J. Den. **28**:227-235, 1958.

Smyd, E. S.: The Role of Tongue, Torsion, and Bending in Prosthodontic Failures, J. Pros. Den. **11**:95-111, 1961.

Yurkstas, A. A.: The Effect of Missing Teeth on Masticatory Performance and Efficiency, J. Pros. Den. **4**:120-123, 1954.

Yurkstas, A., and Curby, W. A.: Force Analysis of Prosthetic Appliances During Function, J. Pros. Den. **3**:82-87, 1953.

Yurkstas, A., Fridley, H. H., and Manly, R. S.: A Functional Evaluation of Fixed and Removable Bridgework, J. Pros. Den. **1**:570-577, 1951.

CLASSIFICATION

Applegate, O. C.: The Rationale of Partial Denture Choice, J. Pros. Den. **10**:891-907, 1960.

Bailyn, M.: Tissue Support in Partial Denture Construction, D. Cosmos **70**:988-997, 1928.

Beckett, L. S.: The Influence of Saddle Classification on the Design of Partial Removable Restoration, J. Pros. Den. **3**:506-516, 1953.

Cummer, W. E.: Partial Denture Service. In Anthony, L. P. (editor): American Textbook of Prosthetic Dentistry, Philadelphia, 1942, Lea & Febiger.

Friedman, J.: The ABC Classification of Partial Denture Segments, J. Pros. Den. **3**:517-524, 1953.

Godfrey, R. J.: Classification of Removable Partial Dentures, J. Am. Col. Den. **18**:5-13, 1951.

Skinner, C. N.: A Classification of Removable Partial Dentures Based Upon the Principles of Anatomy and Physiology, J. Pros. Den. **9**:240-246, 1959.

CLEFT PALATE

Aram, A., and Subtelny, J. D.: Velopharyngeal Function and Cleft Palate Prostheses, J. Pros. Den. **9**:149-158, 1959.

Baden, E.: Fundamental Principles of Orofacial Prosthetic Therapy in Congenital Cleft Palate, J. Pros. Den. **4**:420-433, 1954.

Beder, O. E.: Obturators: A Review, J. Oral Surg. **2**:356-368, 1944.

Beilock, D.: A Congenital Oral Deformity and Its Correction, J.A.D.A. **27**:1627-1631, 1940.

Calvan, J.: The Error of Gustan Passavant, Plast. & Reconstruct. Surg. **13**:275-289, 1954.

Cooper, H. K.: Integration of Service in the Treatment of Cleft Lip and Cleft Palate, J.A.D.A. **47**:27-32, 1953.

Fox, A.: Prosthetic Correction of a Severe Acquired Cleft Palate, J. Pros. Den. **8**:542-546, 1958.

Gibbons, P., and Bloomer, H.: A Supportive-Type Prosthetic Speech Aid, J. Pros. Den. **8**:362-369, 1958.

Graber, T. M.: Oral and Nasal Structures in Cleft Palate Speech, J.A.D.A. **53**:693-706, 1956.

Harkins, C. S.: Role of the Prosthodontist in the Rehabilitation of Cleft Palate Patients, J.A.D.A. **43**:29-33, 1951.

Harkins, C. S.: Modern Concepts in the Prosthetic Rehabilitation of Cleft Palate Patients, J. Oral Surg. **10**:298-312, 1952.

Harkins, C. S., and Ivy, R. H.: Surgery and Prosthesis in the Rehabilitation of Cleft Palate Patients, J. South. California D. A. **19**:16-24, 1951.

Howard, G. D.: Restoring the Lost Vertical Dimension of the Cleft Palate Patient, J.A.D.A. **46**:404-407, 1953.

James, G. J.: Cleft Palate Restoration: An Interpretation of the Fitz-Gibbon Technique, J. Pros. Den. **1**:268-285, 1951.

Landa, J. S.: The Prosthodontist Views the Rehabilitation of the Cleft Palate Patient, J. Pros. Den. **6**:421-427, 1956.

Lazzari, J. B.: A Prosthetic Closure of a Traumatic Palatal Perforation, J. Pros. Den. **2**:831-833, 1952.

Lloyd, R. S., Pruzansky, S., and Subtelny, J. D.: Prosthetic Rehabilitation of a Cleft Palate Patient Subsequent to Multiple Surgical and Prosthetic Failures, J. Pros. Den. **7**:216-230, 1957.

Malson, T. S.: Complete Denture for the Congenital Cleft Palate Patient, J. Pros. Den. **5**:567-578, 1955.

Mansie, J. W.: Intra-Oral Prosthesis in Bilateral Harelip and Cleft Palate, Proc. Roy. Soc. Med., Sec. Odont. **36**:483, 1943.

Martin, B. C., and Trabue, J. C.: The Congenital Cleft of the Palate, J. Pros. Den. **2**:557-561, 1952.

McDonald, E. T.: Speech Considerations in Cleft Palate Prosthesis, J. Pros. Den. **1**:629-637, 1951.

Merkeley, H. J.: Cleft Palate Prosthesis, J. Pros. Den. **9**:506-513, 1959.

Miller, C. W.: Extensive Obturators, J. Pros. Den. **3**:576-581, 1953.

Nidiffer, T. J., and Shipmon, T. H.: The Hollow Bulb Obturator for Acquired Palatal Openings, J. Pros. Den. **7**:126-134, 1957.

Olinger, N. A.: Cleft Palate Prosthesis Rehabilitation, J. Pros. Den. **2**:117-135, 1952.

Rosen, M. S.: Prosthetics for the Cleft Palate Patient, J.A.D.A. **60**:715-721, 1960.

Sharry, J. J.: The Meatus Obturator in Cleft Palate Prosthesis, Oral Surg., Oral Med. & Oral Path. **7**:852-855, 1954.

Sharry, J. J.: Meatus Obturator in Particular and Pharyngeal Impressions in General, J. Pros. Den. **8**:893-896, 1958.

Strain, J. C.: A Simplified Device to Attach the Distal Extension to the Denture of a Cleft Palate Patient, J. Pros. Den. **3**:727-730, 1953.

Strain, J. C.: Cleft Palate Classification, J. Pros. Den. **3**:856-859, 1953.

Torn, D. B.: Speech and Cleft Palate Partial Denture Prosthesis, J. Pros. Den. **2**:413-417, 1952.

Vale, W. A.: Fixed Bridge for a Cleft Palate, Brit. D. J. **96**:65-66, 1954.

Webster, R. C.: Cleft Palate Treatment, Oral Surg., Oral Med. & Oral Path. **1**:647-669, 943-980, 1948; **2**:99-153, 485-542, 1949.

COMPLETE MOUTH AND OCCLUSAL REHABILITATION

Bronstein, B. R.: An Evaluation of Basic Concepts in Mouth Rehabilitation, J. Pros. Den. **1**:560-569, 1951.

Bronstein, B. R.: Rationale and Technique of Biomechanical Occlusal Rehabilitation, J. Pros. Den. **4**:352-367, 1954.

Chestner, S. B.: Cold Cure Acrylic Resin Splints in Occlusal Rehabilitation, J. Pros. Den. **5**:228-231, 1955.

Cohn, L. A.: Occluso-rehabilitation. Principles of Diagnosis and Treatment Planning, D. Clin. North America, pp. 259-281, March, 1962.

Craddock, F. W.: Partial Dentures in Oral Rehabilitation, New Zealand D. J. **49**:6-13, 1953.

Dubin, N. A.: Advances in Functional Occlusal Rehabilitation, J. Pros. Den. **6**:252-258, 1956.

Goldman, I.: The Goal of Full Mouth Rehabilitation, J. Pros. Den. **2**:246-251, 1952.

Goldman, I.: The Art and Science of Full Mouth Rehabilitation, D. Digest **59**:17-22, 1953.

Grewcock, R. J. G.: Oral Rehabilitation, Brit. D. J. **98**:41-49, 1955.

Kazis, H.: Complete Mouth Rehabilitation Through Restoration of Lost Vertical Demension, J.A.D.A. **37**:19-39, 1948.

Kazis, H.: Functional Aspects of Complete Mouth Rehabilitation, J. Pros. Den. **4**:833-841, 1954.

Kornfeld, M.: The Problem of Function in Restorative Dentistry, J. Pros. Den. **5**:670-676, 1955.

Landa, J. S.: An Analysis of Current Practices in Mouth Rehabilitation, J. Pros. Den. **5**:527-537, 1955.

Mann, A. W., and Pankey, L. D.: Oral Rehabilitation. Part I. Use of the P-M Instrument in Treatment Planning and Restoring the Lower Posterior Teeth, J. Pros. Den. **10**:135-150, Jan.-Feb., 1960.

Mann, A. W., and Pankey, L. D.: Oral Rehabilitation Utilizing the Pankey-Mann Instrument and a Functional Bite Technique, D. Clin. North America, pp. 215-230, March, 1959.

Pankey, L. D., and Mann, A. W.: Oral Rehabilitation. Part II. Reconstruction of the Upper Teeth Using a Functionally Generated Path Technique, J. Pros. Den. **10**:151-162, 1960.

Rubinstein, M. N.: Occlusal Rehabilitation in Practice, D. Digest **58**:165-170, 1952.

Rubinstein, M. N.: Mouth Rehabilitation in Practice, D. Digest **59**:207-213, 1953.

Rubinstein, M. N.: Approach to Mouth Reconstruction, D. Digest **61**:24-28, 1955.

Schuyler, C. H.: An Evaluation of Incisal Guidance and Its Influence on Restorative Dentistry, J. Pros. Den. **9**:374-378, 1959.

Schweitzer, J. M.: Open Bite From the Prosthetic Point of View, D. Clin. North America, pp. 269-283, March, 1957.

Simring, M.: Splinting: Theory and Practice, J.A.D.A. **45**:402-414, 1952.

Thompson, M. J.: Hydrocolloid: Its Role in Restorative Dentistry, D. Clin. North America, pp. 101-112, March, 1959.

CROWNS AND FIXED BRIDGE RESTORATIONS

Alexander, P. C.: Analysis of the Cuspid Protective Occlusion J. Pros. Den. 13:309-317, 1963.
Baker, C. R.: Instrumentation for Veneer Crown Preparation, J.A.D.A. 45:550-555, 1952.
Baraban, D. J.: Cementation of Fixed Bridge Prosthesis With Zinc Oxide-Rosin-Eugenol Cements, J. Pros. Den. 8:988-991, 1958.
Bartlett, A. A.: Some Principles of Modern Fixed Bridge Construction, J.A.D.A. 29:2166-2173, 1942.
Boyd, H. R., Jr.: Pontics in Fixed Partial Dentures, J. Pros. Den. 5:55-64, 1955.
Brotman, I. N.: The Roentgenogram as an Aid in Veneer Crown Preparation, J. Pros. Den. 4:349-351, 1954.
Caplan, J.: A Consideration of the Teeth During and Following Their Preparation for Gold Jackets, J. Pros. Den. 3:105-107, 1953.
Caplan, J.: Maintenance of Full Coverage Fixed-Abutment Bridges, J. Pros. Den. 5:852-854, 1955.
Cavanagh, W. D.: Crown and Bridge Prosthesis, J. Canad. D. A. 21:222-226, 1955.
Chestner, S. B.: Cold Acrylic Resin Splints in Occlusal Rehabilitation, J. Pros. Den. 5:228-231, 1955.
Coelho, D. H.: The Ultimate Goal in Fixed Bridge Procedures, J. Pros. Den. 4:667-672, 1954.
Coelho, D. H.: Criteria for the Use of Fixed Prosthesis, D. Clin. North America, pp. 299-311, March, 1957.
Cohn, L. A.: The Acrylic Faced Cast Gold Crown, J. Pros. Den. 1:112-134, 1951.
Cowgen, G. T.: Retention, Resistance and Esthetics of the Anterior Three-Quarter Crown, J.A.D.A. 62:167-171, 1961.
Crown and Bridge Prosthodontics, D. Clin. North America, March, 1959.
Davis, M. C.: Standardized Crown and Bridge Procedure, J. Pros. Den. 3:108-120, 1953.
Davis, M. C., and Klein, G.: Combination Gold and Acrylic Restorations, J. Pros. Den. 4:510-522, 1954.
Ewing, J. E.: Re-evaluation of the Cantilever Principle, J. Pros. Den. 7:78-92, 1957.
Freese, A. S.: Impressions for Temporary Acrylic Resin Jacket Crowns, J. Pros. Den. 7:99-101, 1957.
Gerson, I.: Cementation of Fixed Restorations, J. Pros. Den. 7:123-125, 1957.
Grubb, H. D.: Fixed Bridgework, J. Pros. Den. 3:121-126, 1953.
Hagerman, D. A., and Arnim, S. S.: The Relation of New Knowledge of the Gingiva to Crown and Bridge Procedures, J. Pros. Den. 5:538-542, 1955; D. Abs. 1:44, 1956.
Hamburg, H. L.: Fixed Bridge Assemblage, D. Digest 59:160-161, 1953.
Herschfus, L.: Procedure for Immediate Temporary Bridge, D. Digest 60:550-551, 1954.
Johnston, J. F., Dykema, R. W., Mumford, G., and Phillips, R. W.: Construction and Assembly of Porcelain Veneer Gold Crowns and Pontics, J. Pros. Den. 12:1125-1137, 1962.
Kahn, A. E.: Reversible Hydrocolloids in the Construction of the Unit-Built Porcelain Bridge, J. Pros. Den. 6:72-79, 1956.
Kay, S.: Fixed Splints and Fixed Bridgework Retained by Horizontal Pins, J. Pros. Den. 4:656-666, 1954.
Leff, A.: An Improved Temporary Acrylic Fixed Bridge, J. Pros. Den. 3:245-249, 1953.
Leff, A.: New Concepts in the Preparation of Teeth for Full Coverage, J. Pros. Den. 5:392-400, 1955.
Leff, A.: Reproduction of Tooth Anatomy and Positional Relationship in Full Cast or Veneer Crowns, J. Pros. Den. 6:550-557, 1956.
LeHuche, R.: Preparation of Three-Quarter Crowns, D. Abs. 1:44, 1956.
Ludwick, R. W., Jr., and Lynn, L. M.: A Method to Reduce Pain During Cementation of Restorations, J.A.D.A. 53:563-566, 1956.
Malson, T. S.: Anatomic Cast Crown Reproduction, J. Pros. Den. 9:106-112, 1959.
Miller, C. J.: The Tube Impression, D. Digest 59:171-173, 1953.
Miller, I. F.: Full Coverage Abutment, New York J. Den. 22:339-340, 1952.
Nuttall, E. B.: Clinical and Technical Aspects of Crown and Bridge Prosthesis, Bul. Philadelphia Co. D. Soc. 14:128-133, 1950.
Phillips, B. S., and Price, R. R.: Some Factors Which Influence the Surface of Stone Dies Poured in Alginate Impressions, J. Pros. Den. 5:72-79, 1955.
Phillips, R. W., and Biggs, D. H.: Distortion of Wax Patterns as Influenced by Storage Time, Storage Temperature, and Temperature of Wax Manipulation, J.A.D.A. 41:28-37, 1950.

Phillips, R. W., and Swartz, M. L.: A Study of Adaptation of Veneers to Cast Gold Crowns, J. Pros. Den. **7**:817-822, 1957.

Pound, E.: The Problem of the Lower Anterior Bridge, J. Pros. Den. **5**:543-545, 1955.

Pruden, K. C.: A Hydrocolloid Technique for Pinledge Bridge Abutments, J. Pros. Den. **6**:65-71, 1956.

Retana, J. M.: Pinledges as Bridge Anchorages. Pins and Inlays Combined, D. Abs. **2**:81, 1957.

Rheuben, R. P.: Full Mouth Reconstruction for the General Practitioner, D. Digest **60**:294-301, 1954.

Rubin, M. K.: Full Coverage: The Provisional and Final Restorations Made Easier, J. Pros. Den. **8**:664-672, 1958.

Rubinstein, M. N.: Immediate Acrylic Temporary Crown and Bridge, D. Digest **60**:12-13, 1954.

Saklad, M. J.: An Esthetic Provisional Cast Gold and Acrylic Splint, J. Pros. Den. **4**:653-655, 1954.

Shooshan, E. D.: The Full Veneer Cast Crown, D. Abs. **1**:276-277, 1956.

Shooshan, E. D.: The Reverse Pin-Porcelain Facing, J. Pros. Den. **9**:284-301, 1959.

Sloane, T. S.: Mouth Reconstruction, J. Pros. Den. **3**:127-139, 1953.

Smith, G. P.: The Marginal Fit of the Full Cast Shoulderless Crown, J. Pros. Den. **7**:231-243, 1957.

Smith, G. P.: Objectives of a Fixed Partial Denture, J. Pros. Den. **11**:463-473, 1961.

Sokoloff, A.: The Veneered Full Cast Crown, D. Abs. **1**:165-166, 1956.

Staffanou, R. S., and Thayer, K. E.: Reverse Pin-Porcelain Veneer and Pontic Technique, J. Pros. Den. **12**:1138-1145, 1962.

Stibbs, G. D.: Impression and Pattern Technique for Anterior Three-Quarter Crowns, J. Pros. Den. **6**:558-562, 1956.

Talkov, L.: Lining Up Multiple Abutments, J. Pros. Den. **1**:727-732, 1951.

Talkov, L.: Temporary Acrylic Fixed Bridgework and Splints, J. Pros. Den. **2**:693-702, 1952.

Talkov, L.: The Copper Band Splint, J. Pros. Den. **6**:245-251, 1956.

Terkla, L. G.: Crown Morphology in Relation to Operative and Crown and Bridge Dentistry, D. Abs. **1**:394-396, 1956.

Thompson, M. J.: A Standardized Indirect Technic for Reversible Hydrocolloid, J.A.D.A. **46**:1-18, 1953.

Troxell, R. R.: The Polishing of Gold Castings, J. Pros. Den. **9**:668-675, 1959.

Wallace, F. H.: Resin Transfer Copings, J. Pros. Den. **8**:289-292, 1958.

Wheeler, R. C.: The Implications of Full Coverage Restorative Procedures, J. Pros. Den. **5**:848-851, 1955.

Wheeler, R. C.: Complete Crown Form and the Periodontium, J. Pros. Den. **11**:722-734, 1961.

Willey, R. E.: The Preparation of Abutments for Veneer Retainers, D. Abs. **2**:28, 1957.

Woolson, A. H.: Restorations Made of Porcelain Baked on Gold, J. Pros. Den. **5**:65, 1955.

Wyrick, W.: An Anterior Fixed Bridge Replacing a Missing Tooth Where Abnormally Large Interproximal Spaces Exist, J. Pros. Den. **2**:829-830, 1952.

Yock, D. H.: Indications for the Use of Plastic Resins in Crown and Bridge Prosthesis, J.A.D.A. **46**:505-509, 1953.

Zola, A.: The Acrylic Resin Transfer Pattern, J. Pros. Den. **9**:278-283, 1959.

DENTAL LABORATORY PROCEDURES

Benfield, J. W., and Lyons, G. V.: Precision Dies From Elastic Impressions, J. Pros. Den. **12**:737-752, 1962.

Blanchard, C. H.: Filling Undercuts on Refractory Casts With Investment, J. Pros. Den. **3**:417-418, 1953.

Dirksen, L. C., and Campagna, S. J.: Mat Surface and Rugae Reproduction for Upper Partial Denture Castings, J. Pros. Den. **4**:67-72, 1954.

Enright, C. M.: Dentist-Dental Laboratory Harmony, J. Pros. Den. **11**:393-394, 1961.

Grunewald, A. H.: Dentist, Dental Laboratory, and the Patient, J. Pros. Den. **8**:55-60, 1958.

Grunewald, A. H.: The Role of the Dental Technician in a Prosthetic Service, D. Clin. North America, pp. 359-370, July, 1960.

Grunewald, A. H., Paffenbarger, G. C., and Dickson, G.: The Effect of Molding Processes on Some Properties of Denture Resins, J.A.D.A. **44**:269-284, 1952.

Haszar, G.: Polishing of Artificial Dentures, D. Abs. **1**:680-681, 1956.

Hollenback, G. M., and Skinner, E. W.: Shrinkage During Casting of Gold and Gold Alloys, J.A.D.A. **33**:1391-1399, 1946.

Johnson, H. B.: Technique for Packing and Staining Complete or Partial Denture Bases, J. Pros. Den. **6**:154-159, 1956.

Margetis, P. M., and Hansen, W. C.: Changes in Agar-Agar Type Duplicating Material and Agar-Agar on Heating and Storage, J.A.D.A. **54**:737-745, 1957.

Perlowski, S. A.: Investment Changes During Flasking as a Factor of Complete Denture Malocclusion, J. Pros. Den. **3**:497-499, 1953.

Peyton, F. A.: Packing and Processing Denture Base Resins, J.A.D.A. **40**:520-528, 1950.

Peyton, F. A.: Cast Chromium-Cobalt Alloys, D. Clin. North America, 759-771, Nov. 1958.

Peyton, F. A., and Anthony, D. H.: Evaluation of Dentures Processed by Different Techniques, J. Pros. Den. **13**:269-281, 1963.

Ryge, G., Kozak, S. F., and Fairhurst, C. W.: Porosities in Dental Gold Castings, J.A.D.A. **54**:746-754, 1957.

Schmidt, A. H.: Repairing Chrome-Cobalt Castings, J. Pros. Den. **5**:385-387, 1955.

Smith, G. P.: The Responsibility of the Dentist Toward Laboratory Procedures in Fixed and Removable Partial Denture Prosthesis, J. Pros. Den. **13**:295-301, 1963.

Smyd, E. S.: Wax Refractory Investments and Related Subjects in Dental Technology, J. Pros. Den. **5**:514-526, 1955.

Suffert, L. W., and Mahler, D. B.: Reproducibility of Gold Castings Made by Present Day Dental Casting Technics, J.A.D.A. **50**:1-6, 1955.

Walker, T. J., and Orsinger, W. O.: Palate Reproduction by the Hydrocolloid-Resin Method, J. Pros. Den. **4**:54-66, 1954.

DENTURE ESTHETICS: TOOTH SELECTION AND ARRANGEMENT

Brill, N.: Adaptation and the Hydrid-Prosthesis, J. Pros. Den. **5**:811-824, 1955.

DeVan, M. M.: The Appearance Phase of Denture Construction, D. Clin. North America, pp. 255-268, March, 1957.

Eich, F. A.: The Construction of a Metal Mold for Acrylic Teeth, J. Pros. Den. **1**:594-600,1951.

French, F. A.: The Selection and Arrangement of the Anterior Teeth in Prosthetic Dentures, J. Pros. Den. **1**:587-593, 1951.

Frush, J. P., and Fisher, R. D.: Introduction to Dentogenic Restorations, J. Pros. Den. **5**:586-595, 1955.

Frush, J. P., and Fisher, R. D.: How Dentogenic Restorations Interpret the Sex Factor, J. Pros. Den. **6**:160-172, 1956.

Frush, J. P., and Fisher, R. D.: How Dentogenics Interprets the Personality Factor, J. Pros. Den. **6**:441-449, 1956.

Geiger, E. C. K.: Duplication of the Esthetics of an Existing Immediate Denture, J. Pros. Den. **5**:179-185, 1955.

Hughes, G. A.: Facial Types and Tooth Arrangement, J. Pros. Den. **1**:82-95, 1951.

Krajicek, D. D.: Personalized Acrylic Resin Anterior Teeth, J. Pros. Den. **6**:29-37, 1956.

Krajicek, D. D.: Natural Appearance for the Individual Denture Patient, J. Pros. Den. **10**:205-214, 1960.

Myerson, R. L.: The Use of Porcelain and Plastic Teeth in Opposing Complete Dentures, J. Pros. Den. **7**:625-633, 1957.

Pound, E.: Esthetic Dentures and Their Phonetic Values, J. Pros. Den. **1**:98-111, 1951.

Pound, E.: Lost—Fine Arts in the Fallacy of the Ridges, J. Pros. Den. **4**:6-16, 1954.

Pound, E.: Recapturing Esthetic Tooth Position in the Edentulous Patient, J.A.D.A. **55**:181-191, 1957.

Pound, E.: Applying Harmony in Selecting and Arranging Teeth, D. Clin. North America, pp. 241-258, March, 1962.

Powers, J. L.: Brush on Technique in Natural Coloring of Cured Cross-Linked Plastic Artificial Denture Materials, J. Pros. Den. **3**:350-353, 1953.

Proctor, H. H.: Characterization of Dentures, J. Pros. Den. **3**:339-349, 1953.

Sears, V. H.: Analysis of Art Factors in Full Denture Construction, J.A.D.A. & D. Cosmos **25**:3-12, 1938.

Schopper, A. F.: Esthetic Principles of Partial Denture Prosthesis, Washington Univ. D. J. **5**:112-118, 1939.

Tillman, E. J.: Molding and Staining Acrylic Resin Anterior Teeth, J. Pros. Den. **5**:497-507, 1955; D. Abs. **1**:111, 1956.

Tustison, H. W.: Gold Inlays Cast Into Porcelain Teeth, J. Pros. Den. **3**:181-183, 1953.

Van Victor, A.: Positive Duplication of Anterior Teeth for Immediate Dentures, J. Pros. Den. 3:165-177, 1953.
Van Victor, A.: The Mold Guide Cast—Its Significance in Denture Esthetics, J. Pros. Den. 13:406-415, 1963.
Vig, R. G.: The Denture Look, J. Pros. Den. 11:9-15, 1961.
Wolfson, E.: Staining and Characterization of Acrylic Teeth, D. Abs. 1:41, 1956.
Young, H. A.: Selecting the Anterior Tooth Mold, J. Pros. Den. 4:748-760, 1954.
Young, H. A.: Denture Esthetics, J. Pros. Den. 6:748-755, 1956.

DIAGNOSIS AND TREATMENT PLANNING

Applegate, O. C.: Evaluating Oral Structures for Removable Partial Dentures, J. Pros. Den. 11:882-885, 1961.
Bartels, J. C.: Diagnosis and Treatment Planning, J. Pros. Den. 7:657-662, 1957.
Blatterfein, L.: The Planning and Contouring of Acrylic Resin Veneer Crowns for Partial Denture Clasping, J. Pros. Den. 6:386-404, 1956.
Contino, R. M., and Stallard, H.: Instruments Essential for Obtaining Data Needed in Making a Functional Diagnosis of the Human Mouth, J. Pros. Den. 7:66-77, 1957.
Dunn, B. W.: Treatment Planning for Removable Partial Dentures, J. Pros. Den. 11:247-255, 1961.
Foster, T. D.: The Use of the Face-Bow in Making Permanent Study Casts, J. Pros. Den. 9:717-721, 1959.
Frankel, H. J.: Uses of Antopolymerizing Acrylic Resins in Fixed Partial Prosthesis, J. Pros. Den. 8:1003-1006, 1958.
Frechette, A. R.: Partial Denture Planning With Special Reference to Stress Distribution, J. Pros. Den. 1:700-707 (disc., 208-209), 1951.
Friedman, J.: Cast Analysis of Partial Denture Problems, J. Pros. Den. 4:82-86, 1954.
Friedman, J.: Abutment Sites and Spaces in Partial Denture Case Analysis, J. Pros. Den. 4:803-812, 1954.
Friedman, S.: Effective Use of Diagnostic Data, J. Pros. Den. 9:729-737, 1959.
Gill, J. R.: Treatment Planning for Mouth Rehabilitation, J. Pros. Den. 2:230-245, 1952.
House, M. M.: The Relationship of Oral Examination to Dental Diagnosis, J. Pros. Den. 8:208-219, 1958.
Landa, J. S.: Diagnosis of the Edentulous Mouth and the Probable Prognosis of Its Rehabilitation, D. Clin. North America, pp. 187-201, March, 1957.
McCracken, W. L.: Differential Diagnosis: Fixed or Removable Partial Dentures, J.A.D.A. 63:767-775, 1961.
Moulton, G. H.: The Importance of Centric Occlusion in Diagnosis and Treatment Planning, J. Pros. Den. 10:921-926, 1960.
Payne, S. H.: Diagnostic Factors Which Influence the Choice of Posterior Occlusion, D. Clin. North America, pp. 203-213, March, 1957.
Perry, C. F., and Applegate, S. G.: Study Cast, J. Michigan D. Soc. 28:82-84, 1946.
Sauser, C. W.: Pretreatment Evaluation of Partially Edentulous Arches, J. Pros. Den. 11:886-893, 1961.
Schuyler, C. H.: Elements of Diagnosis Leading to Full or Partial Dentures, J.A.D.A. 41:302-305, 1950.
Seiden, A.: Occlusal Rests and Rest Seats, J. Pros. Den. 8:431-440, 1958.
Wilson, J. H.: The General Principles of Diagnosis and Prognosis of Partial Dentures, D. J. Australia 11:69-77, 1939.
Young, A. C.: Indications and the Diagnosis for Fixed Partial Denture Prosthesis, J.A.D.A. 41:289-295, 1950.
Young, H. A.: Diagnostic Survey of Edentulous Patients, J. Pros. Den. 5:5-14, 1955.

IMPRESSION MATERIALS AND METHODS; THE PARTIAL DENTURE BASE

Applegate, O. C.: The Partial Denture Base, J. Pros. Den. 5:636-648, 1955.
Applegate, O. C.: Stresses Induced by a Partial Denture Upon Its Supporting Structures and Practical Methods of Control, Proc. D. Centenary, pp. 308-319, 1940.
Applegate, O. C.: An Evaluation of the Support for the Removable Partial Denture, J. Pros. Den. 10:112-123, 1960.
Bailey, L. R.: Acrylic Resin Tray for Rubber Base Impression Materials, J. Pros. Den. 5:658-662, 1955.

Bailey, L. R.: Rubber Base Impression Techniques, D. Clin. North America, pp. 156-166, March, 1957.

Beckett, L. S.: Partial Denture Impressions, D. J. Australia **27**:135-138, 1955.

Blanchard, C. H.: Transferring Facial Surfaces From the Impression to the Denture, J. Pros. Den. **4**:621, 1954.

Bollwerk, E. H.: An Improved Impression Technique for Partial Dentures With Distal Extension Saddles, J. Pros. Den. **3**:476-477, 1953.

Boucher, C. O.: A Critical Analysis of Mid-Century Impression Techniques for Full Dentures, J. Pros. Den. **1**:472-491, 1951.

Chase, W. W.: Adaptation of Rubber-Base Impression Materials to Removable Denture Prosthetics, J. Pros. Den. **10**:1043-1050, 1960.

Clark, R. J., and Phillips, R. W.: Flow Studies of Certain Dental Impression Materials, J. Pros. Den. **7**:259-266, 1957.

Davis, M. C.: The Use of Rubber Base Impression Materials in the Construction of Inlays, J. Pros. Den. **8**:123-134, 1958.

Feinberg, E.: Technique for Master Impressions in Fixed Restorations, J. Pros. Den. **5**:663-666, 1955.

Gilmore, W. H., Schnell, R. J., and Phillips, R. W.: Factors Influencing the Accuracy of Silicone Impression Materials, J. Pros. Den. **9**:304-314, 1959.

Heath, V. M.: Lining Paste Impression Technique for Partial Dentures, Brit. D. J. **93**:45-46, 1952.

Hindels, G. W.: Load Distribution in Extension Saddle Partial Dentures, J. Pros. Den. **2**:92-100, 1952.

Hudson, W. C.: Clinical Uses of Rubber Impression Materials and Electroforming of Casts and Dies in Pure Silver, J. Pros. Den. **8**:107-114, 1958.

Johnston, J. F., Cunningham, D. M., and Bogan, R. G.: The Dentist, the Patient, and Ridge Preservation, J. Pros. Den. **10**:288-295, 1960.

Kramer, H. M.: Impression Technique for Removable Partial Dentures, J. Pros. Den. **11**:84-92, 1961.

Mann, A. W.: A Critical Appraisal of the Hydrocolloid Technique: Its Advantages and Disadvantages, J. Pros. Den. **1**:727-732, 1951.

McCracken, W. L.: An Evaluation of Activated Methyl Methacrylate Denture Base Materials, J. Pros. Den. **2**:68-83, 1952.

Morrison, R. D.: An Impression Tray for Rubber Base Materials, D. Abs. **1**:163, 1956.

Myers, G. E.: Electroformed Die Technique for Rubber Base Impressions, J. Pros. Den. **8**:531-535, 1958.

Paffenbarger, G. C.: Hydrocolloid Impression Materials: Physical Properties and a Specification, J.A.D.A. **27**:373-388, 1940.

Perdigon, G. J.: Similarity of Technique for Fixed and Removable Restorations Using Reversible Hydrocolloid, J. Pros. Den. **2**:801-814, 1952.

Peyton, F. A., Shiere, H. B., and Delgado, V. P.: Some Comparisons of Self-Curing and Heat-Curing Denture Resins, J. Pros. Den. **3**:332-338, 1953.

Pfeiffer, K. A.: Clinical Problems in the Use of Alginate Hydrocolloid, D. Abs. **2**:82, 1957.

Phillips, R. W.: Factors Influencing the Accuracy of Reversible Hydrocolloid Impressions, J.A.D.A. **43**:1-17, 1951.

Phillips, R. W.: Factors Affecting the Surface of Stone Dies Poured in Hydrocolloid Impressions, J. Pros. Den. **2**:390-400, 1952.

Phillips, R. W.: Elastic Impression Materials—A Second Progress Report of a Recent Conference, J. South. California D. A. **26**:150-153, 1958.

Phillips, R. W.: Physical Properties and Manipulation of Rubber Impression Materials, J.A.D.A. **59**:454-458, 1959.

Rosenstiel, E.: Rubber Base Elastic Impression Materials, D. Abs. **1**:55, 1956.

Silver, M.: Impressions and Silver-Plated Dies From a Rubber Impression Material, J. Pros. Den. **6**:543-549, 1956.

Skinner, E. W., Cooper, E. N., and Beck, F. E.: Reversible and Irreversible Hydrocolloid Impression Materials, J.A.D.A. **35**:245-256, 1947.

Skinner, E. W., and Hoblit, N. E.: A Study of the Accuracy of Hydrocolloid Impressions, J. Pros. Den. **6**:80-86, 1956.

Steffel, V. L.: Relining Removable Partial Dentures for Fit and Function, J. Pros. Den. **4**:496-509, 1954; J. Tennessee D. A. **36**:35-43, 1956.

Tilton, G. E.: The Denture Periphery, J. Pros. Den. **2**:290-306, 1952.

Wilson, J. H.: Partial Dentures—Relining the Saddle Supported by the Mucosa and Alveolar Bone, J. Pros. Den. **3**:807-813, 1953.

MAXILLOFACIAL PROSTHESIS

Ackerman, A. J.: Maxillofacial Prosthesis, Oral Surg., Oral Med. & Oral Path. **6**:176-200, 1953.

Ackerman, A. J.: The Prosthetic Management of Oral and Facial Defects Following Cancer Surgery, J. Pros. Den. **5**:413-432, 1955.

Appleman, R. M.: The Prosthetic Repair of Defects of the Maxilla Resulting From Surgery, J. Pros. Den. **1**:424-437, 1951.

Appleman, R. M.: Surgical Prosthesis, J. Pros. Den. **2**:401-412, 1952.

Edgerton, M. T., and Pyott, J. E.: Surgery and Prosthesis in Jaw Reconstruction, J. Pros. Den. **4**:257-262, 1954.

Emory, L.: Partial Denture Prosthesis for War Injuries, J.A.D.A. **35**:643-644, 1947.

Grunewald, A. H.: The Prosthodontists's Role in Cranioplasty, J. Pros. Den. **5**:235-243, 1955.

Lazzari, J. B.: A Prosthetic Closure of a Traumatic Palatal Perforation, J. Pros. Den. **2**:831-833, 1952.

Lazzari, J. B.: Intraoral Splint for Support of the Lip in Bell's Palsy, J. Pros. Den. **5**:579-581, 1955.

Olin, W. H.: Maxillofacial Prosthesis, J.A.D.A. **48**:399-409, 1954.

Nadeau, J.: Maxillofacial Prosthesis With Magnetic Stabilizers, J. Pros. Den. **6**:114-119, 1956.

Schork, C. J.: Prosthetic Appliance for Comminuted Fracture of the Nose: Report of a Case, J. Oral Surg. **2**:324-327, 1944.

Smith, E. H., Jr.: Prosthetic Treatment of Maxillofacial Injuries, J. Pros. Den. **5**:112-128, 1955.

Strain, J. C.: A Mechanical Device for Duplicating a Mirror Image of a Cast or Moulage in Three Dimensions, J. Pros. Den. **5**:129-132, 1955.

Strickland, J. M.: Prosthetic Restoration With a Removable Partial Denture After Surgical Removal of a Tumor of the Right Maxillary Antrum, Am. J. Orthodont. & Oral Surg. (Oral. Surg. Sect.) **31**:504-510, 1945.

MISCELLANEOUS

Academy of Denture Prosthetics: Principles, Concepts and Practices in Prosthodontics; Progress Report III, J. Pros. Den. **13**:283-294, 1963.

Anthony, D. H., and Gibbons, P.: The Nature and Behavior of Denture Cleansers, J. Pros. Den. **8**:796-810, 1958.

Applegate, O. C.: Partial Denture in a Program of Preventive Dentistry, J. Michigan D. Soc. **24**:217-219, 1942.

Applegate, O. C.: Conditions Which May Influence the Choice of Partial or Complete Denture Service, J. Pros. Den. **7**:182-196, 1957.

Applegate, O. C.: The Removable Partial Denture in the General Practice of Tomorrow, J. Pros. Den. **8**:609-622, 1958.

Applegate, O. C., and Missle, R. O.: Keeping the Partial Denture in Harmony With Biologic Limitations, J.A.D.A. **43**:409-419, 1951.

Applegate, O. C.: Factors to be Considered in Choosing an Alloy, D. Clin. North America, pp. 583-590, Nov., 1960.

Appleman, R. M.: Why Partial Dentures Fail, D. Digest **54**:490-497, 1948.

Beck, H. O.: A Clinical Evaluation of the Arcon Concept of Articulation, J. Pros. Den. **9**:409-421, 1959.

Beck, H. O.: Alloys for Removable Partial Dentures, D. Clin. North America, pp. 591-596, Nov., 1960.

Beck, H. O., and Morrison, W. E.: Investigation of an Arcon Articulator, J. Pros. Den. **6**:359-372, 1956.

Beckett, L. S.: Some Fundamentals of Partial Denture Construction, Australian J. Den. **44**:363-367, 1940.

Beckett, L. S.: The Influence of Saddle Classification on the Design of Partial Removable Restorations, J. Pros. Den. **3**:506-516, 1953.

Bell, D. H.: Sagittal Balance of the Mandible, J.A.D.A. **64**:486-495, 1962.

Blanchard, C. H.: Eyes in Your Fingers, J. Pros. Den. **2**:36-39, 1952.

Blanchard, C. H.: Repairing a Broken Lingual Bar, J. Pros. Den. **4**:135-136, 1954.

Blatterfein, L.: Role of the Removable Partial Denture in the Restoration of Lost Vertical Dimension, New York Univ. J. Den. **10**:274-276, 1952.

Boucher, Carl O. (editor): Current Clinical Dental Terminology, St. Louis, 1963, The C. V. Mosby Co.

Cole, F. L.: Construction of a Balanced Partial Denture, J. Canad. D. A. **10**:161-163, 1944.

Coomer, O. B.: Attaining and Maintaining Mouth Health, J. Pros. Den. **3**:500-505, 1953.

Cummer, W. E.: Partial Denture Service. In Anthony, L. P. (editor): American Textbook of Prosthetic Dentistry, Philadelphia, 1942, Lea & Febiger, pp. 670-840.

Deck, R. F.: Aspects of Partial Denture Construction, Australian D. Mirror **10**:11-23, 1944.

Dental Materials, D. Clin. North America, 1958.

DeVan, M. M.: The Nature of the Partial Denture Foundation: Suggestions for Its Preservation, J. Pros. Den. **2**:210-218, 1952.

DeVan, M. M.: The Additive Partial Denture: Its Principles and Design (Partial Dentures) North-West Den. **35**:303-307, 312, 1956; D. Abs. **2**:468, 1957.

Elliott, F. C.: Partial Denture Prosthesis as a Health Service, J. Michigan D. Soc. **20**:163-169, 1938.

Elliott, F. C.: Removable Partial Denture Prosthesis, J.A.D.A. **40**:676, 1950.

Elliott, R. W.: The Effects of Heat on Gold Partial Denture Castings, J. Pros. Den. **13**:688-698, 1963.

Ewing, J. E.: Temporary Cementation in Fixed Partial Prosthesis, J. Pros. Den. **5**:388-391, 1955.

Fisher, A. A.: Allergic Sensitization of the Skin and Oral Mucosa to Acrylic Resin Denture Materials, J. Pros. Den. **6**:593-602, 1956.

Flagstad, C. O., and Elliott, F. C.: Problems in Partial Denture Service, J.A.D.A. **29**:1822-1824, 1942.

Fuller, J. F.: Partial Denture Construction, New Zealand D. J. **43**:117-132, 1947.

Gecker, L. M.: Bruxism—A Rationale of Therapy, J.A.D.A. **66**:14-18, 1963.

Giglio, J. J., Lace, W. P., and Arden, H.: Factors Affecting Retention and Stability of Complete Dentures, J. Pros. Den. **12**:848-856, 1962.

Gilbert, A.: Fundamentals of Self-Curing Acrylic Resins, D. Items Interest **74**:420-426, 1952.

Girardot, R. L.: The Physiologic Aspects of Partial Denture Restorations, J. Pros. Den. **3**:689-698, 1953.

Glossary of Prosthodontic Terms, J. Pros. Den. **10**:Nov.-Dec., 1960.

Griffiths, N. H. D.: Partial Denture Prosthesis, Bul. Nat. D. A. **9**:210-214, 1951.

Herlands, R. E.: Removable Partial Denture Terminology, J. Pros. Den. **8**:964-972, 1958.

Hughes, F. C.: The Transition From Natural to Prosthetic Dentures, J. Pros. Den. **1**:145-150, 1951.

Hughes, G. A.: Review of Basic Principles of Removable Partial Denture Prosthesis, Fort. Rev. Chicago D. Soc. **13**:9-13, 23, 1947.

Jankelson, B. H.: Adjustment of Dentures at Time of Insertion and Alterations to Compensate for Tissue Changes, J.A.D.A. **64**:521-531, 1962.

Johnson, O. M.: Some Essentials to be Observed in Partial Denture Service, Baylor D. J. **1**:16-18, 1951.

Johnson, W.: Gold Alloys for Casting Dentures: An Investigation of Some Mechanical Properties, Brit. D. J. **102**:41-49, 1957.

Jones, R. R.: Partial Dentures, Minneapolis Dist. D. J. **23**:28-30, 1939.

Jones, R. R.: Partial Dentures, Minneapolis Dist. D. J. **34**:79-82, 1950.

Jones, R. R.: The Lower Partial Denture, J. Pros. Den. **2**:219-229, 1952.

Jordan, L. G.: Partial Dentures, J.A.D.A. **29**:169-183, 1942.

Jorgensen, N. B.: Premedication in Prosthodontics, J. Pros. Den. **3**:675-681, 1953.

Kaires, A. K.: A Study of Partial Denture Design and Masticatory Pressures in a Mandibular Bilateral Distal Extension Case, J. Pros. Den. **8**:340-350, 1958.

Kelley, E. K.: The Physiologic Approach to Partial Denture Design, J. Pros. Den. **3**:699-710, 1953.

Kessler, B.: An Analysis of the Tongue Factor and Its Functioning Areas in Dental Prosthesis, J. Pros. Den. **5**:629-635, 1955.

Kutscher, A. H.: An Esthetic Masking Cement for Prosthetic Denture Clasps, J. Pros. Den. **3**:715-717, 1953.

Landa, J. S.: Some Fundamental Considerations in Partial Denture Prosthesis, D. Outlook **30**:267-270, 1943.

Landa, J. S.: The Troublesome Transition From a Partial Lower to a Complete Lower Denture, J. Pros. Den. **4**:42-51, 1954.

Lenchner, N. H., Handlers, M., and Weissman, B.: A Modification of a Special Retaining Device for Partial Dentures, J. Pros. Den. **8**:973-980, 1958.

Lew, Isaih: Free-End Saddle Prosthesis, Part 2, D. Digest **63:**456-460, 1957.

Loos, A.: Bio-Physiological Principles in the Construction of Partial Dentures, Brit. D. J. **88:**61-68, 1950.

Main, L. R.: Value of the Roentgen Rays in Partial Denture Prosthesis, J.A.D.A. **28:**766-769, 1941.

Maison, W. G.: Instructions to Denture Patients, J. Pros. Den. **9:**825-831, 1959.

Martone, A. L.: The Fallacy of Saving Time at the Chair, J. Pros. Den. **7:**416-419, 1957.

Martone, A. L.: The Effects of Oral Prostheses on the Production of Speech Sounds, 1956, Ohio State University, D. Abs. **2:**508, 1957.

Martone, A. L.: The Challenge of the Partially Edentulous Mouth, J. Pros. Den. **8:**942-954, 1958.

McLean, D. W.: Factors of Partial Denture Success or Failure, D. Cosmos **77:**256-263, 1935.

McLean, D. W.: Stabilization of Partial Dentures, J.A.D.A. **23:**545-553, 1936.

McLean, D. W.: The Partial Denture as a Vehicle for Function, J.A.D.A. **23:**1271-1278, 1936.

McLean, D. W.: Fundamental Principles of Partial Denture Construction, J. Tennessee D. A. **19:**108-118, 1939.

McCracken, W. L.: A Comparison of Tooth-Borne and Tooth-Tissue-Borne Removable Partial Dentures, J. Pros. Den. **3:**375-381, 1953.

McCracken, W. L.: Auxiliary Uses of Cold-Curing Acrylic Resins in Prosthetic Dentistry, J.A.D.A. **47:**298-304, 1953.

McCracken, W. L.: A Philosophy of Partial Denture Treatment, J. Pros. Den. **13:**889-900, 1963.

Mehringer, E. J.: The Saliva as It Is Related to the Wearing of Dentures, J. Pros. Den. **4:**312-318, 1954.

Merkeley, H. J.: Mandibular Rearmament. Part II. Denture Construction, J. Pros. Den. **9:**567-577, 1959.

Morden, J. F. C., Lammie, G. A., and Osborne, J.: Effect of Various Denture Cleaning Solutions on Chrome Cobalt Alloys, D. Digest **1:**682, 1956.

Mosteller, J. H.: Use of Prednisolone in the Elimination of Postoperative Thermal Sensitivity, J. Pros. Den. **12:**1176-1179, 1962.

Neufeld, J. O.: Changes in the Trabecular Pattern of the Mandible Following the Loss of Teeth, J. Pros. Den. **8:**685-697, 1958.

Öatlund, S. G.: Saliva and Denture Retention, J. Pros. Den. **10:**658-663, 1960.

Osborne, J.: Partial Dentures, D. Practitioner **2:**207-210, 1952.

Osborne, J., and Lammie, G. A.: The Bilateral Free-End Saddle Lower Denture, J. Pros. Den. **4:**640-652, 1954.

Phillips, R. W., and Leonard, L. J.: A Study of Enamel Abrasion as Related to Partial Denture Clasps, J. Pros. Den. **6:**657-671, 1956.

Prosthodontics, D. Clin. North America, March, 1957.

Raybin, N. H.: The Polished Surface of Complete Dentures, J. Pros. Den. **13:**236-239, 1963.

Rothman, R.: Phonetic Considerations in Denture Prosthesis, J. Pros. Den. **11:**214-223, 1961.

Rowlett, A. E.: Oral Hygiene for Partial Denture Wearers, Brit. D. J. **79:**274-275, 1945.

Ryan, E. J.: The Dental Problems of Senescence, J. Pros. Den. **1:**64-70, 1951.

Schnader, Y. E.: Relation Between Partial Dentures and the Living Tissues, Pennsylvania D. J. **49:**29-32, 42, 1946.

Schnadt, H. O.: Removable Partial Prosthesis, D. Abs. **1:**396-397, 1956.

Schole, M. L.: Management of the Gagging Patient, J. Pros. Den. **9:**578-583, 1959.

Schopper, A. F.: Removable Appliances for the Preservation of the Teeth, J. Pros. Den. **4:**634-639, 1954.

Schopper, A. F.: Loss of Vertical Dimension: Causes and Effects: Diagnosis and Various Recommended Treatments, J. Pros. Den. **9:**428-431, 1959.

Schuyler, C. H.: Stress Distribution as the Prime Requisite to the Success of a Partial Denture, J.A.D.A. **20:**2148-2154, 1933.

Schuyler, C. H.: Planning the Removable Partial Denture to Restore Function and Maintain Oral Health, New York D. J. **13:**4-10, 1947.

Sears, V. H.: Comprehensive Denture Service, J.A.D.A. **64:**531-552, 1962.

Sexson, J. C., and Phillips, R. W.: Studies on the Effects of Abrasives on Acrylic Resins, J. Pros. Den. **1:**454-471, 1951.

Silverman, S. I.: The Management of the Trial Denture Base, D. Clin. North America, pp. 231-243, March, 1957.

Skinner, E. W.: Acrylic Denture Base Materials: Their Physical Properties and Manipulation, J. Pros. Den. **1:**161-167, 1951.

Skinner, E. W., Campbell, R. L., and Chung, Paul: A Clinical Study of the Forces Required to Dislodge Maxillary Denture Bases of Various Designs, J.A.D.A. **47**:671-680, 1953.

Skinner, E. W., and Gordon, C. C.: Some Experiments on the Surface Hardness of Dental Stones, J. Pros. Den. **6**:94-100, 1956.

Skinner, E. W., and Jones, P. M.: Dimensional Stability of Self-Curing Denture Base Acrylic Resin, J.A.D.A. **51**:426-431, 1955.

Slack, F. A., Jr.: Experiments in Directional Polymerization, D. Digest **63**:356-359, 1957.

Smith, E. H., Jr.: A Method of Producing Display Models, J. Pros. Den. **5**:563-566, 1955.

Smith, F. W., and Applegate, O. C.: Roentgenographic Study of Bone Changes During Exercise Stimulation of Edentulous Areas, J. Pros. Den. **11**:1086-1097, 1961.

Stahl, D. G.: A Simplified Procedure for Fabricating a Temporary Removable Acrylic Bite Plane, D. Abs. **1**:719, 1956.

Stamoulis, S.: Physical Factors Affecting the Retention of Complete Dentures, J. Pros. Den. **12**:857-864, 1962.

Standard, S. G.: Problems Related to the Construction of Complete Upper and Partial Lower Dentures, J.A.D.A. **43**:695-708, 1951.

Standard, S. G.: Problems Related to the Construction of Complete Upper and Partial Lower Dentures, D. Abs. **1**:196-197, 1956.

Steiger, A. A.: Progress in Partial Denture Prosthesis, Internat. D. J. **2**:542-573, 1952.

Stoner, C.: The Use of Self-Curing Acrylic Resin in the Temporary Splinting of Teeth, D. Digest **61**:296-301, 1955.

Strean, L. P., and Horton, C. P.: Hydrocortisone in Dental Practice, D. Digest **59**:8-16, 1953.

Sweeney, W. T., Myerson, R. L., Rose, E. E., and Semmelman, J. O.: Proposed Specification for Plastic Teeth, J. Pros. Den. **7**:420-424, 1957.

Talkov, L.: Pulp Protection in Crown and Bridge Prosthesis, J. Pros. Den. **4**:288-290, 1954.

Tomlin, H. R., and Osborne, J.: Cobalt-Chromium Partial Dentures; A Clinical Survey, Brit. Den. J. **110**:307-310, 1961.

Van Huysen, G., Fly, W., and Leonard, L.: Artificial Dentures and the Oral Mucosa, J. Pros. Den. **4**:446-460, 1954.

Wilson, J. H.: Some Clinical and Technical Aspects of Partial Dentures, D. J. Australia **26**:176-183, 1954.

Wright, W. H.: Partial Denture Prosthesis: A Preventive Oral Health Service, J.A.D.A. **43**:163-168, 1951.

Young, H. A.: Factors Contributory to Success in Prosthodontic Practice, J. Pros. Den. **5**:354-360, 1955.

Zerosi, C.: A New Type of Removable Splint: Its Indications and Function, D. Abs. **1**:451-452, 1956.

MOUTH PREPARATIONS

Boitel, R. H.: The Parallelometer; A Precision Instrument for the Prosthetic Laboratory, J. Pros. Den. **12**:732-736, 1962.

Brown, H.: Alignment of Abutments for Fixed Partial Dentures, J. Pros. Den. **12**:940-946, 1962.

Glann, G. W., and Appleby, R. C.: Mouth Preparations for Removable Partial Dentures, J. Pros. Den. **10**:698-706, 1960.

Gaston, G. W.: Rest Area Preparations for Removable Partial Dentures, J. Pros. Den. **10**:124-134, 1960.

Heydermann, L.: Occlusal Rests, D. Practitioner **3**:92-94, 1952.

Impaglia, R.: Occlusal Rest in Partial Denture Procedure, Georgetown D. J. **8**:28-29, 1940.

Johnston, J. F.: Preparation of Mouths for Fixed and Removable Partial Dentures, J. Pros. Den. **11**:456-462, 1961.

Kahn, A. E.: Partial Versus Full Coverage, J. Pros. Den. **10**:167-178, 1960.

McCracken, W. L.: Mouth Preparations for Partial Dentures, J. Pros. Den. **6**:39-52, 1956.

Mills, M.: Mouth Preparation for Removable Partial Denture, J.A.D.A. **60**:154-159, 1960.

Perry, C. F., and Applegate, S. G.: Occlusal Rest, An Important Part of a Partial Denture, J. Michigan D. Soc. **29**:24-25, 1947.

Phillips, R. W.: Report of the Committee on Scientific Investigation of the Academy of Restorative Dentistry, J. Pros. Den. **13**:515-535, 1963.

Schorr, L., and Clayman, L. H.: Reshaping Abutment Teeth for Reception of Partial Denture Clasps, J. Pros. Den. **4**:625-633, 1954.

Sollé, W.: The Parallelo-facere: A Parallel Drilling Machine for Use in the Oral Cavity, J.A.D.A. **63**:344-352, 1961.

Yudkoff, I.: Mouth Preparation and Best Design for Partial Dentures, New York D. J. **23**:118-119, 1953.

OCCLUSION; JAW RELATION RECORDS; TRANSFER METHODS

Applegate, O. C.: Loss of Posterior Occlusion, J. Pros. Den. **4**:197-199, 1954.

Augsburger, R. H.: Occlusal Plane Relation to Facial Type, J. Pros. Den. **3**:755-770, 1953.

Baraban, D. J.: Establishing Centric Relation and Vertical Dimension in Occlusal Rehabilitation, J. Pros. Den. **12**:1157-1165, 1962.

Beck, H. O.: A Clinical Evaluation of the Arcon Concept of Articulation, J. Pros. Den. **9**:409-421, 1959.

Beck, H. O.: Selection of an Articulator and Jaw Registration, J. Pros. Den. **10**:878-886, 1960.

Beck, H. O.: Choosing the Articulator, J.A.D.A. **64**:468-475, 1962.

Beckett, L. S.: Accurate Occlusal Relations in Partial Denture Construction, Proc. Cong. Australian D. A. (10th), pp. 456-463, 1939.

Beckett, L. S.: Accurate Occlusal Relations in Partial Denture Construction, J. Pros. Den. **4**:487-495, 1954.

Berman, M. H.: Accurate Interocclusal Records, J. Pros. Den. **10**:620-630, 1960.

Beyron, H. L.: Occlusal Relationship, Internat. D. J. **2**:467-496, 1952.

Beyron, H. L.: Characteristics of Functionally Optimal Occlusion and Principles of Occlusal Rehabilitation, J.A.D.A. **48**:648-656, 1954.

Beyron, H. L.: Occlusal Changes in Adult Dentition, J.A.D.A. **48**:674-686, 1954.

Block, L. S.: Preparing and Conditioning the Patient for Intermaxillary Relations, J. Pros. Den. **2**:599-603, 1952.

Block, L. S.: Tensions and Intermaxillary Relations, J. Pros. Den. **4**:204-207, 1954.

Boos, R. H.: Intermaxillary Relation Established by Biting Power, J.A.D.A. **27**:1192-1199, 1940.

Boos, R. H.: Occlusion From Rest Position, J. Pros. Den. **2**:575-588, 1952.

Boos, R. H.: Basic Anatomic Factors of Jaw Position, J. Pros. Den. **4**:200-203, 1954.

Boos, R. H.: Maxillomandibular Relations, Occlusion, and the Temporomandibular Joint, D. Clin. North America, pp. 19-35, March, 1962.

Borgh, O., and Posselt, U.: Hinge Axis Registration: Experiments on the Articulator, J. Pros. Den. **8**:35-40, 1958.

Boucher, C. O.: Occlusion in Prosthodontics, J. Pros. Den. **3**:633-656, 1953.

Brandrup-Wognsen, T.: The Face-Bow, Its Significance and Application, J. Pros. Den. **3**:618-630, 1953.

Brown, S. W.: Disharmony Between Centric Relation and Centric Occlusion as a Factor in Producing Improper Tooth Wear and Trauma, D. Digest **52**:434-440, 1946.

Cerveris, A. R.: Vibracentric Equilibration of Centric Occlusion, J.A.D.A. **63**:476-483, 1961.

Christensen, P. B.: Accurate Casts and Positional Relation Records, J. Pros. Den. **8**:475-482, 1958.

Christiansen, R. L.: Rationale of the Face-Bow in Maxillary Cast Mounting, J. Pros. Den. **9**:388-398, 1959.

Cohn, L. A.: Factors of Dental Occlusion Pertinent to the Restorative and Prosthetic Problem, J. Pros. Den. **9**:256-277, 1959.

Cohn, R.: The Relationship of Anterior Guidance to Condylar Guidance in Mandibular Movement, J. Pros. Den. **6**:758-767, 1956.

Collett, H. A.: Balancing the Occlusion of Partial Dentures, J.A.D.A. **42**:162-168, 1951.

Craddock, F. W.: The Accuracy and Practical Value of Records of Condyle Path Inclination, J.A.D.A. **38**:697-710, 1949.

Craddock, F. W., and Thompson, J. R.: Functional Analysis of Occlusion, J.A.D.A. **39**:404-406, 1949.

Craddock, F. W., and Wymmons, H. F.: Evaluation of the Face-Bow, J. Pros. Den. **2**:633-642, 1952.

D'Amico, A.: Functional Occlusion of the Natural Teeth of Man, J. Pros. Den. **11**:899-915, 1961.

Draper, D. H.: Forward Trends in Occlusion, J. Pros. Den. **13**:724-731, 1963.

Eberle, W. R.: A Study of Centric Relation as Recorded in a Supine Rest Position, J.A.D.A. **42**:15-26, 1951.

Emmert, J. H.: A Method for Registering Occlusion in Semiedentulous Mouths, J. Pros. Den. **8**:94-99, 1958.

Fedi, P. F.: Cardinal Differences in Occlusion of Natural Teeth and That of Artificial Teeth, J.A.D.A. **62**:482-485, 1962.

Fountain, H. W.: Seating the Condyles for Centric Relation Records, J. Pros. Den. **11**:1050-1058, 1961.

Frank, L.: The Opening Axis of the Jaw, D. Digest **62**:16-19, 1956.

Freese, A. S.: Stable Occlusion With Rubber Impression Material, J. Pros. Den. **6**:756-757, 1956.

Gilson, T. D.: A Theoretic Method of Occlusal Correction. A Theory of Principles for and Their Application in a Technique for Correction by Grinding of Disharmonies in Functional Occlusion of the Human Dentition, J. Pros. Den. **3**:478-492, 1953.

Gilson, T. D.: Theory of Centric Correction in Natural Teeth, J. Pros. Den. **8**:468-474, 1958.

Granger, E. R.: Centric Relation, J. Pros. Den. **2**:160-171, 1952.

Granger, E. R.: The Articulator and the Patient, D. Clin. North America, pp. 527-539, Nov., 1960.

Hardy, I. R.: The Developments in the Occlusal Patterns of Artificial Teeth, J. Pros. Den. **1**:14-28, 1951.

Harris, E.: Occlusion, J. Pros. Den. **1**:301-306, 1951.

Hausman, M.: Interceptive and Pivotal Occlusal Contacts, J.A.D.A. **66**:165-171, 1963.

Hindels, G. W.: Occlusion in Removable Partial Denture Prosthesis, D. Clin. North America, pp. 137-146, March, 1962.

Hughes, G. A., and Regli, C. P.: What is Centric Relation? J. Pros. Den. **11**:16-22, 1961.

Jaffe, V. N.: The Functionally Generated Path in Full Denture Construction, J. Pros. Den. **4**:214-221, 1954.

Jamieson, C. H.: Mandibular Position and the Partial Denture, J.A.D.A. **27**:3-10, 1940.

Jankelson, B.: Considerations of Occlusion on Fixed Partial Dentures, D. Clin. North America, pp. 187-203, March, 1959.

Jeffreys, F. E., and Platner, R. L.: Occlusion in Removable Partial Dentures, J. Pros. Den. **10**:912-920, 1960.

Kapur, K. K.: The Comparison of Different Methods of Recording Centric Relation, 1956, Tufts University, D. Abs. **2**:508, 1957.

Kingery, R. H.: A Review of Some of the Problems Associated With Centric Relation, J. Pros. Den. **2**:307-319, 1952.

Kurth, L. E.: Balanced Occlusion, J. Pros. Den. **4**:150-167, 1954.

Kyes, F. M.: Alginate Impressions as an Aid in Occlusal Equilibration, J.A.D.A. **49**:568-569, 1954.

Launitzen, A. G., and Bodner, G. H.: Variations in Location of Arbitrary and True Hinge Axis Points, J. Pros. Den. **11**:224-229, 1961.

Lazzari, J. B.: Application of the Hanau Model "C" Face-Bow, J. Pros. Den. **5**:626-628, 1955.

Lindblom, G.: The Significance of "Bite Analysis" in Modern Dentistry, D. Record **68**:254-262, 1948.

Lindblom, G.: Balanced Occlusion With Partial Reconstructions, Internat. D. J. **1**:84-98, 1951.

Lindblom, G.: The Value of Bite Analysis, J.A.D.A. **48**:657-664, 1954.

Lucia, V. O.: Centric Relation—Theory and Practice, J. Pros. Den. **10**:849-956, 1960.

Lucia, V. O.: The Gnathological Concept of Articulation, D. Clin. North America, pp. 183-197, March, 1962.

Mann, A. W., and Pankey, L. D.: The P. M. Philosophy of Occlusal Rehabilitation, D. Clin. North America, pp. 621-636, Nov., 1963.

Mann, W. R., and Applegate, O. C.: Acrylic Teeth as a Means of Obtaining Balanced Functional Occlusion in Partial Denture Prosthesis, J.A.D.A. **31**:505-514, 1944.

McCollum, B. B.: The Mandibular Hinge Axis and a Method of Locating It, J. Pros. Den. **10**:428-435, 1960.

McCracken, W. L.: Functional Occlusion in Removable Partial Denture Construction, J. Pros. Den. **8**:955-963, 1958.

McCracken, W. L.: Impression Materials in Prosthetic Dentistry, D. Clin. North America, pp. 671-684, Nov., 1958.

McCracken, W. L.: Occlusion in Partial Denture Prosthesis, D. Clin. North America, pp. 109-119, March, 1962.

Meyer, F. S.: A New, Simple and Accurate Technic for Obtaining Balanced and Functional Occlusion, J.A.D.A. **21**:195-203, 1934.

Meyer, F. S.: Balanced and Functional Occlusion in Relation to Denture Work, J.A.D.A. **22**:1156-1164, 1935.

Meyer, F. S.: The Generated Path Technique in Reconstruction Dentistry. Parts I and II, J. Pros. Den. 9:354-366, 432-440, 1959.

Moore, A. W.: Ideal Versus Adequate Dental Occlusion, J.A.D.A. 55:51-56, 1957.

Moses, C. H.: The Significance of Some Natural Laws in the Practice of Preventive and Restorative Dentistry, J. Pros. Den. 3:304-322, 1953.

Moses, C. H.: Human Tooth Form and Arrangement From the Anthropologic Approach, J. Pros. Den. 9:197-212, 1959.

Moulton, G. H.: The Importance of Centric Occlusion in Diagnosis and Treatment Planning, J. Pros. Den. 10:921-926, 1960.

Myerson, S.: Occlusal Forms and Nature's Plan, D. Digest 59:65-70, 1953.

Nuttall, E. B.: Establishing Posterior Functional Occlusion for Fixed Partial Dentures, J.A.D.A. 66:341-348, 1963.

Olsson, A., and Posselt, U.: Relationship of Various Skull Reference Lines, J. Pros. Den. 11:1045-1049, 1961.

Payne, S. H.: A Comparative Study of Posterior Occlusion, J. Pros. Den. 2:661-666, 1952.

Payne, S. H.: Combined Vulcanite and Acrylic Denture, J. Pros. Den. 3:323-325, 1953.

Payne, S. H.: Selective Occlusion, J. Pros. Den. 5:301-304, 1955.

Pearson, W. D.: Reducing Frictional Resistance in the Occlusion of Dentures, J. Pros. Den. 5:338-341, 1955.

Porter, C. G.: The Cuspless Centralized Occlusal Pattern, J. Pros. Den. 5:313-318, 1955.

Pruden, W. H.: Occlusion Related to Fixed Partial Denture Prosthesis, D. Clin. North America, pp. 121-136, March, 1962.

Rapp, R.: The Occlusion and Occlusal Patterns of Artificial Posterior Teeth, J. Pros. Den. 4:461-480, 1954.

Robinson, M. J.: Centric Position, J. Pros. Den. 1:384-386, 1951.

Robinson, S. C.: Equilibrated Functional Occlusions, J. Pros. Den. 2:462-476, 1952.

Robinson, S. C.: Hydraulic Equilibration in Complete and Partial Artificial Dentures, D. Record 74:114-119, 1954.

Schireson, S.: Grinding Teeth for Masticatory Efficiency and Gingival Health, J. Pros. Den. 13:337-345, 1963.

Schultz, A. W.: Comfort and Chewing Efficiency in Dentures, J. Pros. Den. 1:38-48, 1951.

Schuyler, C. H.: Intra-Oral Method of Establishing Maxillomandibular Relation, J.A.D.A. 19:1012-1019, 1932.

Schuyler, C. H.: Fundamental Principles in the Correction of Occusal Disharmony—Natural and Artificial (Grinding), J.A.D.A. 22:1193-1202, 1935.

Schuyler, C. H.: Correction of Occlusal Disharmony of the Natural Dentition, New York D. J. 13:445-462, 1947.

Schuyler, C. H.: Factors of Occlusion Applicable to Restorative Dentistry, J. Pros. Den. 3:772-782, 1953.

Schuyler, C. H.: Discussion: Human Tooth Form and Arrangement From the Anthropologic Approach by Dr. C. H. Moses, J. Pros. Den. 9:213-214, 1959.

Schuyler, C. H.: An Evaluation of Incisal Guidance and Its Influence in Restorative Dentistry, J. Pros. Den. 9:374-378, 1959.

Schuyler, C. H.: Factors Contributing to Traumatic Occlusion, J. Pros. Den. 11:708-715, 1961.

Sears, V. H.: Occlusion: The Common Meeting Ground in Dentistry, J. Pros. Den. 2:15-21, 1952.

Sears, V. H.: Mandibular Condyle Migrations as Influenced by Tooth Occlusions, J.A.D.A. 45:179-192, 1952.

Sears, V. H.: Occlusal Pivots, J. Pros. Den. 6:332-338, 1956.

Sears, V. H.: Centric and Eccentric Occlusions, J. Pros. Den. 10:1029-1036, 1960.

Sears, V. H.: Mandibular Equilibration, J.A.D.A. 65:45-55, 1962.

Shanahan, T. E. J.: Physiologic and Neurologic Occlusion, J. Pros. Den. 3:631-632, 1953.

Shanahan, T. E. J., and Leff, A.: Interocclusal Records, J. Pros. Den. 10:842-848, 1960.

Shapiro, M.: The Equilibration of Occlusion, D. Digest 58:206-209, 1952.

Shore, N. A.: Equilibration of the Occlusion of the Natural Dentition, J.A.D.A. 44:414-427, 1952.

Silverman, M. M.: The Speaking Method in Measuring Vertical Dimension, J. Pros. Den. 3:193-199, 1953.

Silverman, M. M.: Determination of Vertical Dimension by Phonetics, J. Pros. Den. 6:465-471, 1956; D. Abs. 2:221, 1957.

Soltis, E. D.: The Three Dimensions in the Occlusal Forms of Teeth, J. Pros. Den. **6:**57-64, 1956.

Stuart, C. E.: Accuracy in Measuring Functional Dimensions and Relations in Oral Prosthesis, J. Pros. Den. **9:**220-236, 1959.

Tench, R. W.: Interpretation and Registration of Mandibulomaxillary Relations and Their Reproduction on an Instrument, J.A.D.A. **13:**1675-1691, 1926.

Thompson, M. J.: Cuspal Coordination, J. Pros. Den. **4:**183-195, 1954.

Trapozzano, V. R.: Occlusal Records, J. Pros. Den. **5:**325-332, 1955.

Trapozzano, V. R.: An Analysis of Current Concepts of Occlusion, J. Pros. Den. **5:**764-782, 1955.

Trapozzano, V. R.: Occlusion in Relation to Prosthodontics, D. Clin. North America, pp. 313-325, March, 1957.

Trapozzano, V. R.: Laws of Articulation, J. Pros. Den. **13:**34-44, 1963. Discussion by C. O. Boucher follows.

Ulip, E. J.: Articulator Mounting by Functional Maxillomandibular Records, J. Pros. Den. **5:**756-763, 1955.

Weinberg, L. A.: The Transverse Hinge Axis: Real or Imaginary, J. Pros. Den. **9:**775-787, 1959.

Weinberg, L. A.: An Evaluation of the Face-Bow Mounting, J. Pros. Den. **11:**32-42, 1961.

Weinberg, L. A.: Arcon Principle in the Condylar Mechanism of Adjustable Articulators, J. Pros. Den. **13:**263-268, 1963.

Weinberg, L. A.: An Evaluation of Basic Articulators and Their Concepts. Parts I and II, J. Pros. Den. **13:**622-663, 1963.

Williams, C. H. M.: Occlusion on Partial Dentures—How Can It Be Controlled? J. Canad. D. A. **7:**187, 1941.

Wilson, J. H.: The Use of Partial Dentures in the Restoration of Occlusal Standards, Australian D. J. **1:**93-101, 1956; D. Abs. **1:**634, 1956.

Winslow, M. B.: The Preventive Role of Occlusal Balancing of the Natural Dentition, J.A.D.A. **48:**293-296, 1954.

PARTIAL DENTURE DESIGN

Atkinson, H. F.: Partial Denture Problems. Designing About a Path of Withdrawal, Australian J. Den. **57:**187-190, 1953.

Blatterfein, L.: A Systematic Method of Designing Upper Partial Denture Bases, J.A.D.A. **47:**110, 1953.

Boyd, L.: The Important Factors to Be Considered in the Correct Design and Construction of Partial Dentures, Illinois D. J. **9:**352-356 (disc. 356-357, 372), 1940.

Chick, A. O.: Correct Location of Clasps and Rests on Dentures Without Stress-Breakers, Brit. D. J. **95:**303-309, 1953.

Collett, H. A.: Principles of Partial Denture Design, D. Digest **57:**24-29, 1951.

Collett, H. A.: Biologic Approach to Clasp Partial Dentures, D. Digest **61:**309-313, 1955.

Craddock, F. W.: Labial Bar Partial Denture, New Zealand D. J. **42:**67, 1946.

Craddock, F. W., and Bottomley, G. A.: Second Thoughts on Clasp Surveying, Brit. D. J. **96:**134-137, 1954.

Elliott, F. C.: A Method That Simplifies the Design of Partial Dentures, J.A.D.A. **27:**1263-1268, 1940.

Fish, E. W.: A New Principle in Partial Denture Design, Brit. D. J. **92:**135-144, 1952.

Frechette, A. R.: Partial Denture Planning With Special Reference to Stress Distribution, J. Ontario D. A. **30:**318-329, 1953.

Giradot, R. L.: History and Development of Partial Denture Design, J.A.D.A. **28:**1399-1408, 1941.

Granger, E. R.: Biologic Factors in Partial Denture Design, J. 2nd Dist. D. Soc. **31:**5-12, 47, 1945.

Jordan, L. G.: Designing Removable Partial Dentures With External Attachments (Clasps), J. Pros. Den. **2:**716-722, 1952.

Kelly, E. K.: The Physiologic Approach to Partial Denture Design, J. Pros. Den. **3:**699-710, 1953.

Lammie, G. A., and others: Use of Onlays in Partial Denture Construction, Brit. D. J. **100:**33-42, 1956.

Lazarus, A. H.: Partial Denture Design, J. Pros. Den. **1:**438-442, 1951.

Mansie, J. W.: Design and Construction of Partial Dentures, Brit. D. J., **66**:704-713, 1939.
MacKinnon, K. P.: Indirect Retention in Partial Denture Construction, D. J. Australia **27**:221-225, 1955.
McCracken, W. L.: Contemporary Partial Denture Designs, J. Pros. Den. **8**:71-84, 1958.
McCracken, W. L.: Survey of Partial Denture Designs by Commercial Dental Laboratories, J. Pros. Den. **12**:1089-1110, 1962.
Moore, D. S.: Some Fundamentals of Partial Denture Design to Conserve the Supporting Structures, J. Ontario D. A. **32**:238-240, 1955.
Neurohr, F. G.: Health Conservation of the Periodontal Tissues by a Method of Functional Partial Denture Design, J.A.D.A. **31**:58-70, 1944.
Osborne, J., and Lammie, G. A.: The Bilateral Free-End Saddle Lower Denture, J. Pros. Den. **4**:640-653, 1954.
Perry, C.: Philosophy of Partial Denture Design, Bul. St. Louis D. Soc. **25**:48-49, 1954 (Digest); J. Pros. Den. **6**:775-784, 1956.
Ryan, J.: Technique of Design in Partial Denture Construction, J.D.A. South Africa **9**:123-133, 1954.
Rybeck, S. A., Jr.: Simplicity in a Distal Extension Partial Denture, J. Pros. Den. **4**:87-92, 1954.
Schmidt, A. H.: Planning and Designing Removable Partial Dentures, J. Pros. Den. **3**:783-806, 1953.
Schmidt, A. H.: Planning and Designing Removable Partial Dentures, J. Canad. D. A. **20**:415-422, 1954.
Schmidt, A. H.: Partial Dentures: Planning and Designing, J.A.D.A. **35**:562-569, 1947.
Schmidt, A. H.: Planning and Designing Partial Dentures, D. Digest **54**:444-450, 498-502, 544-546, 1948; **55**:18, 1949.
Schmidt, A. H.: Part I. Planning and Designing Removable Partial Dentures, U. S. Armed Forces M. J. **1**:1465, 1950.
Schmidt, A. H.: Part II. Planning and Designing Removable Partial Dentures, U. S. Armed Forces M. J. **3**:1313, 1952.
Schmidt, A. H.: Planning and Designing Removable Partial Dentures, D. Practitioner **3**:2-7, 47-52, 76-77, 109-110, 1952.
Schuyler, C. H.: The Partial Denture as a Means of Stabilizing Abutment Teeth, J.A.D.A. **28**:1121-1125, 1941.
Scott, D. C.: Suggested Designs for Metal Partial Dentures, D. Technician **2**:21, 26, 1954.
Steffel, V. L.: Simplified Clasp Partial Dentures Designed for Maximum Function, J.A.D.A. **32**:1093-1100, 1945.
Steffel, V. L.: Fundamental Principles Involved in Partial Denture Designs—With Special Reference to Equalization of Tooth and Tissue Support, Australian J. Den. **54**:328-333, 1950; D. J. Australia **23**:68-77, 1951.
Steffel, V. L.: Fundamental Principles Involved in Partial Denture Design, J.A.D.A. **42**:534-544, 1951.
Tench, R. W.: Fundamentals of Partial Denture Design, J.A.D.A. **23**:1087-1092, 1936.
Weinberg, L. A.: Lateral Force in Relation to the Denture Base and Clasp Design, J. Pros. Den. **6**:785-800, 1956.
Wills, N. G.: Practical Engineering Applied to Removable Partial Denture Designing, Proc. D. Centenary, pp. 319-331, 1940.

PERIODONTAL CONSIDERATIONS

Amsterdam, M., and Fox., L.: Provisional Splinting—Principles and Technics, D. Clin. North America, pp. 73-99, March, 1959.
Applegate, O. C.: The Interdependence of Periodontics and Removable Partial Denture Prosthesis, J. Pros. Den. **8**:269-281, 1958.
Bauer, W. H.: Effect of a Faultily Constructed Partial Denture on a Tooth and Its Supporting Tissue, With Special Reference to Formation of Fibrocartilage in the Periodontal Membrane as Result of Disturbed Healing Caused by Abnormal Stresses, Am. J. Orthodont. & Oral Surg. (Oral Surg. Sect.) **27**:640-651, 1941.
Berkson, R.: Dental Cement: A Study of Its Property of Adhesion, Am. J. Orthodont. **36**:701-710, 1950.
Bush, S. H., and Peyton, F. A.: The Effect of Section Size on the Mechanical Properties of Wrought Gold Wires, J. Dent. Res. **30**:745-752, 1951.
Fish, E. W.: Periodontal Diseases: Occlusal Trauma and Partial Dentures, Brit. D. J. **95**:199-206 (disc. 206-210), 1953.

Glickman, I. J.: Periodontal Structures and Removable Partial Denture Prosthesis, J.A.D.A. **37**:311-316, 1948.
Glickman, I. J.: Interrelation of Local and Systemic Factors in Periodontal Disease: Bone Factor Concept, J.A.D.A. **45**:422-429, 1952.
Glickman, I. J.: The Role of Systemic Therapy in the Treatment of Periodontal Disease, J.A.D.A. **62**:414-423, 1961.
Ivancie, G. P.: Interrelationship Between Restorative Dentistry and Periodontics, J. Pros. Den. **8**:819-830, 1958.
Jordan, L. G.: Treatment of Advanced Periodontal Disease by Prosthodontic Procedures, J. Pros. Den. **10**:908-911, 1960.
Kimball, H. D.: The Role of Periodontia in Prosthetic Dentistry, J. Pros. Den. **1**:286-294, 1951.
Krogh-Poulsen, W.: Partial Denture Design in Relation to Occlusal Trauma in Periodontal Breakdown, Acad. Rev. **3**:18-23, 1955; Internat. D. J. **4**:847-867, 1954.
McCall, J. O.: Periodontist Looks at the Clasp Partial Denture, J.A.D.A. **43**:439-443, 1951.
McKenzie, J. S.: Some Periodontal Considerations in Partial Denture Planning, J.A.D.A. **45**:314-318, 1952.
McKenzie, J. S.: Mutual Problems of the Periodontist and Prosthodontist, J. Pros. Den. **5**:37-42, 1955.
Morris, M. L.: Artificial Crown Contours and Gingival Health, J. Pros. Den. **12**:1146-1155, 1962.
Nevin, R. B.: Periodontal Aspects of Partial Denture Prosthesis, J. Pros. Den. **5**:215-219, 1955.
Orban, B. S.: Biologic Principles in Correction of Occlusal Disharmonies, J. Pros. Den. **6**:637-641, 1956.
Osborne, J.: Free-End Saddle and the Periodontal Patient, D. Practitioner **4**:287-297, 1954.
Overby, G. E.: Esthetic Splinting of Mobile Periodontally Involved Teeth by Vertical Pinning, J. Pros. Den. **11**:112-118, 1961.
Peyton, F. A., Shiere, B. A., and Delgado, V. P.: Some Comparisons of Self-Curing Resins, J. Pros. Den. **3**:332-338, 1953.
Rubinstein, M. N.: Splinting: Periodontal and Prosthetic Support, D. Digest **60**:342-348, 1954.
Schopper, A. F.: Partial Denture and Its Relation to Periodontics, J.A.D.A. **45**:415-421, 1952.
Schuyler, C. H.: The Partial Denture and a Means of Stabilizing Abutment Teeth, J.A.D.A. **28**:1121-1125, 1941.
Smith, S. B.: Partial Denture Construction and Periodontia, Bul. Nat. D. A. **6**:12-13, 1947.
Souder, W., and Paffenbarger, G. C.: Physical Properties of Dental Materials, Circular of the National Bureau of Standards C433, Washington, 1942, United States Government Printing Office.
Sternlicht, H. C.: Prosthetic Treatment Planning for the Periodontal Patient, D. Abs. **2**:81-82, 1957.
Talkov, L.: Survey for Complete Periodontal Prosthesis, J. Pros. Den. **11**:124-131, 1961.
Thomas, B. O. A., and Gallager, J. W.: Practical Management of Occlusal Dysfunctions in Periodontal Therapy, J.A.D.A. **46**:18-31, 1953.
Trapozzano, V. R., and Winter, G. R.: Periodontal Aspects of Partial Denture Design, J. Pros. Den. **2**:101-107, 1952.
Ward, H. L., and Weinberg, L. A.: An Evaluation of Periodontal Splinting, J.A.D.A. **63**:48-54, 1961.

PHYSIOLOGY; MANDIBULAR MOVEMENT

Brandrup-Wognsen, T.: Present Conceptions of the Movements and Functional Positions of the Human Lower Jaw. An Articulator Construction Based on These Principles, J. Pros. Den. **2**:780-793, 1952.
Brekke, C. A.: Jaw Function. Part I. Hinge Rotation. J. Pros. Den. **9**:600-606, 1959.
Brekke, C. A.: Jaw Function. Part II. Hinge Axis, Hinge Axes, J. Pros. Den. **9**:936-940, 1959.
Brekke, C. A.: Jaw Function. Part III. Condylar Placement and Condylar Retrusion, J. Pros. Den. **10**:78-85, 1960.
Brotman, D. N.: Contemporary Concepts of Articulation, J. Pros. Den. **10**:221-230, 1960.
Clapp, G. W.: Accurate Tracings of Mandibular Movements, J. Pros. Den. **4**:179-182, 1954.
Emig, G. E.: The Physiology of the Muscles of Mastication, J. Pros. Den. **1**:700-707, 1951.
Hesse, F.: The Mechanics of the Chewing Movements of the Human Jaw, J. Pros. Den. **4**:175-178, 1954.
Jankelson, B., Hoffman, G. M., and Hendron, J. A., Jr.: The Physiology of the Stomatognathic System, J.A.D.A. **46**:375-386, 1953.

Jankelson, B.: Physiology of Human Dental Occlusion, J.A.D.A. **50**:664-680, 1955.
Kurth, L. E.: Mandibular Movements in Mastication, J.A.D.A. **29**:1769-1790, 1942.
Kurth, L. E.: Mandibular Movement and Articulator Occlusion, J.A.D.A. **39**:37-46, 1949.
Kurth, L. E.: Centric Relation and Mandibular Movement, J.A.D.A. **50**:309-315, 1955.
Messerman, T.: A Concept of Jaw Function With a Related Clinical Application, J. Pros. Den. **13**:130-140, 1963.
Naylor, J. G.: Role of the External Pterygoid Muscles in Temporomandibular Articulation, J. Pros. Den. **10**:1037-1042, 1960.
O'Rourke, J. T.: Significance of Tests for Biting Strength, J.A.D.A. **38**:627-633, 1949.
Posselt, U.: Studies in the Mobility of the Human Mandible, Acta Odont. Scandinavica **10**:19-160 (Supp. 10), 1952.
Posselt, U.: Movement Areas of the Mandible, J. Pros. Den. **7**:375-385, 1957.
Posselt, U.: Terminal Hinge Movement of the Mandible, J. Pros. Den. **7**:787-797, 1957.
Schweitzer, J. M.: Masticatory Function in Man, J. Pros. Den. **11**:625-647, 1961.
Shanahan, T. E. J.: Dental Physiology for Dentures. The Direct Application of the Masticatory Cycle to Denture Occlusion, J. Pros. Den. **2**:3, 1952.
Sicher, H.: Positions and Movements of the Mandible, J.A.D.A. **48**:620-625, 1954.
Söstenbö, H. R.: C. E. Luce's Recordings of Mandibular Movement, J. Pros. Den. **11**:1068-1073, 1961.
Thompson, J. R.: The Rest Position of the Mandible and Its Significance to Dental Science, J.A.D.A. **33**:151-180, 1946.
Ulrich, J.: The Human Temporomandibular Joint: Kinematics and Actions of the Masticatory Muscles, J. Pros. Den. **9**:399-406, 1959.
Vaughan, H. C.: The External Pterygoid Mechanism, J. Pros. Den. **5**:80-92, 1955.
Yippo, A.: The Effect of Dentures on Speech, D. Abs. **1**:42-43, 1956.

REBASING AND RELINING

Blatterfein, L.: Rebasing Procedures for Removable Partial Dentures, J. Pros. Den. **8**:441-467, 1958.
Steffel, V. L.: Relining Removable Partial Dentures for Fit and Function, J. Pros. Den. **4**:496-509, 1954.
Steffel, V. L.: Relining Removable Partial Dentures for Fit and Function, J. Tennessee D. A. **36**:35-43, 1956.
Wilson, J. H.: Partial Dentures—Rebasing the Saddle Supported by the Mucosa and Alveolar Bone, D. J. Australia **24**:185-188, 1952.
Wilson, J. H.: Partial Dentures—Relining the Saddle Supported by the Mucosa and Alveolar Bone, J. Pros. Den. **3**:807-813, 1953.

STRESSBREAKER DESIGNS

Cody, L. G.: Broken Stress and Splinting in the Field of Partial Dentures, J. Colorado D. A. **23**:87-92, 1945.
Hekneby, M.: The "Spring Slide Joint," a New Attachment for Lower Partial Dentures, D. Abs. **1**:679-680, 1956.
Hirschtritt, E.: Removable Partial Dentures With Stress-Broken Extension Bases, J. Pros. Den. **7**:318-324, 1957.
James, A. G.: Stress Breakers Which Automatically Return the Saddle to Rest Position Following Displacement. Mandibular Distal Extension Partial Dentures, J. Pros. Den. **4**:73-81, 1954.
Jones, R. R.: Procedures for Making a Lower Partial Denture With a Spring Stress-Breaker, J.A.D.A. **29**:2154-2161, 1942.
Kabcenell, J. L.: Stress Breaking for Partial Dentures, J.A.D.A. **63**:593-602, 1961.
Lane, R. P.: Practical Stress Breaking in Partial Dentures, D. J. Australia **19**:314-322, 1947.
Levitch, H. C.: Physiologic Stress-Equalizer, J. Pros. Den. **3**:232-238, 1953.
Marris, F. N.: The Precision Dowel Rest Attachment, J. Pros. Den. **5**:43-48, 1955.
McGee, G. F.: The Use of Stressbreakers in Tissue Borne Partial Dentures, J.A.D.A. **39**:387-392, 1949.
Neill, D. J.: The Problem of the Lower Free-End Removable Partial Denture, J. Pros. Den. **8**:623-634, 1958.
Schopper, A. F.: Value of Stressbreakers for Unilateral Partial Denture With Free-End Saddles, J.A.D.A. **38**:183-187, 1949.

Schopper, A. F.: Value of Stress Breaker for Universal Partial Dentures With Free-End Saddles, J. South. California D. A. **23**:34-36, 1955.

Simpson, D. H.: Considerations for Abutments, J. Pros. Den. **5**:375-384, 1955.

Terrell, W. H.: Split Bar Technic Applicable to Both Precision Attachment and Clasp Cases, J. South. California D. A. **9**:10-14, 1942.

Turkheim, H. J.: Modified Stress-Breaker, D. Practitioner **3**:197-198, 1953.

Van Minden, F.: Ideal Stressbreaking for Partial Dentures, J.A.D.A. **30**:657-669, 1943.

SURVEYING

Applegate, O. C.: Use of the Paralleling Surveyor in Modern Partial Denture Construction, J.A.D.A. **27**:1317-1407, 1940.

Atkinson, H. F.: Partial Denture Problems. Surveyors and Surveying, Australian J. Den. **59**:28-31, 1955.

Bolatin, L.: Surveying and Practical Clasp Designing, New York J. Den. **23**:170-172, 1953.

Chestner, S. G.: A Methodical Approach to the Analysis of Study Cases, J. Pros. Den. **4**:622-624, 1954.

Katulski, E. M., and Appleyard, W. N.: Biological Concepts of the Use of the Mechanical Cast Surveyor, J. Pros. Den. **9**:629-634, 1959.

Sollé, W.: An Improved Dental Surveyor, J.A.D.A. **60**:727-731, 1960.

Index

Connectors, minor—cont'd
  form and location, 150
  functions, 149
  rigid, preparing areas for, 108
Consultation, records for, 41
Continuous clasps, definition, 25
  description, 214
Contouring wax patterns, 245
  surveyor used for, 92
Contours, tooth, unfavorable, reduction of, 37
Convex surfaces in partial denture design, rule, 133
Convexity, tooth, area of greatest, 168, 170
Cooling hydrocolloid mold, 378
Copper band impressions, 293-296
Correction, occlusal, remounting and, 430-433
Crib clasp, 194
Crown, single, establishing functional occlusion on, 360-361
Crowns, abutment, ledges on, 246-262
  cast, abutment preparations using, 255-256
    to fit existing partial denture clasps, 273, 274
    making of, 272-275
  and fixed bridge restorations, references, 495
  temporary, cementation of, 271-272
    preparation of, 266-270
    where partial is being worn, 270-272
  veneer, for support of clasp arms, 262-263
Crozat-type clasp, modified, 193, 194
Cummer's classification of partial dentures, 73-74

D

D-E hinge-type stress breaker, 231
Definitions, prosthodontic, 21
Delivery, adjustment, and servicing of partial denture, 437-448
Density, bone, value of interpreting, 44-45
Dental casting, factors influencing excellence of, 397-398
  disease, signs of, 35, 36
  prosthesis, definitions, 22, 23
  stones, definition, 27
    improved, for master casts, 47
  surveyor (*see* Surveyor)
  vocabulary, 21, 27
Dentatus articulator and face-bow, 50, 55
  face-bow, 339
Dentistry, prosthetic, definition, 22
Dentition, natural and artificial, adjustment of occlusion in harmony with, 439-443
Denture areas, tooth-borne, relining, 474-477
  base(s), 218-229
    adjustments to bearing surfaces of, 439
    definition, 23
    facial surfaces, 434

Denture base(s)—cont'd
  free-end (*see* Free-end base)
  ideal, requirements, 220-221
  and impression trays, making of, 412-416
  materials, 429, 430
    according to type, 114
  metal, advantages, 221-223
    use, 328
  movements, 208
  processed to functional and to anatomic form, comparison, 126
  purposes, 218
  references, 498
  resurfacing, 23
  retention of, forces resulting in, 165
  tissue conditioning prior to relining, 480
  tooth-supported, functions, 218
  waxing, 424-426
  clasps, existing, making crowns and inlays to fit, 272-275
  framework, making with blockout ledges and ready-made pattern forms, 381
    occlusal interference from, 438
    tooth-borne, outlined on master cast, 118
  peripheries, 433, 434
  prosthesis, complete and partial differentiated, 22
    kinds, 23
  repair by soldering, 486-488
  rocking, correction of, 446
  rotation about axis, 208-209
  support, factors in, 300
  splint bar for, 146-149
Dentures, complete and partial, choice between, 70-72
  occlusion compared, 338
  definitions, 22, 23
  finishing, Frush's instructions and instruments, 436
  partial (*see* Partial dentures)
Design, clasp, any given, advantages and disadvantages, 173
  basic principles of, 175-177
  differences in, 115-117
  partial denture, essentials, 117-122
    factors influencing, 128
    principles, 113-127
    references, 507
    rigid, advantages and disadvantages, 237
    rule about convex surfaces, 133
    treatment planning and, 29-31
DeVan clasp, 116, 194
Diagnosis, recording of data, 61-63
  and treatment planning, 35-72
    references, 498
    surveying study cast, 92
    record chart, 42
Die, electroformed, method of making, 292